FRONTIERS OF INFECTIOUS DISE
NEW ANTIVIRAL STRATEGIES

FRONTIERS OF INFECTIOUS DISEASES

NEW ANTIVIRAL STRATEGIES

PROCEEDINGS OF AN INTERNATIONAL SYMPOSIUM,
BROCKET HALL, HERTFORDSHIRE
24-26 APRIL 1988

EDITED BY

S. R. NORRBY

University of Lund,
Sweden.

CO-EDITORS

J. MILLS

San Francisco General Hospital,
USA.

E. NORRBY

Karolinksa Institute,
Stockholm, Sweden.

L. J. WHITTON

Scripps Clinic,
La Jolla, USA.

ORGANISING COMMITTEE

S. R. NORRBY	P. K. PETERSON	J. VERHOEF	K. P. W. J. McADAM	H. C. NEU
Lund,	Minneapolis,	Utrecht,	London,	New York,
Sweden	USA	Netherlands	UK	USA

CHURCHILL LIVINGSTONE
EDINBURGH LONDON MELBOURNE AND NEW YORK 1988

Proceedings of a symposium sponsored by an educational grant from Glaxo Research.

Distributed in the United States of America by Churchill Livingstone Inc., 1560 Broadway, New York, N.Y. 10036, and by associated companies, branches and representatives throughout the world.

First Edition 1988

ISBN 0-443-04165-2

British Library Cataloguing in Publication Data
New anti-viral strategies: proceedings of an international symposium, Brocket Hall, Hertfordshire, 24–26 April, 1988.
   1. Virology
   I. Norrby, S. R. II. Mills, John, 1940
   III. Norrby, Erling. IV. Whitton, L. J.
   V. Series.
   576'.64

Library of Congress Cataloging in Publication Data
New anti-viral strategies: proceedings of an international symposium, Brocket Hall, Hertfordshire, 24–26 April 1988/edited by S. R. Norrby; co-editors, John Mills, E. Norrby, L. J. Whitton.
      p.   cm. — (Frontiers of infectious diseases)
ISBN 0 443 04165 2
1. Virus diseases—Congresses. 2. Virus diseases—Chemotherapy—Congresses. 3. Antiviral agents—Congresses. 4. Viral vaccines—Congresses. I. Norrby, Ragnar. II. Series.
[DNLM: 1. Antiviral Agents—therapeutic use—congresses. 2. Viral Diseases—drug therapy—congresses. 3. Viral Proteins—immunology—congresses. 4. Viral Vaccines—congresses. WC 500 N5317 1988]
RC114.5.N48 1988
616.9'2506—dc19 88 28553

Printed in Great Britain at The Bath Press, Avon

Preface

These proceedings are the first of a series of small symposia entitled Frontiers of Infectious Diseases. When deciding on the theme for the first symposium, held in April 1988 at Brocket Hall in England, the choice naturally fell on virology. Boosted by the inventions of new biological methods for example, techniques for production of monoclonal antibodies, nucleic acid base sequence analysis, and DNA and RNA hybridization, basic virology has undergone a striking evolution during the last decade. The practical consequencies of this rapid evolution can be exemplified by the research done on HIV and AIDS. When the consequences of the AIDS epidemic became apparent to the scientific community and, for once, adequate economical resources were placed at its disposition, an unparalleled scientific activity was initiated all over the world. Today it is clear that with no disease, infectious or other, has such rapid progress been made in such a short time as with HIV infections and AIDS. That would not have been possible a decade ago when we lacked access to the new techniques.

These proceedings of the Brocket Hall symposium exemplify the rapid development within three different fields of virology; antiviral chemotherapy, viral pathogenesis to diseases other than the classical infections and viral vaccines. As an introduction to these themes, Tyrrell summarizes his unique experiences within the field of the common cold. Again, the rapid evolution during the last decade is well exemplified. Following a long period during which Tyrrell and his group systematically studied the aetiology, natural course and epidemiology of these infections, new insights into the molecular and sterical structure of the causative agents, especially rhinoviruses, now offer possibilities for development of specific therapy, for example by blocking the 'canyon' in the capsid.

Clumeck and Mills discuss the various approaches now being investigated for therapy of HIV infections. Clearly zidovudine is not going to be the final solution to antiviral treatment in patients with HIV infections. With the complex pathogenesis of this infection and the time required for evaluation of efficacy and safety of new drugs, it is clear that a final solution to the problem of treatment of HIV is unlikely to be found in the near future. Similarly, with human papilloma virus infections, a growing problem within the field of sexually transmitted diseases, no final solution to therapy has yet been found, as reviewed by Reichmann et al and Becker. Within the field of antiviral therapy of chronic hepatitis, Thomas et al and Perillo present data indicating that some patients with hepatitis B or hepatitis non-A, non-B infections will benefit from interferon treatment while others will not. The best results with antiviral chemotherapy are still those with acyclovir in the treatment of infections caused by herpes simplex virus as summarized by Fiddian and Whitley. Considering the pathogenesis of these infections, especially the fact that they remain latent after the primary infection, and the high degree of efficacy and safety of acyclovir, it seems doubtful if any major further progress can be made within this field.

The part of the proceedings dealing with pathogenesis starts with an extensive presentation by Prusiner and a subsequent comment by Carlson on the role of prions as causative agents of 'slow virus infections' such as Creutzfeld-Jakob's disease and kuru. Although there are still scientists who refuse to accept the concept that an organism without nucleic acid can be reproduced in a host organism, the tremendous amount of factual information supporting the view that prions cause these slow progressing neurological infections, should now reverse the burden of proof; that is, the non-believers will have to offer an alternative explanation to the aetiology of these infections.

A novel approach to the consequences of viral infections is presented by Fujinami and Dyrberg. They both present strong experimental evidence for the possibility that autoimmune conditions may be caused by viral infections. Special consideration should be given to the finding that autoimmune reactions can be induced by synthetic peptides representing epitopes which are shared by known autoantigens and viral proteins.

Plotz et al, in their paper, give experimental evidence for a picornavirus causing chronic inflammatory disease. This is followed up by Cohen who also reviews the evidence for a viral aetiology of at least some cases of diabetes mellitus.

Several of the above mentioned papers emphasize the importance of inter-action between immunity and infections as causes of clinical syndromes. This is further pursued by Kozinowski and Whitton in their articles on the role of cytolytic T-lymphocytes in response to experimental infections with cytomegaloviruses.

The section of the proceedings dealing with new viral vaccines brings us back to HIV, against which an intensive search for an effective vaccine is ongoing. Bolognesi and Weiss, in their papers, summarize the knowledge of the immune response to HIV envelope glycoproteins and the possible approaches to production of an HIV vaccine. As pointed out by both of them, the solution is not readily to hand and there are tremendous logistic problems in large-scale testing of an HIV vaccine.

One of the most fascinating sections of this book is that containing the paper on poliovaccines by Almond et al and the discussion by Racaniello. Of special interest is Almond's description of the possibilities of modifying the Sabin type 1 attenuated poliovirus strain and incorporate other genes in its capsid. Thus, it has been possible to produce a chimaera strain containing antigenic determinants of both polio 1 and polio 3. The strain is neutralized by antibodies to polio 1 or polio 3 and offers a possibility to overcome the problems with polio 3 vaccines reverting to wild type characteristics and increased neuropathogenicity. By recombination technique it has also been possible to include antigens of other organisms, for example Chlamydia, in the polio 1 capsid, thus producing a vaccine offering protection not only against polio 1 but also against a second pathogen.

Rotavirus infection continues to be the most important cause of intestinal infections in children and is also a major cause of mortality in infants in the developing world. Kapikian and Wadell, in their contributions discuss the result with rotavirus vaccines obtained so far. Kapikian favours the 'Jennerian' approach, i.e. to use a rhesus rotavirus strain with reduced infectivity in man while others aim at producing an attenuated, polyvalent vaccine derived from human rotavirus strains.

Plotkin and Just present data on the attenuated varicella vaccines now introduced in several countries. Although the vaccines have now been proven to be effective and safe and without producing increased frequencies of herpes zoster, the main question still remains to be answered: how long will immunity after childhood vaccination last and will such vaccinations increase the frequency of varicella in adults? If that should be the case, re-vaccinations may become necessary to avoid the more serious forms of varicella often seen in adults.

The last paper in this book brings us back to clinical reality and deals with the practical problems of handling patients with confirmed or suspected Lassa fever. Dr Glover describes in an excellent way the medical consequences of governmental decisions taken on the basis of poor information about how an infection spreads in the society. The lessons to be learned from his paper are several and should be carefully studied by those who still think that HIV infections spread by normal contacts with infected individuals.

Finally, as editor of these proceedings I would like to extend my sincere thanks to the authors and to the participants of the symposium for their excellent submissions, to my co-editors for taking the responsibility for the scientific contents, and, above all, to Glaxo Group Research who sponsored this symposium.

S.R.N.
1988

List of participants

Organising Committee:

McADAM, Keith PWJ, London School of Hygiene and Tropical Medicine, London, United Kingdom

NEU, Harold C, Department of Medicine, Columbia University, New York, NY, United States of America.

NORRBY, S. Ragnar, Department of Infectious Diseases, University of Lund, Lund, Sweden

PETERSON, Phillip K, Department of Medicine, Hennepin County Medical Center, Minneapolis, Minnesota, United States of America.

VERHOEF, Jan, Department of Clinical Microbiology, University Hospital, GV Utrecht, The Netherlands.

Chairmen:

MILLS, John, Division of Infectious Diseases, San Francisco General Hospital, San Francisco, California, United States of America (Also Discussant).

NORRBY, Erling, Department of Virology, Karolinska Institute, Stockholm, Sweden

WHITTON, J. Lindsay, Research Institute of Scripps Clinic, La Jolla, California, United States of America (Also Discussant).

Speakers:

ALMOND, Jeffrey W, Department of Microbiology, University of Reading, Reading, United Kingdom.

BOLOGNESI, Dani P, Surgical Virology Laboratory, Duke University Medical Center, Durham, North Carolina, United States of America.

CLUMECK, Nathan, Department of Infectious Diseases, Hospital Saint Pierre, Brussels, Belgium

FIDDIAN, Paul, Wellcome Research Laboratories, Beckenham, Kent, United Kingdom.

FUJINAMI, Robert S, Department of Pathology, University of California, California, United States of America.

GLOVER, Stuart C, Infectious Diseases Unit, Ham Green Hospital, Bristol, United Kingdom.

KAPIKIAN, Albert Z, Laboratory of Infectious Diseases, National Institutes of Health, Bethesda, Maryland, United States of America.

KOSZINOWSKI, Ulrich, Department of Virology, University of Ulm, Ulm, West Germany

PLOTKIN, Stanley A, Children's Hospital of Philadelphia, Philadelphia, Pensilvania, United States of America.

PLOTZ, Paul H, National Institute of Arthritis, Musculoskeletal & Skin Diseases, National Institutes of Health, Bethesda, Maryland, United States of America.

PRUSINER, Stanley, Department of Neurology, University of California, San Francisco, California, United States of America.

REICHMAN, Richard, Infectious Disease Unit, University of Rochester Medical Center, School of Medicine & Dentistry, Rochester, New York, NY, United States of America.

THOMAS, Howard C, Chairman of Medicine, St Mary's Medical School, London, United Kingdom.

TYRELL, David A J, MRC Common Cold Unit, Harvard Hospital, Salisbury, Wiltshire, United Kimgdom.

Discussants:

BECKER, Thomas M, Department of Medicine, University of New Mexico School of Medicine, Albuquerque, New Mexico, United States of America.

CARLSON, George A, The Jackson Laboratory, Bar Harbor, Maine, United States of America.

COHEN, Stuart, Division of Infectious Diseases, University of California, Sacramento, California, United States of America.

DYRBERG, Thomas, Hagedorn Research Laboratory, Gentofte, Denmark.

JUST, Max, Basles Kinderhospital, Basel, Switzerland.

PERRILLO, Robert, VA Medical Center, St Louis, Missouri, United States of America.

RACANIELLO, Vincent R, Department of Microbiology, Columbia University College of Physicians and Surgeons, New York, NY, United States of America.

WADELL, Göran, Virology Laboratory, Regionsjukhuset, Umea, Sweden.

WEISS, Robin A, Chester Beatty Laboratories, Institute of Cancer Research, Royal Cancer Hospital, Fulham Road, London, United Kingdom.

WHITLEY, Richard, Department of Clinical Virology, The Childrens Hospital Towers, Birmingham, Alabama, United States of America.

Contents

Guest Lecture

1. What can we learn from the common cold?   3
   David A. J. Tyrrell

Section I: Antiviral Chemotherapy: The Future

Chairman: *John Mills*

2. Antiviral chemotherapy of HIV infection   15
   Nathan Clumeck and Philippe Hermans
   Discussant: *John Mills*

3. Human papillomaviruses and treatment of condyloma   36
   acuminatum with intralesionally administered interferon
   Richard C. Reichman, Mark H. Stoler and David Oakes
   Discussant: *Thomas M. Becker*

4. Management of chronic hepatitis virus infection   52
   Howard C. Thomas
   Discussant: *Robert Perrillo*

5. Herpes group viruses   72
   Paul Fiddian
   Discussant: *Richard Whitley*

Section II: Interaction Between Virus Proteins and the Host Immune System

Chairman: *J. Lindsay Whitton*

6. Prions causing slow infections   99
   Stanley Prusiner
   Discussant: *George A. Carlson*

7. Viral determinants and autoimmunity   135
   Robert S. Fujinami
   Discussant: *Thomas Dyrberg*

8. Picornavirus-initiated chronic inflammation   145
   Paul H. Plotz, Mary E. Cronin, Lori A. Love, Frederic W. Miller,
   Patrick McClintock and David W. Smith
   Discussant: *Stuart Cohen*

9. The cytolytic T lymphocyte response to murine   158
   cytomegalovirus infection
   Ulrich Koszinowski
   Discussant: *J. Lindsay Whitton*

Section III: New Viral Vaccines
Chairman: *Erling Norrby*

10. The immunobiology of the HIV envelope   187
    Dani P. Bolognesi
    Discussant: *Robin A. Weiss*

11. Redesigning poliovirus for vaccine purposes   205
    Jeffrey W. Almond, Karen L. Burke, Michael A. Skinner,
    Morag Ferguson, Eric D. A. D'Souza, Glynis Dunn,
    Vincent R. Racaniello and Philip D. Minor
    Discussant: *Vincent R. Racaniello*

12. Prospects for development of a rotavirus vaccine against rotavirus   217
    diarrhoea by a Jennerian and a modified Jennerian strategy
    Albert Z. Kapikian, Jorge Flores, Kim Y. Green,
    Yasutaka Hoshino, Mario Gorziglia, Kazuo Nishikawa,
    Robert M. Channock and Irene Perez-Schael
    Discussant: *Göran Wadell*

13. Vaccination against varicella   240
    Stanley A. Plotkin, Stuart E. Starr, Anne A. Gershon,
    Barbara Zajc and Barbara J. Kuter
    Discussant: *Max Just*

Guest Lecture

14. Lessons from Lassa—A brief review and perspective   263
    Stuart C. Glover

Guest Lecture

1. What can we learn from the common cold?

David A. J. Tyrrell

INTRODUCTION

Virus infection of the respiratory tract is a significant disease problem and is for most people the main reason for being unwell and performing below normal. Study of the common cold also provides a number of guidelines for understanding viral infectious diseases in general.

DEFINITIONS

In the United Kingdom this group of shortlived non-bacterial respiratory infections has been classified according to the site at which the main clinical signs and symptoms are observed i.e. the nose, the pharynx and so on (Miller, 1973). Subsequent aetiological studies have shown that the relationship between the causative virus and these clinical patterns is quite complex (see Chanock & Parrott, 1965; Chanock et al, 1965). For example, an adenovirus may typically cause pharyngitis but it can also cause pneumonia or conjunctivitis. These relationships were not immediately obvious but have been worked out by carefully planned combined clinical and laboratory studies (Tyrrell, 1963) which documented, first, the exact disease pattern, secondly the presence of virus infection and, thirdly, that virus was present in a higher proportion of cases than of a comparison group such as siblings who formed 'healthy controls' (Working Party, 1965). When the epidemiological data were inconclusive and the expected disease was mild, it was ethical and scientifically efficient to inoculate viruses into volunteers and show that a typical disease was produced and that it was significantly associated with infection (Tyrrell & Bynoe, 1958, 1969; Tyrrell et al, 1959). These experiments played an important role in the 1950s and 1960s in determining which viruses caused colds and which did not (Buckland et al, 1959).

It therefore makes sense only to discuss acute upper respiratory infections as a whole, with emphasis perhaps being placed on the mildest and commonest, namely common colds. In many respects this has all been done before and there are excellent reviews focusing on the clinical condition (Couch, 1984), on the

3

viruses e.g. rhinoviruses (MacNaughton, 1982) or coronaviruses (Siddell et al, 1983) at the biological level. We are now learning the molecular genetics and structure of these viruses at an amazing speed (e.g. Rossman et al, 1985). This paper discusses how our present understanding was arrived at, how it interrelates with other aspects of science and medical practice and what might be the next steps forward.

PRESENT KNOWLEDGE

The impact of colds
The full effects of these diseases and these viruses on the population is unknown. In experimental infections only half of those infected develop colds, even mild ones and as family studies show that adults have about four colds per year (Dingle et al, 1964), an estimate of about eight infections per year can be made. Alternatively it appears that, by about 20 years of age, two thirds of subjects have antibodies against any one rhinovirus and as all rhinoviruses seem to be similarly infectious and pathogenic, and as there are about 100 serotypes, an adult of 20 must have had about 70 infections, or 3.5 per year without counting colds due to other viruses—probably at least twice as many. A study from the Royal College of General Practitioners shows how these infections are distributed (Table 1.1) but while they probably contribute to fatal disease there is no accurate assessment. Furthermore we have little measure of how they influence performance, e.g. ability to study or carry out a job. For commercial purposes the present market in cold remedies has been estimated to total about £100M in the UK or £2 per head of the population per year and $6 billion in the USA, which is an index of how much the average person thinks it is worth to try and get rid of colds. If they knew a treatment was effective they might be willing to spend more. All in all it has to be admitted that we have only a rough idea of the social and economic effect of common colds and related diseases.

Natural history and transmission
The common cold viruses are well adapted and adjusted organisms and propagate without causing serious harm to most of their hosts. Many of them do, however, induce symptoms in a high proportion of infected subjects, and successful transmission depends on the host producing excessive nasal discharge and sneezing in order to disperse the virus.

These are relatively easy generalizations but it is difficult to provide well-founded data on how viruses are transmitted. There are excellent laboratory data that a typical respiratory virus like influenza is only infectious if introduced into the respiratory tract, and for many years it was accepted that colds were transmitted through the air (Lovelock et al, 1952). The group at Charlottesville were impressed with their finding that rhinoviruses remained infectious on fingers and inanimate objects and could be transferred by this route, and from fingers to the conjunctiva or nasal mucosa. Nevertheless, respiratory viruses can be transmitted to man by aerosol. The problem is which route is the more important quantitatively in any specific circumstance. Dick and his colleagues studied a poker game model in which a rhinovirus was being transmitted and showed that, although virus got onto the cards and fingers, transmission was not prevented by restraining the players' hands with splints or collars so that they could not touch their eyes or nose; so presumably it was travelling through the air, though the amount of airborne virus was clearly very small (Dick et al, 1987). However the amount need not be large—the tidal air is about 10 litres per minute and the nasal mucosa removes airborne particles of a suitable size very efficiently, so one infectious particle in 6,000 litres would transmit infections after an hour.

Table 1.1 RCGP weekly returns service (242,000)

	Mean weekly incidence for 1986 per 100/000	
	Total	0–4 years
Asthma	19	52
Bronchitis	99	247
Chickenpox	11	49
Common cold	153	741
Hay fever	21	14
Hepatitis	0.26	0.30
Herpes zoster	5.6	0.6
Intestinal infections	45	247
Epidemic influenza	9.7	6.7
Influenza-like disease	53	194
Laryngitis and tracheitis	22	44
Measles	4.0	35
Meningitis/encephalitis	0.1	0.3
Infectious mononucleosis	1.6	0.45
Mumps	5.7	39
Otitis media	62	450
Pneumonia and pneumonitis	4.1	7.9
Rubella	6.1	38
Sinusitis	32	8.3
Sore throat/tonsillitis	90	207
Whooping cough	2.5	24

Finding the correct answer to the question of transmission is central to the thorough exploration of the possible control of these diseases. There is some evidence that respiratory infections are more common in more crowded homes, and in urban as compared with rural areas, but complex variables are hidden in these associations and it is unlikely that the incidence could be markedly reduced by improved housing conditions. It could be conclusive proof of the point and valuable in practice if the transmission of colds in the home or factory could be reduced by treating fingers or the air. Unfortunately a thorough study in families in Virginia (Farr et al, 1988) shows little or no benefit from using viricidal nasal tissues which suggests that the virus was often travelling through the air.

Immunity to common colds
Rhinovirus antibody measurements have recently been refined using a new ELISA test (Barclay & Al-Nakib, 1987). It appears that the presence of circulating antibody protects against disease while secretory antibody is particularly effective in preventing infection.

Such new information encourages us to review again the possibility of an antirhinovirus vaccine. Early experiments using formalin-inactivated virus harvested from infected tissue cultures induced some antibody response. Unselected volunteers given vaccine by injection were protected against disease induced by a small dose of homologous virus, but selected volunteers given vaccine parenterally were not protected against a large dose of virus though intranasal vaccine gave some protection (Scientific Committee, 1965; Douglas & Couch, 1972).

These results were equivocal but the question was not pursued because it was becoming clear that numerous serotypes of rhinoviruses existed and, with the technology of the day, it would not have been possible to produce a sufficiently polyvalent vaccine. However, we are now in the middle of a collaborative study with the group at Wellcome Biotechnology under Dr F Brown, with the initial objective of understanding the determinants of immunity at the molecular level, using infection with human rhinovirus type 2 (RV2) as a model. Three epitopes have been identified on the surface of this virus which are recognized by mouse monoclonal antibodies. By using these monoclonals and antipeptide sera as blocking reagents it has been possible to detect specific antibody in volunteers directed against these epitopes, and also to investigate which one is associated with resistance to infections. It is interesting that the most important site 'seen' by the human immune system seems to be less important to the mouse (Barclay et al, 1988). We already know that antisera prepared against a peptide mimicking one epitope shows low level neutralizing activity against the virus. Virus escape mutants that resist neutralization by the monoclonal antibodies are also being prepared and when sequenced it should be possible to decide which are the most 'protective sites' on the virus (Francis et al, 1987). We can then plan to prepare a specific peptide antigen which might protect against RV2 infection in volunteers, just as vaccination with peptides that copy the epitopes of foot-and-mouth disease virus protect animals against infection and disease (Bittle et al, 1981).

It is interesting that most of this work was modelled on studies done in quite different fields—for instance the proof that an oligopeptide antigen selected from a single picornavirus peptide could protect against infection was obtained from experiments on infections of guinea-pigs with foot-and-mouth disease virus which resembles rhinoviruses closely at the molecular level, but causes very different diseases and epizootics.

However, the problem of immunity and resistance to colds must not be oversimplified and, in real life, viruses attack individuals in a great variety of immune states. Nevertheless, it is possible to analyse the separate roles of the different elements by studying a varied group of volunteers and analysing their immune, virological and clinical response to a standard virus challenge.

We have done a study of this sort in volunteers exposed to a coronavirus (Callow, 1985). The results showed that both circulating and secretory antibody contributed to protection against infections and disease but that IgA reduced the period of virus shedding. Male volunteers or those who had had recent cold were more resistant to infections and illness and they also had more specific antibodies and nasal secretion proteins than females and those who had not had a cold recently. Some earlier studies showed that the personality of a volunteer and the presence of stress altered susceptibility to colds, so we are now in the middle of a large collaborative study with Dr Sheldon Cohen of Pittsburgh, in which he is looking in more detail at the psychological parameters, and we are also measuring systematically a number of indices of immune status in case the psychological effects are mediated through the immune system.

All this emphasizes an important difference from other virus infections. Although the initial infection, say of the intestinal mucosa by polioviruses, is no doubt similar, the fate of the individual can be largely predicted from the presence or absence of neutralizing antibody in the circulation. Thus, the target for the development of a vaccine was clearer and simpler than is the case with respiratory viruses. As we understand immunity better it should be possible to set up similar objectives for the development of vaccines against colds defining what antibodies should react with peptide epitopes, what their biological effects should be and where they should be found.

We must, however, be careful about over-simplifying. For instance, as is well known, vaccines made with formalin-inactivated paramyxoviruses (RSV or measles) enhanced disease, probably because the critically important fusion protein was made non-antigenic by the formalin used in production. Similarly naturally induced immune responses may make colds worse—this is suggested by the finding that high concentrations of IgE in the circulation or nasal secretions are associated with worse disease in coronavirus infections (Callow et al, 1988).

What induces symptoms?

Rhinoviruses destroy many ciliated epithelial cells in *in vitro* infections of organ cultures but, during a cold, the damage in the human nose is relatively mild. Mucociliary transport is slowed during symptomatic colds and influenza B infections and this can be correlated with the loss of cilia from superficial epithelial cells (Wilson et al, 1987). However, this has also been ascribed to a reduction in ciliary beat frequency, change in the amount and consistency of mucus or ultrastructural defects in the cilia (Pedersen et al, 1983; Sakkakura, 1983; Carson et al, 1985). There is also nasal congestion and increased blood flow and a large increase in nasal secretion, apparently derived in part from an increase in vascular permeability (Bende et al, 1988). We and others have looked for inflammatory mediators such as arachidonic acid derivatives—leukotrienes and prostaglandin—or histamine but no substantial or convincing increases have been found (Callow et al, 1988), except in bradykinins (Naclerio et al, 1985). Nedocromil, a drug that blocks release of leukotrienes, histamine, etc., provided some benefit in rhinovirus colds, which may support the idea that these play a role even though their concentration in the secretion is not raised. It will be interesting to see if any benefits derive from bradykinin inhibitors which are now becoming available.

Cytokines and lymphokines are also likely to be produced in a membrane in which inflammation and immune responses are going on. There is some evidence that interleukin 1 (IL–1) is produced, since even in mild colds an increase of serum amyloid A protein (SAA) is found at the time of marked symptoms (Whicher et al 1985) and this presumably means that IL–1 released by local cells, such as macrophages, induces the synthesis of SAA, as a typical part of the acute phase

7

reaction. Systemic involvement is particularly prominent in experimental influenza, and in these illnesses, unlike colds, interferon alpha (IFN–α) can be found in the circulation. This is known to have systemic effects often called 'toxic' (Scott, 1982), and that small doses produce malaise, fever, tachycardia, etc. It is plausible that the molecule is the cause of at least some of these symptoms of influenzal illnesses.

THE CONSEQUENCES OF COLDS

The fact that the patient with a cold also feels ill has attracted little attention, but it has recently been shown that not only are there real effects on human performance during colds, but that these are much more specific and long lasting than might have been expected (Smith et al, 1987). Volunteers infected with influenza virus were found to perform less well on tasks requiring visual attention, and the effects were still present (though less marked) if they were infected and without symptoms than if they had clinical influenza. Volunteers with colds produced by various viruses, performed less well than normal on tasks requiring hand–eye co-ordination but performed normally on tasks that demanded attention. These effects were not large but were as great as those seen following amounts of alcohol or lack of sleep which are known to be significant in real life situations. It is also now known that defects of performance can still be detected after the clinical signs of infection have disappeared. Observations like this need to be extended out into the community to discover whether road accidents, school performance, etc., are affected by these viral infections.

In the same way information is accruing on psychological make-up and response to viral infection. For example, Broadbent and colleagues (1984) have shown that volunteers with introverted personalities are more susceptible, as are subjects showing evidence of 'stress'.

COMMON COLDS AND OTHER DISEASES

It is clear, when examining full clinical records of patients with respiratory virus infections, that nasal symptoms are present in the large majority, although this may not be obvious in the diagnostic label. In this sense the common cold is a part of most virus infections of the lower airways, either preceding or accompanying the presenting illness (Hope-Simpson & Miller, 1973).

Secondly, virus infections may predispose to or accompany bacterial infections. It is now clear that the influenza virus impairs resistance in several ways, e.g. by damaging the mucociliary escalator and impairing phagocytosis. There is little evidence that common cold viruses do the same. Nevertheless it may be that, in developing countries, where there is a high mortality from bacterial pneumonia, and all the common respiratory viruses are also prevalent, the mild damage done by the viruses does predispose (along with malnutrition, high carrier rates, air pollution and other factors of course) to the development of pneumonia in certain children (Pio et al, 1985).

Colds can also exacerbate chronic diseases though it may be quite difficult to prove. In early (unpublished) studies we failed to show that rhinoviruses were infecting patients suffering from relapses of chronic bronchitis. However, when arrangements were made to test them very early in the relapse it was found that these and other common respiratory viruses did apparently initiate the process of relapse (e.g. Stenhouse, 1967). In children with Still's disease there was a highly significant connection between a minor respiratory illness and the reactivation of their disease in the succeeding weeks, due perhaps to the infection 'jolting' the immune system out of a precarious balance (De-Vere Tyndall et al, 1984).

APPROACHES TO MANAGEMENT AND TREATMENT

Vaccine
A common cold vaccine seemed at one time to be a likely target once 'the common cold virus' had been cultured in the laboratory, until it was realised that there were so many viruses that a vaccine would have to be impossibly polyvalent. More recent data indicate that circulating antibody plays a major role in protecting against disease in rhinovirus common colds, raising new hopes for a rhinovirus vaccine. In the case of the biologically similar virus, foot-and-mouth disease virus, it is known that neutralizing antibody is stimulated by injection of a peptide mimicking an epitope on the surface of the virus and protects against experimental infection. If it is also possible to protect man against a rhinovirus by vaccinating with a peptide antigen, it might be possible to produce a multiple component vaccine which would protect against a useful proportion of the viruses and the illnesses they cause.

Antiviral molecules
Antiviral therapy was at first regarded as impossible, partly because it was thought not possible to find molecules which were sufficiently active and non-toxic when administered intra-nasally. However in 1973 it was shown that human interferon sprayed up the nose prevents colds, and recently we showed that a spray of a sufficiently potent synthetic antirhinovirus drug can prevent colds produced by a sensitive rhinovirus (Al-Nakib et al, 1987). Putting these facts together with the effectiveness of amantadine and related drugs in influenza, we can see that prevention or treatment of colds with antiviral drugs is not impossible in principle, even though it is still not achievable in practice.

Correcting physiology
The effectiveness of oral rehydration to compensate for the physiological disturbances induced by an infection has been proven in cholera and other diarrhoeal diseases. It is probable that it is also good physiological management in the intensive care unit that has reduced the mortality from RSV infection in infants. On the other hand, the use of drugs to reduce nasal secretion or obstruction in colds is widely regarded as symptomatic treatment. This may be because the present drugs used are not really satisfactory or free of unwanted

effects, nor able to prevent serious sequelae. If the important mediators of the symptoms and signs of colds were known it might be possible to develop specific inhibitors; since it has recently been suggested that kinins may be important in this regard, anti-kinins might prove useful.

SOME BROAD CONCLUSIONS

Colds and other infections are typical broad medical problems

(1)   There is no single virus causing a single disease syndrome, but numerous pathogens to detect, analyse and understand.

(2)   To understand the disease close attention must be paid to the immune status and response of the host.

(3)   A clinical research 'hunt' should be in progress for the key molecules involved in the disease processes.

(4)   The study of infection is much more than microbiology alone.

(5)   While animal studies are very valuable, in the end the answer can only be obtained by studying man.

Colds and infections include an element of interaction with the CNS

(1)   Common colds provide an opportunity for ethical and quite rigorous experiments to find some of the rules by which life situations and personality play a part in organic and in psychosomatic disease.

(2)   Colds also offer an opportunity to investigate the nature and mechanism of changes in behaviour and human performance in response to infectious disease.

Colds illustrate the range of options there are for managing infections

(1)   It was naive to think that colds might be prevented by a simple vaccine, but it was also premature to think, in the 1960s, that a multivalent vaccine would never be possible.

(2)   As the mechanism of the increase of nasal secretion in colds is unknown there is, as yet, no really logical way of controlling the symptoms.

New science or new techniques may give insight or solutions to problems which seemed quite insoluble

(1)   Interferon for clinical trials is now available with the advent of recombinant DNA and associated techniques.

(2)   The combination of molecular virology and crystallography has now provided a rational approach to defining the peptides of rhinoviruses which stimulate immunity to infection.

REFERENCES

Al-Nakib W, Higgins P G, Tyrrell D A J et al 1987 Tolerance and prophylactic efficacy of a new antirhinovirus compound R61837. Seventh International Congress of Virology Edmonton Abstract R32.3

Barclay W S et al 1988 In preparation

Barclay W S, Al-Nakib W 1987 An ELISA for the detection of rhinovirus specific antibody in serum and nasal secretion. Journal of Virological Methods 15: 53–64

Bende M, Barrow I, Heptonstall J et al 1988 Changes in human nasal mucosa during experimental coronavirus common colds Acta Otolaryngologica, in press

Bittle J L, Houghten R A, Alexander H et al 1981 Protection against foot and mouth disease by immunization with a chemically synthesized peptide predicted from the viral nucleotide sequence. Nature London 298: 30–33

Broadbent D E, Broadbent M H P, Phillpotts R J, Wallace J 1984 Some further studies on the prediction of experimental colds in volunteers by psychological factors. Journal of Psychosomatic Research 28: 511–523

Buckland F E, Bynoe M L , Philipson L et al 1959 Experimental infection of human volunteers with the U virus—a strain of ECHO virus type 11. Journal of Hygiene Cambridge 57: 274–284

Callow K A 1985 Effect of specific humoral immunity and some non-specific factors on resistance of volunteers to respiratory coronavirus infection. Journal of Hygiene Cambridge 95: 173–189

Callow K A, Tyrrell D A J, Shaw R J et al 1988 The influence of atopy on the clinical manifestations of coronavirus infection in adult volunteers. Clinical Allergy 18: 119–129

Carson J L, Collier A M, Hu S S 1985 Acquired ciliary defects in nasal epithelium of children with acute viral upper respiratory in fections. New England Journal of Medicine 312: 463–468

Chanock R M, Mufson M A, Johnson K M 1965 Comparative biology and ecology of human virus and mycoplasma respiratory pathogens. Progress in Medical Virology 7: 208–252

Chanock R M, Parrott R H 1965 Acute respiratory disease in infancy and childhood: present understanding and prospects for prevention. Pediatrics 36: 21–39

Couch R B 1984 The common cold: control. Journal of Infectious Diseases 150: 167–173

De-Vere Tyndall A, Bacon T, Parry R, Tyrrell D A J, Denman A M, Ansell B M 1984 Infection and interferon production in systemic juvenile chronic arthritis: a prospective study. Annals of the Rheumatic Diseases 43: 1–7

Dick E C, Jennings L C, Mink K A et al. 1987 Aerosol transmission of rhinovirus colds. Journal of Infectious Diseases, 156: 442–448

Dingle J H, Badger G F, Jordan W S Jr 1964 Illness in the Home. Western Reserve University, Cleveland, Ohio, pp1–398

Douglas R G Jr, Couch R B 1972 Parenteral inactivated rhinovirus vaccine: minimal protective effect. Proceedings of the Society for Experimental Biology and Medicine 139: 899–902

Farr B M, Hendley J O, Kaiser D L et al 1988 Two randomized controlled trials of virucidal nasal tissues in the prevention of natural upper respiratory tract infections. American Journal of Epidemiology, in press

Francis M J, Hastings G Z, Sangar D V et al 1987 A synthetic peptide which elicits neutralizing antibody against human rhinovirus type 2. Journal of General Virology 68: 2687–2691

Hope-Simpson R E, Miller D L 1973 The definition of acute respiratory illnesses in general practice. Postgraduate Medical Journal 49: 763–770

Lovelock J E, Porterfield J S, Roden A T et al 1952 Further studies on the natural transmission of the common cold. Lancet ii: 657–660

MacNaughton M R 1982 The structure and replication of rhinoviruses. Current Topics in Microbiology and Immunology 987: 1–26

Miller D L 1973 Collaborative studies of acute respiratory disease in patients seen in general practice and in children admitted to hospital. Aim, field methods and morbidity rates. Postgraduate Medical Journal 49: 749–762

Naclerio R M, Gwaltney J M, Kendley K O et al 1985 Kinins are generated during rhinovirus colds. Clinical Research 33: 613A

Pedersen M, Sakkakura Y, Winther B, Brofeldt S, Mygino N 1983 Nasal mucociliary transport, number of ciliated cells and beating pattern in natural acquired colds. European Journal of Respiratory Disease 64 (Suppl 128) 355–364

Pio A, Leowski J, Ten Damm H G 1985 IN: Douglas RM, Derby-Eatan E (eds) The magnitude of the problem of acute respiratory infection in ARI in childhood. Department of Community Medicine, Adelaide, South Australia, pp 3–16

Rossmann M J, Arnold E, Erickson J W et al 1985 Structure of a human common cold virus and functional relationship to other picornaviruses. Nature London 317: 145–153

Sakkakura Y 1983 Changes of mucociliary function during colds. European Journal of Respiratory Diseases 64 (Suppl 128) 348–354

Scientific Committee on Common Cold Vaccines 1965 Prevention of cold by vaccination against a rhinovirus. British Medical Journal 1: 1344–1349

Scott G M. 1982 Interferon: pharmacokinetics and toxicity. Philosophical Transactions of the Royal Society of London, Series B 299: 91–107

Siddell S G, Wege H, ter Meulen V 1983 The biology of coronaviruses. Journal of General Virology 64: 761–776

Smith A P, Tyrrell D A J, Coyle K, Willman J S. 1987 Selective effects of minor illnesses on human performance. British Journal of Psychology 78: 183–188

Stenhouse A C 1967 Rhinovirus infection in acute exacerbations of chronic bronchitis: a controlled prospective study. British Medical Journal 3: 461–463

Tyrrell D A J 1963 Discovering and defining the etiology of acute respiratory viral disease. American Review of Respiratory Diseases, 88: 77–84

Tyrrell D A J, Bynoe M L 1958 Inoculation of volunteers with JH strain of a new respiratory virus. Lancet 2, 931–933

Tyrrell D A J, Bynoe M L 1969 Studies on parainfluenza type 2 and 4 viruses obtained from patients with common colds. British Medical Journal 1: 471–474

Tyrrell D A J, Bynoe M L, Peterson K B et al 1959 Inoculation of human volunteers with parainfluenza viruses types 1 and 3 (HA2 and HA1). British Medical Journal 2: 909–911

Whicher J T, Chambers R E, Higginson J, Nashef L and Higgins P G 1985 Acute phase response of serum amyloid A protein and C-reactive protein to the common cold and influenza. Journal of Clinical Pathology 38: 312–316

Wilson R, Alton E, Rutman A et al 1987 Upper respiratory tract infection and mucociliary clearance. European Journal of Respiratory Disease, 7: 272–279

Working Party on Acute Respiratory Virus Infections 1965 A collaborative study on the aetiology of acute respiratory infections in Britain 1961–1964, British Medical Journal 2: 319–366

Section I:
ANTIVIRAL CHEMOTHERAPY: THE FUTURE

Chairman: John Mills

2. Antiviral chemotherapy of HIV infection

Nathan Clumeck and Phillippe Hermans

INTRODUCTION

Infections with human immunodeficiency virus (HIV) may be treated with antiviral or immunomodulatory drugs. Antiviral drugs could act at a number of points in viral replication: by blocking the absorption and penetration; by inhibiting reverse transcriptase (RT); by preventing the integration of viral DNA into the host genome, blocking transcription or translation of viral DNA into viral messenger RNA (mRNA) and proteins; by interfering with glycosylation steps, assembly and budding. The immunomodulatory approach seeks to improve immune function by stimulating T-cells through various cytokines or by enhancing replacement of depleted cells through bone marrow or thymus transplantation. It is almost certain that combination of both antiviral and immunomodulatory approaches will be necessary to achieve long-term effective therapy of AIDS. Because HIV infects the central nervous system (CNS) and can remain clinically dormant in the host for a protracted period, the ideal anti-HIV drug or combination of drugs should be of low cost, be administered orally, be non-toxic enough to take over an extended period of time, be able to cross the blood–brain barrier, and be active on every target cell.

To date, only zidovudine has been shown to be an effective, although not an ideal antiretroviral drug. This review deals with antiviral drugs (Table 2.1) which have shown some promise *in vitro*, but which require further extended clinical investigations before a determination of their place in the treatment of HIV infection can be made.

ADSORPTION AND PENETRATION BLOCKERS

CD4-analogues (rs-T4)
Soluble forms of CD4 analogues (rs-T4) have been produced using recombinant DNA technology. Like the CD4 molecule of T lymphocytes they have a high affinity for the HIV-envelope glycoprotein gp120. Soluble CD4 is not a true antiviral drug since it does not inhibit replication or destroy the virus. It probably interferes with the binding of HIV to lymphocytes by covering the gp120. This

soluble CD4 analogue has been demonstrated to neutralize the infectivity of HIV_1 *in vitro*. When incubated with virus infected cells, soluble CD4 prevented the growth of HIV_1. Although there is a potential to interfere with normal immunological functions, preliminary evaluation in chimpanzee of rs-T4 failed to show adverse immunological effects (Abrams et al, 1988; Smith et al, 1987).

Table 2.1 Name and mode of action of anti-HIV drugs

  I. *Adsorption and penetration blockers*
    a. CD4-analogues (rs-T4)
    b. Dextran-sulphate and other sulphated polysaccharides
    c. Peptide T
    d. Al-721

 II. *Reverse transcriptase inhibitors*
    a. Nucleoside analogues—zidovudine
    —dideoxycytidine
    b. Suramin
    c. HPA 23
    d. Foscarnet
    e. Rifabutine

III. *Transcription inhibitor*
    a. Ribavirin

IV. *Glycosylation inhibitors*
    a. Castanospermine

  V. *Assembly blockers*
    a. Interferons or interferon inducers
    b. Ampligen
    c. ABPP

VI. *Undetermined mechanisms*
    a. Avarol
    b. Isoprinosine
    c. Gamma interferon
    d. Fusidic acid

Dextran sulphate
Developed in the 1950s, dextran sulphate is a sulphated polysaccharidic anion of low toxicity, clinically administered for its anticoagulant properties.

As an anti-HIV drug dextran sulphate has been demonstrated to inhibit RT activity and formation of syncytial giant cells. By its anionic charge, dextran sulphate also alters viral binding to the host cell. If added to the culture medium, viral adsorption is totally inhibited. If confirmed, its cumulative properties with zidovudine could be attractive considering the lack of meaningful toxicity of dextran sulphate. Phase I clinical trials are underway among AIDS/ARC patients (Abrams et al 1987, Center for Diseases Control AIDS 1987, Ueno & Kuno 1987).

Derivatives of this class without anticoagulant properties are now being developed and investigated for antiretroviral activity.

Peptide T
Peptide T is a synthetic octapeptide sequence which is similar for five terminal amino acids to a peptide sequence of the HIV_1 envelope glycoprotein (gp120).

The proposed mode of action of peptide T is the blocking of host-cell T_4-receptor by competing with the envelope glycoprotein (gp120) of HIV. Inhibition of HIV replication has also been reported. Enormous controversy exists in the literature concerning peptide T. Indeed, *in vitro* effectiveness of peptide T initially reported by Pert was confirmed by only one other laboratory. Under various experimental conditions, nine laboratories were unable to detect any anti-HIV activity to peptide T. At narrow concentration range, it is possible that peptide T has potent biological effects perhaps mediated by receptors other than T4. Expression of the Ia histocompatibility antigen in mouse macrophages has also been reported. Peptide T has a very short half-life in experimental animals and is also unlikely to cross the blood–brain barrier. Despite these uncertainties, a clinical trial of peptide T has now begun in 36 AIDS patients in Sweden. A preliminary study reported some improvement in four male AIDS patients who received peptide T intravenously for four weeks on a compassionate use basis (Barnes, 1987; Ruff et al, 1987).

AL-721

AL-721 is a mixture of neutral glyceride-phosphatidylcholine-phosphatidyl-ethanolamine activated lipids in a 7:2:1 ratio, hence its name. These components are extracted from the egg yolks of hens. *In vitro*, high concentrations are required to inhibit HIV replication and no data on serum concentrations achieved with oral administration are available. AL-721 is thought to work by fluidizing the virus membrane making it impossible for it to attach to the T4 receptor of host cell. Thus, both cell-to-cell and virion-to-cell virus transmission could be blocked.

Preliminary human trials showed no side-effects attributable to AL-721 with oral doses up to 60 g daily. After an eight-week phase I pilot study involving eight patients with persistent generalized lymphadenopathy (PGL) taking 10 g twice a day, a marked reduction of reverse transcriptase activity in viral co-cultivation assays has been noted in five of seven subjects and an increased lymphoproliferative response to mitogens in four of five patients with immunological deficiency. However, no improvement in CD4 lymphocyte count was observed and one patient developed a generalized CMV infection and cerebral toxoplasmosis several weeks after treatment. Large scale double-blind placebo-controlled trials of AIDS/ARC and PGL patients with AL-721, possibly combined with thymic humoral factor, will start in Israel and New York (Abrams et al, 1987; Abrams et al, 1988; Grieco et al, 1987; Sandstrom & Kaplan, 1987).

REVERSE TRANSCRIPTASE INHIBITORS

Nucleotide analogues

Zidovudine (AZT)

Many investigational inhibitors belonging to the family of nucleoside analogues have been tested for activity against HIV, mostly *in vitro* (De Clercq, 1986). Reduction or removal of a hydroxyl group by substituting halo or amino groups at the 3'-carbon position of purine or pyrimidine bases leads to an anti-HIV activity.

Zidovudine, a thymidine analogue, is phosphorylated intracellularly to the 5'-triphosphate form which is a potent and selective inhibitor of HIV encoded reverse transcriptase. Incorporation of zidovudine triphosphate into proviral DNA blocks any further elongation. A phase I human study revealed that 60% of administered zidovudine was metabolized to glucuronide conjugates and eliminated by renal excretion. Following oral administration, bioavailability was 65%. The ability of zidovudine to cross the blood–brain barrier is confirmed by the CFS/plasma concentration which is approximately 0.5 (Klecker et al, 1987). Macrophage cells could be unable to phosphorylate zidovudine. A first, phase I, pharmacokinetic and tolerance study in 19 patients with advanced HIV infection showed clinical and immunological benefits: 15 of the 19 patients had increased CD_4 lymphocyte numbers, six patients recovered delayed type hypersensitivity in skin test reactions, two fungal nailbed infections improved without specific therapy, six patients had other clinical improvement and weight gain on the whole group was 2.2 kg (Yarchoan et al, 1986).

A double-blind, placebo-controlled multicentre trial, started in February 1986, was prematurely terminated in September 1986 due to a markedly increased survival in treated patients, both those with severe ARC as well as those with AIDS (within three months of their first episode of *Pneumocystis carinii* pneumonia). There was only one death in the 145 patients who received AZT compared with 19 in the 137 patients of the placebo arm. During the placebo-controlled period, opportunistic infections occurred in only 18% of the zidovudine recipients and in 36% of the placebo recipients. The mortality rate among patients receiving AZT for 36 weeks was 6.2% compared with 39.3% among the placebo group (Fischl et al, 1987). No apparent benefit of zidovudine was found in patients with Kaposi's sarcoma. Another study suggested that zidovudine administration was associated with a five-fold reduction in the mortality rates at one year in a population of AIDS patients with cerebral toxoplasmosis (Hermans et al, 1988).

The major toxicity of AZT reported in these studies was bone marrow suppression. One or more blood transfusions were given to 31% of the zidovudine group versus 11% of the placebo arm (Richman et al, 1987). While there have been reports of neurological improvement under zidovudine therapy, neurological disease attributed to zidovudine has also been noted—specifically headaches and seizures.

Co-administration of drugs such as probenecid, aspirin, indomethacin or acetaminophen, inhibiting glucuronidation, must be avoided as well as nephrotoxic or myelotoxic agents. Presently, trends in zidovudine treatment are the following:

(1)   Association with immunomodulatory or other antiviral drugs (Yarchoan et al, 1988) (Table 2.2).

(2)   Modification of mode of administration. Early results with zidovudine administered six hourly have shown that it was as efficacious as four–hourly administration, well tolerated and made compliance easier for the patient (Weerts et al, 1988).

(3)   Use of zidovudine very early in the evolution of HIV infection (when T4-cells are greater than 400/mm³, asymptomatic stage) in order to prevent evolution to ARC or AIDS. These multicentric placebo-controlled studies are presently underway with around 2000 patients in Europe and in USA.

Table 2.2 Likely interactions among antiretroviral drugs

Effect	Drug concentrations
Cumulative	Zidovudine—Dextran sulphate Zidovudine—DDC
Synergistic	Purine analogues + Ribavirin Zidovudine + alpha interferon Zidovudine + GM-CSF Zidovudine + Acyclovir
Antagonist	Zidovudine + Ribavirin Pyrimidine analogues + Ribavirin

Acyclovir, another DNA polymerase inhibitor commonly used in the treatment of herpes viruses infections, acts as a competitor of the deoxyguanosine triphosphate and has been shown to be synergistic with AZT *in vitro*. Clinical trials are presently underway to evaluate the relevance of this observation. Trials using AZT combined to alpha-interferon of DDC are also ongoing (Mitsuya & Broder, 1987).

Other compounds, such as CS-87, seem to be at least as active as AZT and maybe less toxic in experiments using human granulocyte-macrophage precursor cells. Pre-clinical studies are underway.

2'–3'-Dideoxycytidine (DDC)

2'–3'-Dideoxycytidine (DDC) is a nucleoside analogue developed at the National Cancer Institute, and is more active by weight than zidovudine *in vitro* (Mitsuya et al, 1987). Preliminary clinical trials in 70 AIDS/ARC patients have shown clinical and immunological improvement. There was no suppression of erythropoiesis, which is the major adverse reaction encountered with AZT, but severe dose-related peripheral neurotoxicity has been reported (Abrams et al, 1987; Abrams et al, 1988). Another point of concern is the poor diffusion of DDC through the blood–brain barrier. A two arm phase I trial with lower doses (0.03 mg/kg every four or eight hours) is ongoing. So far, no significant side-effects have been reported among the 12 patients enrolled. Combined therapy with AZT and DDC at lower doses is now proposed with the hope of diminishing their respective dose-related side-effects and maybe increase their antiviral potency (Yarchoan et al, 1988). Thus, a phase I study of DDC in severe HIV infection as a single agent or alternating with zidovudine has been performed in patients with AIDS or AIDS-related complex. By week two, 10 of the 15 patients receiving 0.03–0.09 mg/kg every four hours increased their T4-cells. After six weeks, their mean absolute number was grossly similar to the mean T4-cell count at the entry. Moreover, DDC induced a transient fall in serum p24 antigen. Dose-related side-effects included fever, rash, mouth sores, neutro- and thrombocytopenia and a reversible, severe neuropathy occurred in 10 patients.

This data suggested that DDC, as an anti-HIV agent *in vivo*, has a different toxicity profile than zidovudine.

The alternating regimen administered to five patients (oral AZT, 200 mg every four hours for seven days; DDC, 0.03 mg/kg every four hours for seven days) was well tolerated. Patients sustained beneficial effects on CD_4 lymphocyte counts or serum p24 antigen concentrations. Larger controlled studies are needed to determine whether such alternating regimens with AZT and DDC at lower doses might provide good antiviral effect and lower toxicity.

Suramin

Used for over 50 years for the treatment of protozoan infections, suramin sodium has been known to be a potent reverse transcriptase inhibitor since 1979. Its virustatic activity was further demonstrated against HIV. A preliminary clinical trial suggested a potential dose-related antiviral activity among AIDS patients and some enthusiastic results in a non-controlled trial were published among African patients (Rouvroy et al, 1985). No improvement of immune function was noted.

However, an extended multicentre trial of 98 AIDS/ARC patients who received 0.5, 1.0 or 1.5 g/week for six weeks followed by maintenance therapy with 0.5 or 1.0 g weekly intravenously for a maximum of one year, showed no immunologic improvement, only one clinical remission and seven minor clinical responses. Many severe and even fatal toxic effects occurred including nausea, neurological impairments, neutropenia and thrombocytopenia, proteinuria, liver function alterations, adrenal insufficiency, fever, rash and malaise, and a possible keratopathy seen in 12–34% of the treated patients. Interestingly, the drug did have an antiviral effect as 40% of the patients became HIV-culture negative, but this was without any correlation between virus recovery and serum suramin concentration.

The conclusions of the U.S. Suramin Working Group are: 'Suramin as currently administered cannot be recommended as effective therapy for AIDS' (Cheson et al, 1987).

Antimoniotungstate (HPA-23)

Heteropolyanion-23 is tri-amonium-21-tungsto-9-antimoniate, a cryptate mineral which was proposed, without conclusive results, as a treatment for Creutzfeld-Jacob disease. *In vitro*, HPA-23 inhibits HIV-replication by acting as a competitive inhibitor of the reverse transcriptase.

The first report of the use of this compound in four AIDS or ARC patients suggested a slight clinical improvement and a marked decrease of the virus reverse transcriptase activity. A further study of 69 AIDS patients who intravenously received dosages of 0.25 to 2 mg/kg showed a dose-dependent reduction of reverse transcriptase activity without any significant change in immunological parameters and in clinical symptoms. In a 15-subject clinical trial using 3 mg/kg/day, response was poor in patients with previous HIV neurological disease or in those who experienced an opportunistic infection. Side-effects of HPA-23 are dose-related and consist of a transient thrombocytopenia, an increase of hepatic enzymes or renal toxicity. More data are needed to assess the doubtful place of HPA-23 as a potential therapy for AIDS (Moskovitz, HPA-23 Cooperative Study Group, 1987; Vittecocq et al, 1987).

Foscarnet (phosphonoformate)

The virustatic activity of phosphonoformic acid has been demonstrated against animal or human retroviruses and also against hepatitis B and herpes viruses, including cytomegalovirus (CMV). This pyrophosphate analogue acts as a non-competitive inhibitor of the reverse transcriptase or DNA polymerase. The drug has to be administered by intravenous infusion to maintain plasma drug levels at about 150 mg/l; adjustments of the rate of infusion according to serum creatinine levels is necessary.

Another hallmark of the drug is its ability to concentrate in bone and to be eliminated very slowly over one year, thus excluding the long-term use of this drug as an anti-HIV agent. Moreover, anti-HIV activity is obtained only from high dosages, which fall within the toxic range, and in vitro, high doses of foscarnet induced some human cell growth suppression. Due to its activity against CMV, clinical trials have focused on patients with suspected CMV infection and AIDS. A British pilot study with eight patients and suspected CMV pneumonitis has started. After one to four weeks of treatment with intravenous infusions of foscarnet, three patients were cured of pneumonia and four others improved, under therapy. Minor thrombophlebitis, impairment of the renal function, anaemia, nausea, headache, fatigue and several neurological signs have been noted (Anderson et al, 1987; Bergdahl et al, 1987; Deray et al, 1987; Vaghefi et al, 1986).

Rifabutine (Ansamycin)

Rifabutine is a semi-synthetic rifamycin S derivative currently used to treat *Mycobacterium avium* intracellular (MAI) infections among AIDS patients. The anti-HIV effect (inhibition of RT) of rifabutine was not suspected until recently.

An oral dosage of 300–600 mg daily among patients with HIV encephalopathy revealed that 30–40% of the drug crosses the blood–brain barrier (Davidson et al 1987). Previous liver diseases increase the risk of hepatotoxicity and reversible neutropenia may occur.

In a dose-escalating trial, no clinical, immunological or antiviral responses have been reported in five ARC patients at dosage of 450 mg daily, but at this dosage, the drug plasma level was below the in vitro effective dose. Clinical data on the possible anti-HIV effectiveness of rifabutine among patients are presently lacking, and its use as antiviral therapy remains doubtful (Burger et al, 1987).

TRANSCRIPTION INHIBITOR

Ribavirin

The aerosol form of this synthetic guanosine analogue is currently used for the treatment of respiratory syncytial virus infections. Antiviral activity against influenza viruses and herpes viruses have also been shown. The drug inhibits inosine monophosphate dehydrogenase. Messenger RNA priming and elongation are altered by the decrease of the guanosine triphosphate pool. The azidothymidine phosphorylation step could be inhibited by this mechanism of action which explains its potential antagonism with zidovudine. More than 60% of the plasma drug level is found in the CSF.

Aside from one heavily critized study involving patients with persistent generalized lymphadenopathy (PGL), no clinical or immune improvement has been reported in a multicentre phase I double-blind placebo-controlled trial with 212 ARC patients. Moreover, preliminary data suggested that patients receiving ribavirin presented with more deaths or medical problems than the placebo group. One non-comparative study involving AIDS/ARC patients showed equivocal results: six of nine patients with a previous HIV-positive culture became HIV-negative; lymphoproliferative responses increased in nine of 14 patients; four of eight AIDS/ARC patients enrolled for the one-year study were alive at the end of the study. Minor side-effects were reported including headache, insomnia, irritability, gastrointestinal symptoms, liver function impairments and mild anaemia. Nevertheless, the lack of proven efficacy and safety led the U.S. FDA to reject the use of ribavirin as treatment of AIDS patients (Connor et al, 1987; Mansell et al, 1987; Spector et al, 1987; Vernon & Schulof, 1987).

GLYCOSYLATION INHIBITORS

Castanospermine
The 1,6,7,8, tetrahydroxyoctahydroindolizine compound is an alkaloid derivative of an Australian chestnut tree. *In vitro* studies have shown that this molecule acts by interfering with post-translational glycosylation, inhibiting the transformation of gp160 into gp120 and affecting the HIV env glycoprotein and not the CD4 molecule. The drug also prevents the uptake of modified virions into cells and syncytium formation, accounting for a likely reduced infectiousness of the newly formed particles. The effectiveness of the drug *in vitro*, suggests that it should be moved rapidly into clinical trials (Walker et al, 1987a; Walker et al, 1987b). Other compounds such as 2-deoxy-D-glucose or deoxynojirimycin could have antiviral properties but unusual dosages are required (De Clercq, 1988 personal communication).

ASSEMBLY BLOCKERS

Interferons

Alpha interferon
Alpha interferons are a group of closely related proteins, one of the three major classes of interferons (alpha, beta and gamma). Interferon (IFN) is now produced by recombinant genetic techniques and these interferons have the same biological activity as the natural forms. Alpha interferon has antiviral, immunomodulating and antiproliferative effects.

After binding to IFN receptors, IFN acts in the HIV infected cell by inducing production of several enzymes that probably interfere with transcription–translation of the mRNA, protein synthesis, assembly and release of the virion.

Alpha interferon was first used in AIDS patients with Kaposi's sarcoma (KS) (Volberding et al, 1987). Tumour regressions have been noted in 20% to 50% of these patients and viral isolation was less frequently noted in the responders than in the non-responder group of KS patients. In a placebo-controlled trial testing the anti-HIV effects of high doses of 35 MU per day of alpha interferon in asymptomatic HIV-culture-positive men, four of the five subjects treated with IFN, and one of the five in the placebo group, became HIV-culture negative. In patients with KS the anti-HIV effects of alpha IFN were noted in only those patients with a mean CD4 count of $445/mm^3$ and who had not yet lost immunocompetence. The possible effects of alpha IFN as an immunomodulating drug are less clear. In a study of 35 KS patients who received human lymphoblastoid interferon ($20mg/m^2/day$) for eight weeks, natural killer cell activity and CD4 counts significantly increased among those patients with less extensive disease. However, another randomised double-blind placebo-controlled study among 67 AIDS patients without KS failed to demonstrate any improvement of immunological parameters.

Side-effects of alpha IFN include 'flu-like symptoms, CNS disturbances, leucopenia, thrombocytopenia, liver function abnormalities and alopecia. They are dose-dependent but high doses of alpha interferon are relatively well tolerated by HIV-infected patients.

Since a synergism between alpha IFN and zidovudine has been demonstrated *in vitro* against HIV, phase I trials involving 23 AIDS patients with KS are ongoing to test the combination of alpha IFN (9 MU/day) and zidovudine (600 mg/day).

After four weeks, haematological and hepatic tolerance were good. Eight patients receiving 9 MU/day of alpha IFN and 1200 mg of zidovudine for three weeks developed more severe haematological toxicity. Further studies are needed to assess adequately the usefulness and tolerance of such association (Fischl et al, 1987; Friedland et al, 1987; Kovacs et al, 1987; Krown et al, 1987).

Beta interferon
Beta interferon is produced by viral induction of fibroblasts. Recombinant beta interferon is now used for experimental purposes. Like alpha interferon, beta interferon has an anti-HIV and anti-tumour activity but the specific mechanism of action still remains unclear. Adverse reactions to beta interferon are grossly similar to those observed with alpha interferon. Ongoing trials are proposed with dosages varying from 45 to 450 MU daily, alone or in combination with zidovudine (Miles et al, 1987).

Ampligen
Ampligen is a polynucleotide derivative of poly(I)-poly(C) with several uracil groups which are composed of a synthetic, mismatched, double stranded RNA, and acts as an interferon inducer. The antiviral activity of Ampligen could also

be due to an activation of some intracellular enzymes such as an RNA polymerase-L or to an enhancement of natural killer cell activity. Ampligen has been given intravenously at dosages of 100 up to 500 mg twice a week and the antiviral effects were observed with the higher doses. Both *in vitro* and *in vivo* studies have demonstrated strong anti-HIV properties without significant adverse reactions, except transient myalgia. In a pilot study of 10 patients, those with ARC or lymphadenopathy syndrome showed improvement of T and B cell function.

Another study with 25 ARC and five AIDS patients with positive culture for HIV were given 100–250 mg IV infusion twice weekly for two to 12 months. Within 12 months of treatment, delayed type hypersensitivity increased among 80% of the patients. At high doses, anti-HIV properties were shown and immune or clinical improvement were noted in 10 ARC patients treated for more than 12 weeks. In spite of antiviral therapy, Kaposi's sarcoma progressed in four cases. To date, none of the ARC patients have progressed to AIDS. The clinical immune improvement and the HIV inhibition suggest that it could be wise to use ampligen in combination with zidovudine which is synergistic (Abrams et al, 1987; Abrams et al, 1988; Henriques et al, 1987a; Henriques et al, 1987b). Further trials with this drug are underway.

ABPP

The 2-amino-5-bromo-6-phenyl-3(H)-pyrimidine (ABPP) has been tested as an antiviral agent against various RNA and DNA viruses. ABPP induces interferon production and exhibits antiviral, antitumour and immunomodulatory activity. ABPP increases natural killer activity, macrophage-mediated cytotoxicity and the lymphoproliferative responses to mitogens (Wierenga, 1985).

The oral route of administration favours its clinical use but further *in vivo* studies are needed to assess its efficacy. Orthostatic hypotension, nausea, vomiting and leg cramp have been reported in phase I trial in patients with AIDS and KS (Abrams et al, 1987).

UNDETERMINED MECHANISMS

Avarol

Avarol is a quinone derivative from a murine sponge *Dysidea avara*. *In vitro* preliminary data have shown a dose-dependent inhibition of HIV replication and a possible immunomodulating effect. The antiviral mechanism of action is to be determined. Animal trials showed a low toxicity and a good penetration in the central nervous system. Clinical trials with AIDS/ARC patients are ongoing but so far no results are available (Abrams et al, 1987; Sarin, 1987).

Isoprinosine

In vitro, isoprinosine, a synthetic inosine derivative, has demonstrated antiviral but mostly immunomodulating activity. Isoprinosine has been proposed as treatment of a broad spectrum of diseases including condyloma, cytomegalovirus carrier, herpes viruses infections or multifocal leucoencephalitis. At usual doses

(50–100 mg/kg daily), toxicity appears to be limited to a transient rise of the serum uric acid level.

The mitogen reponses, natural-killer cell activity, macrophage activation, T-rosette formation, gamma interferon and IL2 production have been increased *in vitro* when cells cultured from an ARC patient were exposed to isoprinosine. In a preliminary placebo-controlled trial in patients at risk of AIDS, treated with 1 to 3 g daily for one month, immunological improvements as mentioned above were noted. Larger phase II or III double-blind, placebo-controlled trials are now being conducted in Scandinavia, Australia and the USA in ARC/PGL or symptom-free patients (Abrams et al, 1987; Fischl et al, 1987; Pompidou et al, 1986; Wallace & Bekesi, 1986). Results are not yet available.

Gamma interferon
Gamma IFN lacks the anti-HIV activity of alpha IFN and beta IFN. Since AIDS/ARC patients have been found to be deficient in gamma IFN, gamma IFN has been administered in patients with AIDS, ARC and KS but no benefits have been found. Combination of gamma IFN and tumour-necrosis-factor (TNF) demonstrated, *in vitro*, strong anti-HIV effects by reducing expression of viral antigens and RNA and by killing cells acutely infected by HIV. Clinical studies are currently underway involving gamma interferon in combination with TNF in ARC patients. Neutralising antibodies against gamma IFN are rarely found.

Drug-related 'flu-like symptoms frequently occurred such as a mild neutropenia or hepatic enzyme dysfunction (Wong et al, 1987).

Fusidic acid
Anecdotal reports suggested anti-HIV properties of fusidic acid among four out of eight ARC patients with circulating p24 antigen. Adverse reactions were not common and recent data suggests that the apparent antiviral properties of the drug can only be obtained with toxic doses, the mechanism of action is still unclear. Sodium fusidate could interfere with the intracellular phosphorylation steps (De Clercq 1986).

CONCLUSION

Since the discovery of HIV as a new pathogen outstanding progress has been made in research and development of new antiviral drugs. Presently, among the many compounds available, no single agent is ideal. However most important from the clinical point of view, mortality and morbidity of HIV infection is now decreasing under antiviral therapy.

One can expect in the future worthwhile development in this new field which has already mobilized government agencies, basic scientists, clinicians and pharmaceutical companies throughout the world.

REFERENCES

Abrams D, Gottlieb M, Grieco M, Speer M, Berstein S 1987 In: Amfar Directory of Experimental Treatments for AIDS & ARC. Mary Ann Liebert, New York 1: 1–53

Abrams D, Gottlieb M, Grieco M, Speer M, Berstein S 1988 In: Amfar Directory of Experimental Treatments for AIDS & ARC. Mary Ann Liebert, New York January suppl. 1–14

Anderson M G, Farthing C, Ellis M E, Gazzard B G, Chanas A 1987 Treatment of cytomegalovirus pneumonitis with foscarnet (trisodium phosphonoformate) in patients with AIDS. III International Conference on AIDS, Washington, USA, June 1–5, Abstract;THP. 237: 203

Barnes D M 1987 Debate over potential AIDS drug. Science 237: 128–130

Bergdahl S, Biberfeld G, Julander I, Lernestedt J O, Morfeldt-Manson L, Asjo B 1987 Foscarnet-treatment in HIV-infected homosexual men. III International Conference on AIDS, Washington, USA, June 1–5, Abstract;THP. 238: 203

Burger H, Weiser B, Neff S et al 1987 An antiviral trial of Rifabutin in patients with ARC. III International Conference on AIDS, Washington, USA, June 1–5, Abstract;THP. 233: 202

Center for Disease Control AIDS Weekly 1987 November 2, 21.

Cheson B D, Levine A M, Mildvan D et al 1987 Suramin therapy in AIDS and related disorders. Journal of the American Medical Association 258 10: 1347–1351

Connor E, Morrison S, Minnefor A, et al 1987 Preliminary data from a phase I study of oral Ribavirin (RIB) in children with AIDS-related complex (ARC) III International Conference on AIDS, Washington, USA, June 1–5, Abstract;TP. 226: 100

Davidson B P, Siegal F P, Reife R A et al 1987 Ansamycin (Rifabutin), an inhibitor of HIV in vitro, crosses the blood–brain barrier. III International Conference on AIDS, Washington, USA, June 1–5, Abstract;THP. 228: 201

De Clercq E 1986. Chemotherapeutic approaches to the treatment of the acquired immune deficiency syndrome (AIDS). Journal of Medicinal Chemistry 29: 1516–1569

Deray G, Cacoub P, Le Hoang P et al 1987 Foscarnet-induced acute renal failure and effectiveness of haemodialysis. Lancet 2: 216

Fischl M A, Patrone-Reese J, Dearmas L, Uttamchandani R 1987 Phase I study of the combination of alpha interferons and Zidovudine in patients with AIDS-associated Kaposi's sarcoma. Annual Meeting of the ISIR, Washington, November 2–6; Abstract II–47: 774

Fischl M A, Richman D D, Grieco M H et al 1987 The efficacy of azidothymidine (AZT) in the treatment of patients with AIDS and AIDS-related complex. New England Journal of Medicine 317: 185–191

Friedland G H, Landesman S H, Crumpacker C S et al 1987 A clinical trial of recombinant alpha-interferon in patients with AIDS. III International Conference on AIDS, Washington, USA, June 1–5, Abstract;TH.4.6: 156

Grieco M H, Lange M, Klein E B et al 1987 Open study of AL-721 in HIV-infected subjects with generalized lymphadenopathy syndrome (LAS). III International Conference on AIDS, Washington, USA, June 1–5, Abstract;TP.223: 99

Henriques HF, Simon GL, Strayer DR, Carter WA, Einck L, Schulof RS 1987a Ampligen therapy for HIV related immunodeficiency. III International Conference on AIDS, Washington, USA, June 1–5, Abstract;MP.216: 46

Henriques H F, Simon G L, Parenti D M et al 1987b Effects of Ampligen doses in HIV-infected patients. ICAAC, October 4–7 Abstract 374: 162

Hermans P, Magrez P, De Wit S, Weerts D, Cauchie E, Clumeck N 1988 The benefit of Zidovudine in the treatment of AIDS patients with cerebral toxoplasmosis. IV International Conference on AIDS, Stockholm, Sweden, June 12–16, Abstract C3667: 183

Klecker R W, Collins J M, Yarchoan R et al 1987 Plasma and cerebrospinal fluid pharmacokinetics of 3'-azido-3'-deoxythymidine: a novel pyrimidine analogue with potential application for the treatment of patients with AIDS and related diseases. Clinical Pharmacology and Therapeutics 41: 407–412

Kovacs J, Lane HC, Masur H, Herpin B, Feinberg J, Fauci AS 1987. In vivo anti-retroviral properties of recombinant alpha interferon in AIDS with Kaposi's sarcoma and healthy HIV-seropositive homosexual men. III International Conference on AIDS, Washington, USA, June 1–5, Abstract;MP.228: 48

Krown S E, Bundow D, Tong W P et al 1987 Interferon-alpha plus azidothymidine (AZT) in AIDS-associated Kaposi's sarcoma. Annual Meeting of the ISIR, Washington, November 2–6 Oral Presentations: 688

Mansell P W A, Heseltine P N R, Roberts R B et al 1987 Ribavirin delays progression of the lymphadenopathy syndrome (LAS) to the acquired immunodeficiency syndrome (AIDS). III International Conference on AIDS, Washington, USA, June 1–5, Abstract 1987;T.5: 58

Miles S A, Cortes E, Marcus S G, Carden J, Rudo R, Mitsuyasu R T 1987 A phase II study of beta-interferon given subcutaneously to patients with AIDS related Kaposi's sarcoma. III International Conference on AIDS, Washington, USA, June 1–5, Abstract;TP.227.

Mitsuya H, Broder S 1987 Strategies for antiviral therapy in AIDS. Nature 325: 773–778

Mitsuya H, Jarrett R F, Matsukura M et al 1987 Long-term inhibition of human T-lymphotropic virus type III/lymphadenopathy-associated virus (human immunodeficiency virus) DNA synthesis and RNA expression in T cells protected by 2',3'-dideoxynucleosides in vitro. Proceedings of the National Academy of Sciences of the USA 34: 2033–2037

Moskovitz BL 1987 HPA-23 Cooperative Study Group Phase I tolerance study of HPA-23 in patients with AIDS and preliminary data of anti-HIV activity. III International Conference on AIDS, Washington, USA, June 1–5, Abstract;THP.222: 99

Pompidou A, Telvi L, Delsaux M C, Fouquet F, Platel C, Sarin P 1986 Influence of immunomodulators on T lymphocytes differentiation and resistance to LAV/HTLV-III infection. II International Conference of AIDS, Paris, France, June 23–25; Abstract 592: 93

Richman D D, Fischl M A, Grieco M H et al 1987 The toxicity of azidothymidine (AZT) in the treatment of patients with AIDS and AIDS-related complex. New England Journal of Medicine 317: 192–197

Rouvroy D, Bogaerts J, Habyarimana J B, Nzaramba D, Van de Perre P 1985 Short-term results with ueramin for AIDS-related conditions. Lancet 1: 878–879

Ruff M, Hallberg P L, Hill J M, Pert C B 1987 Peptide T(4–8) is core HIV envelope sequence required for CD4 receptor attachment Lancet 2: 751

Sandstrom E G, Kaplan J C 1987 Antiviral therapy in AIDS. Clinical Pharmacological Properties and Therapeutic Experience to Date. Drugs 34: 372–390

Sarin P S 1987 Inhibition of replication of the ethiologic agent of acquired immunodeficiency syndrome by Avarol and Avarone. Journal of the National Cancer Institute 78 4: 663–6

Smith D H et al 1987 Blocking of HIV-1 infectivity by a soluble, secreted form of the CD4 antigen. Science 238: 1704–1707

Spector S A, Kennedy G, McCutchan J A, et al 1987 Antiviral effect of Zidovudine (AZT) and Ribavirin in clinical trials. ICAAC, October 4–7 Abstract 389: 164

Ueno R, Kuno S 1987 Anti-HIV synergism between dextran sulphate and zidovudine. Lancet 2: 796–797

Vaghefi M M, McKernan P A, Robins R K 1986 Synthesis and antiviral activity of certain nucleoside 5'-phosphonoformate derivatives. Journal of Medical Chemistry 29: 1389–1393

Vernon A, Schulof R S 1987 Serum HIV core antigen in symptomatic ARC patients taking oral Ribavirin or placebo. III International Conference on AIDS, Washington, USA, June 1–5, Abstract;T.8.6.: 58

Vittecocq D, Modai J, Woerle R, Barre-Sinoussi F, Chermann J C 1987 Reverse transcriptase activity (RTA) in lymphocyte cultures of patients infected by HIV treated with short course of HPA-23. ICAAC, October 1–7 Abstract 376: 162

Volberding P A, Mitsuyasu R T, Golando J P, Speigel R J 1987 Treatment of Kaposi's sarcoma with interferon alfa-2b. Cancer 59: 620–625

Walker B D, Kowalski M, Goh W C, Rohrschneider L, Haseltine W A, Sodroski J 1987[a] Anti-HIV properties of Castanospermine. III International Conference on AIDS, Washington, USA, June 1–5, Abstract; T.4.3: 54

Walker B D, Kowalski M, Goh W C, Rohrschneider L, Haseltine W A, Sodroski J 1987[b] Inhibition of HIV syncytium formation and replication by Castanospermine. ICAAC, October 1–7 Abstract 373: 162

Wallace J, Bekesi J G 1986 A double-blind clinical trial of the effects of Inosine Pranobex in immunodepressed patients with prolonged generalized lymphadenopathy. Clinical Immunology and Immunopathology 39: 179–186

Weerts D, Cauchie E, De Wit S, Hermans P, Van Laethem Y. Clumeck N 1988 One year experience of Azidothymidine (AZT) administered six hourly in 40 patients with AIDS or AIDS- related complex. Abstract, IV International Conference on AIDS, Stockholm June 12–16.

Wierenga W 1985 Antiviral and other bioactivities of pyrimidinones. Pharmacology and Therapeutics 30: 67–89

Wong G H W, Krowka J, Stites D P, Goeddel D V 1987 Tumor necrosis factor-alpha and Interferon-gamma have anti-HIV activity. III International Conference on AIDS, Washington, USA, June 1–5, Abstract;T.4.5: 54

Yarchoan R, Klecker R W, Weinhold K J et al 1986 Administration of 3'-azido-3'deoxythymidine, an inhibitor of HTLV-III/LAV replication, to patients with AIDS or AIDS-related complex. Lancet 1: 575–580

Yarchoan R, Thomas R V, Allain J P et al 1988 Phase I studies of 2',3'-dideoxycytidine in severe human immunodeficiency virus infection as a single agent and alternating with Zidovudine (AZT). Lancet 1: 76–81

Discussion of paper presented by Nathan Clumeck

Discussant: John Mills

Drs Clumeck and Hermans have provided us with a scholarly and comprehensive overview of the field of antiretroviral chemotherapy to date. Rather than reiterating what has already been said, I would like to discuss specific aspects of the therapy of human immunodeficiency virus (HIV) infection, some practical and others theoretical, which have implications for therapy in the future.

No discussion of the therapy of HIV infection would be complete without an exposition of some of the potential problems that are likely to be faced in the management of this disease. There is a very long latent period between infection with HIV and the onset of AIDS; current estimates are that the median incubation period may be nearly a decade (Moss et al, 1988). The state of HIV during this long incubation period is currently unknown, although the subject of intense investigation; the results will have direct bearing on the approach to chemotherapy during the incubation period. Although HIV is commonly described as being 'latent' during the incubation period, individuals studied during this interval have detectable virus in blood (Gallo et al 1984), and their secretions and blood are infectious for others by a variety of routes. Although infection of quiescent cultured lymphocytes with HIV results in latent infection which reactivates when the cells are activated by exposure to mitogens or recall antigens, it is not clear whether this phenomenon is important *in vivo*. On the contrary, current evidence suggests that the monocyte–macrophage may be the major site of replication of HIV (Crowe et al, 1987) and in these cells the replication of HIV tends to be chronic and non-cytocidal (Crowe et al, 1987). Hence, a more likely model of HIV infection is that it is a true chronic viral infection in which the disease does not develop until years after infection, for unknown reasons. This model of HIV infection makes the justification for beginning chemotherapy in the pre-symptomatic stage somewhat more plausible; however, with either the 'latent' or 'chronic' infection model, chemotherapy will not eradicate the virus. Hence, as with chemosuppression of recurrences of herpes simplex virus infection, lifelong therapy will be required for continued suppression of HIV replication.

Current chemotherapeutic agents such as zidovudine are relatively toxic, and only partially inhibit the progression of HIV infection (Richman et al, 1987a; Fischl et al, 1987). Given the slow, overall progress in antiviral chemotherapy during the past three decades, it is excessively optimistic to suppose that highly effective, non-toxic antiretrovirals will be developed in the near future. Hence, therapy of HIV infection will require combinations of drugs, necessary to achieve less toxicity and greater efficacy than can be achieved with a single agent. Studies with dideoxycytidine, alpha interferon, foscarnet and acyclovir in combination with zidovudine are already underway in the first attempts to evaluate this concept (Yarchoan et al, 1988).

We believe that foscarnet shows particular promise as an agent to combine with zidovudine. The drug is an effective antiretroviral in HIV-infected patients (Farthing et al, 1987; Asjo et al, 1987; Bergdahl et al, 1987; Gaub et al, 1987) and *in vitro* is synergistic with zidovudine (Mills et al, unpublished data; Oberg et al, personal communication). Foscarnet is non-toxic and is also effective for the concomitant herpes simplex virus and cytomegalovirus infections which are common in AIDS patients (Jacobson et al, 1988; Mills et al, unpublished data). Although foscarnet must be given intravenously, it may only need to be administered intermittently (e.g. for two weeks every two months) to be effective against HIV when combined with continuous zidovudine therapy.

The other implication of the inevitable toxicity of antiretroviral chemotherapy is that the improved well-being and prolongation of life which results from therapy will be accompanied by morbidity associated with adverse reactions, which in turn will increase the cost of caring for AIDS patients. This problem is already upon us. The major toxicity of zidovudine is anaemia and many of the treated patients require transfusions to maintain a tolerable haematocrit (Richman et al, 1987a; Walker et al, 1988); the resulting increased demand for blood has strained the resources of blood banks in some communities (Costello et al, 1987).

All of these considerations—whether HIV is latent during the incubation period, how to employ combination chemotherapy to optimize efficacy and decrease toxicity, and the relationship between the health benefits of antiretroviral therapy and the inevitable toxicity and increased cost which result—will come together as studies are performed to assess where in the course of HIV infection chemotherapy should be initiated. Although simple risk–benefit considerations would suggest that therapy with toxic and expensive drugs should not be initiated until after the patient is symptomatic, the irreversible nature of some of the manifestations of HIV infection (specifically, the neurological disease) points towards beginning therapy in the presymptomatic phase. Only long-term clinical trials will answer these questions.

Although the efficacy of zidovudine for treatment of HIV infection has been established unequivocally (Fischl et al, 1987), the single study on which this determination was based was a short term investigation in a well-defined subgroup of HIV-infected patients. Numerous studies are underway to assess the role of zidovudine therapy for longer periods of time and in other conditions. Many of these trials are being performed by the AIDS Clinical Trials Group (ACTG) of the National Institutes of Allergy and Infectious Diseases of the U.S. National Institutes of Health. ACTG protocol number 001 is a comparison of zidovudine with placebo in patients with early Kaposi's sarcoma; the study has been underway for about nine months and has not yet been terminated by the

Data Monitoring and Safety Board (as it would be if definite evidence of efficacy or unacceptable toxicity were observed). This study may confirm the apparent lack of efficacy of zidovudine for Kaposi's sarcoma which was observed in the original studies (Fischl et al, 1987; Yarchoan et al, 1986). ACTG study 002, a comparison of two doses of zidovudine (100 mg vs 200 mg taken every four hours) in patients who have had one episode of *Pneumocystis carinii* pneumonia, has also not yet been terminated by the Data Monitoring and Safety Board. The most disturbing observation from this study is the high frequency of recurrent *Pneumocystis carinii* pneumonia in the study patients—nearly 50% of subjects developed a recurrence within nine to 12 months of beginning therapy (Fischl et al, unpublished data). For this reason, the Opportunistic Infection Committee of the ACTG has recommended routine *Pneumocystis carinii* chemoprophylaxis for patients after their first episode of pneumocystosis, regardless of whether they are receiving antiretroviral chemotherapy. A study of the efficacy of high doses of zidovudine in patients with neurological disease (ACTG 005) has not had sufficient accrual of patients to permit data analysis. However, the question asked in this trial—whether zidovudine therapy reverses central nervous system disease due to HIV—remains an important one.

Possibly the most important zidovudine study being conducted by the ACTG is protocol 019 (principal investigator, Paul Volberding, MD), a comparison of zidovudine with placebo in asymptomatic HIV infected subjects. Despite enrolment of over 1500 patients, this study is expected to last over three years before a clinical endpoint is reached—i.e. whether zidovudine therapy significantly delays progression of HIV infection to AIDS Related Complex (ARC) or AIDS. No efficacy data are available from this study; however, the drug appears to be better tolerated in this asymptomatic population than it was in patients with AIDS or severe ARC (Richman et al, 1987a); this might have been predicted given the observation in the study of Richman et al that the risk of toxicity increased with decreasing CD4 lymphocyte numbers. If this study (ACTG 019) shows that zidovudine therapy delays progression of HIV infection, long-term placebo controlled studies with new candidate antiretrovirals will become unethical to conduct.

Another important and unanswered question with zidovudine is whether therapy begun shortly after infection will completely prevent infection. In experimental animal retroviral infection, treatment with zidovudine beginning at the time of infection or shortly thereafter will completely prevent infection. Whether a similar prophylactic strategy will be effective in humans infected with HIV (e.g. following a needlestick exposure) is unknown. However, a study to answer that question is being considered by Burroughs Wellcome (Lehrman, personal communication).

Although zidovudine was orginally reported to delay the onset of opportunistic infections in patients with AIDS or ARC and to prolong survival, recent anecdotes have suggested that it may benefit some of the other manifestations of HIV infection. Letters and case reports suggest that HIV-related thrombocytopenia may be improved with zidovudine therapy (even though the drug itself may cause thrombocytopenia) (Hymes et al, 1988; Gottlieb et al, 1987). Severe psoriasis is a feature of HIV infection and there are several reports of remission of psoriasis with zidovudine therapy (Feeney & Frazier, 1988; Ruzicka et al, 1987; Duvic et al, 1987). Whether these anecdotal clinical observations will hold up under the scrutiny of controlled clinical trials remains to be seen.

In the experience that has accumulated on the use of zidovudine subsequent to the publication of the placebo-controlled trial (Fischl et al, 1987; Richman et al, 1987a), the adverse reactions noted in that study—anaemia, neutropenia, nausea and headache—have continued to be the adverse reactions most commonly noted by clinicians caring for treated patients. However, some additional adverse reactions have been reported. Nail pigmentation is common in treated subjects (Panwalker, 1987; Furth & Kazakis, 1987). Neurotoxicity, rarely severe, has also been noted in some cases (Davtyan & Vinters, 1987; Jacobson et al, unpublished data). A few patients have developed fever, with or without a rash, following several months of therapy with zidovudine which may be due to anti-drug antibodies (Lehrman, personal communication; Jacobson et al, unpublished data). The observation that the risk of adverse reactions (especially anaemia and neutropenia) appears to increase with decreasing CD4 lymphocyte counts has held up (Richman et al, 1987a); in addition, there appears to be an increasing risk of adverse reactions with increased patient age (Lehrman, personal communication).

What does the future hold for therapy of HIV infection. Many of the drugs currently under study, such as zidovudine, dideoxycytidine and foscarnet (Fischl et al, 1987; Yarchoan et al, 1988; Äsjo et al, 1987) are reverse transcriptase inhibitors. Although these drugs will probably have some clinical benefit, they will not be effective in chronically-infected cells where abundant viral DNA (either integrated or unintegrated) has already been formed (Smith et al, 1987; Crowe et al, unpublished observations). In cell culture, and possibly in patients, the therapeutic efficacy of zidovudine tends to wane with time (Smith et al, 1987). A report that zidovudine was not effective in HIV-infected macrophages (Richman et al, 1987b) has not been confirmed (Bolognesi, personal communication; Crowe et al, unpublished data). New molecular targets for antiretroviral drugs are desperately needed, to increase the likelihood of synergy with reverse transcriptase inhibitors and to offer the promise of efficacy in chronically-infected cells. Binding or neutralizing extracellular virus with dextran or soluble CD4 (Traunecker et al, 1988; Hussey et al, 1988; Fisher et al, 1988; Smith et al, 1987) is a method of treating chronic viral infections which has not yet previously been tested; the agents proposed are at least likely to be non-toxic. Replication of HIV is absolutely dependent upon function of the viral protease (Debouck et al, 1987; Pearl & Taylor, 1987) as well as at least two transactivating genes ('tat' and 'trs/art') (Knight et al, 1987); blockade of any of these viral functions by a selective inhibitor would likely result in an effective chemotherapuetic agent.

In summary, the treatment of HIV infection presents formidable challenges to the chemist, virologist and clinician. Much work—both in the laboratory and in the clinic—will have to be done before we have a relatively safe and highly effective drug (or combination of drugs) to treat HIV infection. These studies will require imagination, persistence and hard work by investigators at all levels if we are to achieve success.

REFERENCES

Äsjo B, Marfeldt-Manson L, Bergdahl S et al 1987 Phosphonoformic acid (foscarnet) treatment and the effect on human immunodeficiency virus. III International Conference on AIDS. Washington DC, (Abstract) THP 13

Bergdahl S, Biberfield G, Julander I, Lernestedt J O, Morfeldt-Manson L, Asjo B 1987 Foscarnet treatment in HIV-infected homosexual men. III International Conference on AIDS. Washington DC, (Abstract) THP 238

Costello C, Mir N, Luckit J 1987 The blood transfusion service and zidovudine treatment for AIDS. British Medical Journal 295: 1486

Crowe S, Mills J, McGrath M 1987 Quantitative immunocytofluorographic analysis of CD4 surface antigen expression and HIV infection of human peripheral blood monocyte/macrophages. AIDS Research and Human Retroviruses 3: 135–145

Davtyan D G, Vinters H V 1987 Wernicke's encephalopathy in AIDS patients treated with zidovudine. Lancet 1: 890–891

Debouck C, Gorniak J G, Strickler J E, Meek T D, Metcalf B W, Rosenberg M 1987 Human immunodeficiency virus protease expressed in *Escherichia coli* exhibits autoprocessing and specific maturation of the gag precursor. Proceedings of the National Academy of Sciences USA 84: 903–906

Duvic M, Rios A, Breweton G W 1987 Remission of AIDS-associated psoriasis with zidovudine. Lancet 2: 627

Farthing C D, Dalgleish A G, Clark A, McClure M, Chanas A, Gazzard B G 1987 Phosphonoformate (foscarnet): a pilot study in AIDS and AIDS related complex. AIDS 1: 21–25

Feeney G F, Frazier I 1988 AIDS-associated psoriasis responds to azidothymidine. Medical Journal of Australia 148: 155

Fischl M A, Richman D D, Grieco M H, Gottlieb M S, Volberding P A, Laskin O L, Leedom J M, Groopman J E, Mildvan D, Schooley R T et al 1987 The efficacy of azidothymidine (AZT) in the treatment of patients with AIDS and AIDS-related complex. A double-blind, placebo-controlled trial. New England Journal of Medicine 317: 185–191

Fisher R A, Bertonis J M, Meier W, Johnson V A, Costopoulos D S, Liu T, Tizard R, Walker B D, Hirsch M S, Schooley R T et al 1988 HIV infection is blocked in vitro by recombinant soluble CD4. Nature 331: 76–78

Furth P A, Kazakis A M 1987 Nail pigmentation changes associated with azidothymidine (zidovudine). Annals of Internal Medicine 107: 350

Gallo R C, Salahuddin S Z, Popovic M et al 1984 Frequent detection and isolation of cytopathic retroviruses (HTLV-III) from patients with AIDS and at risk of AIDS. Science 224: 500–503

Gaub J, Pederson C, Poulsen A G et al 1987 The effect of foscarnet (phosphonoformate) on human immunodeficiency virus isolation, T-cell subsets and lymphocyte function in AIDS patients. AIDS 1: 27–33

Gottlieb M S, Wolfe P R, Chafey S 1987 Response of AIDS-related thrombocytopenia to intravenous and oral azidothymidine. AIDS Research on Human Retroviruses 3: 109–114

Hussey R E, Richardson N E, Kowalski M et al 1988 A soluble CD4 protein selectively inhibits HIV replication and syncytium formation. Nature 331: 78–81

Hymes K B, Greene J B, Karpatkin S 1988 Expression of the art/trs protein of HIV and study of its role in viral envelope synthesis. Science 236: 837–40

Jacobson M A, Crowe S, Levy J et al 1988 Effect of foscarnet on HIV infection. Journal of Infectious Diseases, in press

Knight DM, Flomerfelt FA, Ghrayeb J 1987 Expression of the art/trs protein of HIV and study of its role in viral envelope synthesis. Science 236: 837–40

Moss A R, Bacchetti P, Osmond D et al 1988 Seropositivity for HIV and the development of AIDS or AIDS related condition: three year follow up of the San Francisco General Hospital cohort. British Medical Journal 296: 745

Panwalker A P 1987 Nail pigmentation in the acquired immunodeficiency syndrome (AIDS). Annals of Internal Medicine 107: 943–944

Pearl L H, Taylor W R 1987 A structural model for the retroviral proteases. Nature 329: 351–354

Richman D D, Fischl M A, Grieco M H et al 1987a The toxicity of azidothymidine (AZT) in the treatment of patients with AIDS and AIDS-related complex. A double-blind, placebo-controlled trial. New England Journal of Medicine 317: 192–197

Richman D D, Kornbluth R S, Carson D A 1987b Failure of dideoxynucleosides to inhibit human immunodeficiency virus replication in cultured human macrophages. Journal of Experimental Medicine 166: 1144–1149

Ruzicka T, Froschl M, Hohnleutner U, Holzmann H, Braun-Falco O 1987 Treatment of HIV-induced retinoid-resistant psoriasis with zidovudine. Lancet ii: 1469–1470

Smith D H, Bryn R A, Masters S A, Gregory T, Groopman J E, Capon D J 1987 Blocking of HIV-1 infectivity by a soluble, secreted form of the CD4 antigen. Science 238: 1704–1707

Traunecker A, Luke W, Karjalainen K 1988 Soluble CD4 molecules neutralize human immunodeficiency virus type 1. Nature 331: 84–66

Walker R E, Parker R I, Kovacs J A, Masur H, Lane H C, Carleton S, Kirk L E, Gralnick H R, Fauci A S 1988 Anemia and erythropoiesis in patients with the acquired immunodeficiency syndrome (AIDS) and Kaposi's sarcoma treated with zidovudine. Annals of Internal Medicine 108: 372–6

Yarchoan R, Klecker R W, Weinhold K J et al 1986 Administration of 3'-azido-3'-deoxythymidine, an inhibitor of HTLV-III/LAV replication, to patients with AIDS or AIDS-related complex. Lancet i: 575

Yarchoan R, Perno C F, Thomas R V et al 1988 Phase I studies of 2'-3'-dideoxycytidine in severe human immuodeficiency virus infection as a single agent and alternating with zidovudine (AZT). Lancet i: 76–81

Discussion: Antiviral chemotherapy of HIV infection

Nathan Clumeck and John Mills

The discussion period began with a lively interchange regarding the mechanism of bone marrow toxicity of AZT, whether it is less in HIV-infected patients who are asymptomatic compared with those with AIDS or ARC, and the effect of GMCSF therapy on AZT-induced myelosuppression. Known variables which increase the risk of anaemia or neutropenia include pre-therapy anaemia or neutropenia and low CD4 lymphocyte numbers. In at least one study, low serum B12 levels increased the risk of toxicity and this was reduced when B12 supplements were given. Preliminary data from the studies of AZT in patients with asymptomatic HIV infection suggest better drug tolerance than in patients with AIDS or ARC. However, there are reports of some AZT-treated asymptomatic patients requiring transfusions, so the degree of tolerance is still an open question. Preliminary studies with GM-CSF suggest that it will at least partially reverse AZT-induced myelosuppression. *In vitro* studies which suggest that GM-CSF may augment HIV replication have not been confirmed to date.

No one was aware of the mechanism of AZT-induced myelosuppression, or why erythrocyte precursors are affected preferentially. A possible differential effect of AZT on erythrocyte thymidylate synthetase which would permit uridine rescue needs to be explored.

It was proposed that the beneficial effect of foscarnet on HIV infection might be attributable to its inhibition of CMV infection. However, this seems unlikely as ganciclovir, which is about as effective for CMV infections as foscarnet, has no effect on HIV p24 antigenaemia. The antigen levels tend to rise during therapy with ganciclovir and the reverse is true with foscarnet.

There was some discussion of what would constitute a valid endpoint for determination of drug efficacy in antiretroviral trials in asymptomatic HIV-infected patients. Although there was hope that early laboratory endpoints (e.g. maintenance of normal CD4 lymphocyte numbers) could be employed, it is not clear that they will be adequate, and some clinical endpoint may have to be used. Given the prognostic implications of some 'minor' opportunistic infections such as oral candidiasis, waiting for the development of AIDS-defining opportunistic infections may not be required.

With regard to new targets for chemotherapy, the HIV gag protein may have a beta barrel structure similar to that of the rhinoviruses. If that is the case, it would be worthwhile to look at some of the molecules known to be inserted into the beta barrels of picornaviruses (blocking uncoating) to assess their effect on HIV replication.

One participant questioned whether antiviral chemotherapy would reduce the infectiousness of HIV-infected patients. This benefit appears speculative at best. The observed reductions in serum p24 antigen (as a measure of virus load) are only 50–90%, very modest compared with the several-orders-of-magnitude reductions seen with other pathogens. Conversely, if a patient's well-being is improved they may revert to the activities that contributed to transmission of the disease in the first place.

A brief discussion of the relevance of animal models to HIV infection of humans ensued. Other than HIV-infection of chimpanzees, there are three models that have been developed. One is a group of animal retrovirus models of which the simian immunodeficiency virus, murine leukaemia virus and feline retrovirus have been the most popular; the second is transgenic mice which have been transfected with HIV in the embryo stage, and the third model is a haemotransplant in a combined immunodeficiency mouse injected with human fetal liver. The mouse then has the haematopoietic system of the human. The animal retrovirus models have been useful for evaluating anti-retroviral drugs; the utility of the other models remains to be established. As the transgenic mouse begins life with every cell having intracellular HIV cDNA, it will likely not be a good model to assess reverse transcriptase inhibitors. It was also pointed out that in the murine and feline models, you can give AZT or ddc up to seven days after infection with the retrovirus, clear the infection and then stop treatment without a relapse occurring. These observations offer a strong justification for clinical trials of AZT to prevent infection—for example, following a needle-stick exposure. This is the same logic used with respect to herpes simplex virus, that is, the antiviral drug is highly effective as a prophylactic in animal models and therefore it is logical to study it for that indication in humans. However, there are obviously enormous difficulties that will be encountered in designing and conducting trials to assess the prophylactic efficacy of AZT or acyclovir. This is particularly true given the logistic difficulties encountered in the placebo-controlled trials of AZT in asymptomatic HIV-infected patients.

3. Human papillomaviruses and treatment of condyloma acuminatum with intralesionally administered interferon

Richard C. Reichman, Mark H. Stoler and David Oakes

HUMAN PAPILLOMAVIRUS

Human papillomaviruses (HPV) are members of the A genus of Papovaviridae (Shah, 1985). They are non-enveloped viruses approximately 55 nm in diameter with icosahedral capsids and a circular, double-stranded DNA genome, containing approximately 7900 base pairs. At the present time, papillomaviruses (PV) have not been propagated successfully in tissue culture, although some PV can be used to transform tissue culture cells. One such system in particular, bovine PV type 1 (BPV1) transformation of mouse C127 cells, has enabled investigators to determine partially the function of certain parts of the PV genome (Turek et al, 1982). In addition, Kreider has described recently a system in which HPV11 has been grown successfully using genital wart tissue and human foreskin fibroblasts placed under the renal capsule of athymic mice (Kreider et al, 1987). This system has promise for producing relatively large numbers of virion particles, may help to determine mechanisms of pathogenesis, and can be used to evaluate antiviral drugs and possibly other forms of treatment as well.

Typing
In addition to the lack of a suitable tissue culture or animal model system, most HPV-induced lesions contain few intact virion particles. Thus, well characterized antigen preparations are not available, and typing of HPVs is dependent upon determination of degree of polynucleotide sequence homology, rather than on immunological characterization using serological reagents. Using this system, a unique HPV type has a maximum of 50% DNA homology with other classified viruses. HPV subtypes have more than 50%, but less than 100%, homology, and vary with respect to sites of cleavage by bacterial restriction endonucleases.

The genomic organization of PVs is remarkably similar among different virus types, and an example is provided in a schematic diagram of the HPV 6b genome (Fig. 3.1). Structure and function of PV genomes has been reviewed recently by Broker (1987). In general, functions of the different open reading frames (ORFs) have been delineated using site-directed mutagenesis and subsequent effects on transformation assays, such as the BPV1-mouse cell system alluded to above. Thus, certain ORFs have been identified with specific functions. For example,

E1 is involved with extrachromasomal replication of PV DNA, and E2 participates in cell transformation. L1 and L2 products appear to constitute major and minor capsid proteins, respectively.

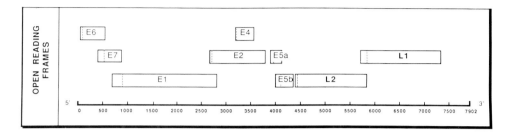

Fig. 3.1 Diagram of HPV 6b genome (provided by Dr William Bonnez). Dotted lines represent potential exon coding start locations

As indicated in Table 3.1, HPV types are associated with disease at specific sites. For example, HPV1 is found in plantar warts, whereas type 2 is most frequently found in common warts. HPV types 6 and 11 are the most common aetiological agents of condyloma acuminatum, and other HPV types, such as 16, 18 and 31, are commonly found in cervical carcinomas and other genital tract malignancies and dysplasias.

Table 3.1 Association of HPV types with specific diseases (modified from Broker, 1987)

Virus type	Disease
1	Plantar and palmar warts
2	Common warts
3, 10, 28, 29	Flat warts
4	Plantar and common warts
5, 8, 9, 12, 14, 15, 17, 19–25, 36, 40	Epidermodysplasia verruciformis
6, 11, 42	Condyloma acuminatum, respiratory papillomatosis
7	Common warts in meat and animal handlers
13, 32	Focal epithelial hyperplasia (Heck's disease)
16, 18, 31, 33, 35, 39	Genital dysplasias and carcinomas
26, 27	Warts in immunosuppressed patients
30, 34, 37, 38, 40, 41	Isolated cases of benign and malignant neoplasms

IMMUNE RESPONSE

Immune responses to HPV are poorly understood. Studies of humoral and cellular immunity to these agents have been conducted, but have generally employed poorly characterized and poorly standardized antigen preparations. Denaturation of partially purified PV particles produces a 'genus specific antigen'. Immunization of rabbits with these preparations induces antisera which detect PV antigens in formalin fixed tissues. Presence of naturally occurring antibodies to this antigen in human sera is uncertain. Some investigators have reported the presence of such antibodies in some patient populations, but others have failed to confirm these findings. Type-specific antigens appear to be located on capsid proteins. However, because of the difficulties associated with obtaining purified antigen preparations, as discussed above, the importance of such antigens in pathogenesis of HPV infections is poorly understood. Recently, several laboratories have begun to produce antigens using DNA recombinant technology to circumvent the lack of a suitable tissue culture system.

CONDYLOMA ACUMINATUM

Natural history

Data from several sources indicate that the incidence of anogenital (venereal) warts is rapidly increasing (Becker et al, 1987; Sexually transmitted diseases, 1985). Several pieces of information indicate that this infection is sexually transmitted. The age of onset of condyloma acuminatum is similar to that of other STDs, and consort studies indicate that sexual partners of infected patients commonly develop genital warts. In addition, these patients often have concomitant STDs, or histories of such infections. In addition, as discussed above, particular HPV types are associated with these lesions and are rarely found at other sites. Approximately two-thirds of sexual contacts of patients with anogenital warts appear to develop the disease, and the infectivity of these lesions is thought to be inversely related to their duration (Oriel, 1984).

With the exception of observations of placebo recipients in recently conducted clinical trials, little systematically collected information is available concerning the natural history of this disease. In men, the most frequent site of involvement is the penis. The urethral meatus may also be involved, and these lesions may be associated with more proximal disease. Perianal warts occur commonly among homosexual/bisexual men, but are observed often among heterosexual men and women as well. The vulva is the most common site of infection in women, with frequent extension into the vagina and cervix. Cervical warts may be present in the absence of external lesions. Morphology of anogenital warts does not appear to be related to natural history of disease or response to therapy. The most common complaints associated with venereal warts are disfiguration and local irritation. Bleeding occurs occasionally, and superinfection is rare. So-called 'giant condyloma' are uncommon lesions which are histologically benign, but which may behave as locally invasive neoplasms. Anogenital warts may enlarge during pregnancy and lead to obstruction of the birth canal, necessitating caesarean section. Recurrent respiratory papillomatosis (RRP) is an uncommon disease which occurs in young children, and in adults as well. Because similar HPV types cause both anogenital warts and RRP, the disease in children may be acquired by passage of the infant through an infected birth canal. Although systematic studies have not been conducted, additional epidemiological information supporting this concept has been provided by studies of children with RRP. Approximately 50% of the mothers of these children have a history of anogenital warts.

Relation to neoplasm

In addition to the rapidly increasing incidence of condyloma acuminatum, interest in HPV has been stimulated recently by several pieces of data which suggest that these viruses may have a role in the development of cervical carcinoma as well as other genital tract neoplasms (Gissmann et al, 1987). The strongest piece of information linking HPV with these lesions is the observation that approximately 90% of biopsies of cervical cancers contain detectable HPV DNA, usually of types 16, 18 and 31. In addition, limited longitudinal studies indicate that 'precursor' lesions which are associated with these same types are more likely to progress than are precursor lesions associated with HPV types which cause benign condylomata (types 6 and 11). Also of interest is the observation that HPV DNA in tumour cells is integrated, rather than located extrachromasomally as is the case in benign lesions. Integration has been shown to occur at specific sites in the HPV genome although insertion into host cell chromosomes appears to occur randomly. In addition, several studies have demonstrated that HPV DNA is transcribed in tumour tissue. A variety of 'immortal' cell lines have also been found to be infected with HPV types, again in an integrated fashion containing specific parts of the HPV genome. Another piece of information suggesting the ability of these viruses to transform human cells, is the observation that transfection of human foreskin fibroblasts with HPV16 DNA produces an extended life span, as well as an increased ability to passage these cells.

Diagnosis

Diagnosis of HPV infection is usually made accurately upon gross physical examination of typical exophytic lesions. However, gross physical examination of anogenital lesions is incorrect approximately 10% of the time when compared to histological examination of biopsy specimens. Sensitivity of physical examination is increased substantially by application of dilute solutions of acetic acid in combination with colposcopy. 'Aceto-white' lesions produced by this procedure frequently contain HPV DNA when biopsy specimens are processed appropriately. In addition to routine histological examination, detection of HPV antigens can be helpful in confirming PV infection. These studies can be conducted utilizing commercially available antisera. The most sensitive method of detecting infection with these viruses is demonstration of HPV nucleic acids using *in situ* or southern hybridization techniques. As discussed previously, well characterized HPV antigens are not available currently, and reliable serological tests are not available.

Treatment

Design, execution, and interpretation of clinical trials of treatments for HPV infections, and condyloma acuminatum in particular, are difficult to perform for several reasons. The lack of adequate natural history data, as discussed above, necessitates a randomized, placebo-controlled design. In addition, several clinical and virological parameters of potential importance must be taken into account. For example, virus type, duration of disease prior to study entry, effects of previous therapies, and immunological status of patients must be established. In addition, sex, and sexual preference of patients may be of importance and must be considered in treatment studies. At the present time, only size and number of lesions can be utilized as objective measurements of disease. Although semi-quantitative estimates of amounts of PV antigens and nucleic acids can be determined using sequential biopsy materials, such biopsies are difficult to obtain and are subject to sampling error. Because condyloma acuminatum is known to recur frequently, adequate periods of follow-up must be included in appropriately conducted clinical trials.

Table 3.2 Some currently available modes of treatment for condyloma acuminatum

(1) Podophyllin, podophyllotoxin
(2) Cryotherapy
(3) Tri- and bichloro-acetic acids
(4) 5-fluorouracil
(5) Immunotherapy
(6) Electrocautery
(7) Surgery
(8) Laser

As indicated in Table 3.2, a variety of different treatment modalities are currently available for patients with condyloma acuminatum. Although investigations of most of these modes of therapy have been reported, they have not been, in general, randomized or placebo-controlled. In addition, the factors described above have usually not been taken into account. In contrast, recent studies of different interferon preparations in the treatment of this disease have been conducted using randomized, placebo-controlled designs. An example of one such recently completed study, supported by the Development and Applications Branch of the National Institute of Allergy and Infectious Diseases, National Institutes of Health, Bethesda, MD, USA, has been performed using intralesional administration of different interferon preparations (Reichman et al, 1988). Patients who participated in these studies were otherwise healthy, and all had disease which was refractory to conventional modes of therapy. Histological confirmation of clinical diagnosis was obtained in all cases. Patients were then randomized to receive either 1×10^6 units of an interferon or placebo, injected intralesionally three times per week for four weeks. Only one lesion per patient was injected. Interferon preparations which were employed included alpha-n1, alpha-2b, and beta interferons. Characteristics of the patients who participated in this study are listed in Table 3.3. As indicated, most patients were white men, with a mean duration of disease of approximately two years. Fig. 3.2 depicts resolution of injected warts only, comparing the combined interferon group to the placebo group using survival analysis. A statistically significant difference between interferon and placebo groups was observed ($p < 0.01$). Effects of the three different interferon preparations were not significantly different from one another, and all were superior to placebo (Fig. 3.3). Results of complete resolution of injected warts are presented in Table 3.4. Approximately 50% of recipients of interferon experienced complete resolution of injected lesions as compared to approximately 20% of placebo recipients.

Table 3.3 Characteristics of patients in a study of intralesionally administered interferons for treatment of condyloma acuminatum

	Study medication			
	Alpha-N1 (n = 15)	Beta (n = 20)	Alpha-2b (n = 23)	Placebo (n = 18)
Sex (No. of patients)				
Men	10	15	16	14
Women	5	5	7	4
Mean age (years)	27	29	27	29
Race (No. of patients)				
Black	2	2	3	4
White	13	18	20	14
Duration of disease prior to therapy (months)	13 ± 10*	27 ± 31	24 ± 30	28 ± 32
Mean lesion areas of injected warts at study entry (Ln area in mm^2)	2.6 ± 1.6*	3.4 ± 1.5	2.6 ± 1.0	2.8 ± 1.6
Types of previous therapy (No. of patients)				
Podophyllin	11	18	20	16
Cryotherapy	5	6	6	5
Surgery	1	1	1	1
Laser 1	2	1	0	0
Other	2	3	5	2

* Mean ± SD

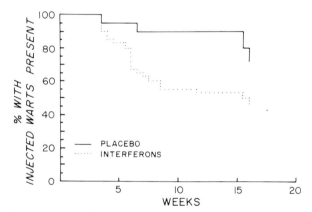

Fig. 3.2 Complete resolution of injected warts. All interferon recipients were combined into one group and this combined interferon group was compared with placebo. Proportions of patients whose injected lesions were present at the indicated timepoint were plotted against weeks of observation after study entry. The difference between the combined interferon group and the placebo group is highly significant (p=0.01 by long rank test)

Table 3.4 Rates of complete resolution of injected warts after 16 weeks of study

Study medication	Rates of resolution
Alpha-N1	6/15 (40%)
Beta	10/20 (50%)
Alpha-2b	11/23 (48%)
All interferons	27/58 (47%)
Placebo	4/18 (22%)

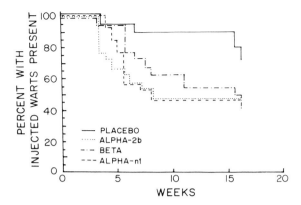

Fig. 3.3 Complete resolution of injected warts. Proportions of patients whose injected warts were present at the indicated timepoint are plotted against weeks of observation after study entry. Statistically significant differences were noted when both the alpha-2b and the beta interferon groups were compared separately with the placebo group (p=0.02 for each comparison by log rank test). In addition, the difference between the alpha-n1 interferon group and the placebo group approached statistical significance (p=0.07). No significant differences were observed among the three different interferon groups (p=0.8)

In a subset of these patients studied at the University of Rochester, patients were evaluated on the basis of histologic and virologic descriptions of pre-treatment biopsies. All lesions were classified into one of two groups:

(1)   HPV infected lesions: (a) characteristic histology including koilocytosis and/or (b) detection of PV antigens by immunocytochemical techniques, or detection of HPV nucleic acids by *in situ* or Southern hybridization (Wilbur et al, 1988).
(2)   Suggestive but not diagnostic of HPV infection: characteristic histological changes of HPV infection but without clearly defined koilocytes or presence of PV antigens or HPV nucleic acids as described above.

In efficacy analyses of this subgroup of patients, rates of complete lesion resolution were determined according to both histological and virological diagnosis and treatment. Using a log-linear model (McCullagh & Nelder, 1983), the significant difference in rate of response between placebo and interferon recipients was strengthened further when attention was restricted to HPV infected lesions (Table 3.5). This observation indicates that in patients with condyloma acuminatum treated with interferon, histological and virological evaluation of pre-therapy biopsies may be of value in predicting response to therapy.

SUMMARY

HPV infections induce several common clinical entities with a variety of clinical manifestations. The natural history and host defense reponses to HPV infection

Table 3.5 Rates of complete lesion resolution according to histological diagnosis and treatment

	Rates of lesion resolution
HPV infected lesions	
Placebo	0/8 (0%)
Interferon	15/28 (54%)
Suggestive but not diagnostic of HPV infection	
Placebo	1/2 (50%)
Interferon	2/5 (40%)

$p < 0.05$* (for the bracketed group: HPV infected lesions Interferon and the Suggestive section)

* Test for interaction between treatment and confirmed HPV infection.

are poorly understood. Recent studies employing modern molecular biological techniques have delineated some of the functions of the HPV genome and should provide appropriate antigens which will all help in conducting epidemiological, pathogenetic, and treatment studies. Among currently available treatment modalities, different interferon preparations are the best studied. Intralesional administration of alpha and beta interferons have been shown definitively to be superior to injections of placebo. Clearly defined virological and histological characterization of pre-therapy biopsies may be of value in interpretation of study results. Additional studies of treatment modalities including definitive evaluations of parenterally administered interferons, other biological response modifiers, and antiviral drugs, with or without conventional methods of local destructive therapy, will be required to determine optimal modes of treatment for this common STD.

Acknowledgement
Supported by PHS CA-43629 and A1-32510, National Institutes of Health, Bethesda, MD, USA.

REFERENCES

Becker T M, Stone K M, Alexander E R 1987 Genital human papillomavirus infection. Obstetrics & Gynecology Clinics of North America 14: 389–396

Broker T R 1987 Structure and Genetic Expression of Papillomaviruses. Obstetrics & Gynecology Clinics of North America 14: 329–348

Kreider J W, Howett M K, Leure-Dupree A E, Zaino R J, Weber J A 1987 Laboratory production in vivo of infectious human papillomavirus type II. Journal of Virology 61: 590–593

Gissmann L, Durst M, Oltersdorf T, von Knebel Doeberitz M 1987 Human papillomaviruses and cervical cancer. Cancer Cells 5/Papillomaviruses. Cold Spring Harbor Laboratory pp 275–380

McCullagh P, Nelder J A 1983 Log-linear models: Generalized Linear Models. Cox D R, Hinkley D V (eds) University Press, Great Britain pp 127–148

Oriel J D 1984 Genital Warts. In: Sexually Transmitted Diseases, Holmes K K et al (eds) McGraw Hill, New York pp 496–507

Reichman R C, Oakes D, Bonnez W et al 1988 Treatment of condyloma acuminatum with three different interferons administered intra-lesionally: A multicentered, placebo-controlled trial. Annals of Internal Medicine 108: 675–679

Sexually transmitted diseases 1985. Genitourinary Medicine 61: 204–207

Shah K V 1985 Papovaviruses In: Virology, Fields B N et al (eds) Raven Press, NY pp 371–391

Turek L P, Byrne J C, Lowy D R, Dvoretzky I, Freidman R M, Howley P M 1982 Interferon induces morphologic reversion with elimination of extrachromosomal viral genomes in bovine papillomavirus-transformed mouse cells. Proceedings of the National Academy of Sciences USA 79: 7914–7918

Wilbur D C, Reichman R C and Stoler M H 1988 Detection of infection by human papillomavirus in genital condylomata. American Journal of Clinical Pathology 69: 505–510

Discussion of paper presented by Richard Reichman

Discussant: Thomas M. Becker

GENITAL HUMAN PAPILLOMAVIRUS INFECTION: AN
EPIDEMIOLOGICAL PERSPECTIVE

Introduction
Genital human papillomavirus infections (HPV) are among the most common
sexually transmitted diseases (STDs) in the world and, like other sexually
transmitted viral diseases, the number of cases appears to be increasing (Becker
et al, 1985; Becker et al, 1986a; 1986b; 1987; Chuang et al, 1983; Centers for
Disease Control, 1987; World Health Organization, 1987). In addition, strong
links have been observed between papillomavirus infections and genital cancers,
and these infections pose numerous diagnostic and therapeutic challenges. To
define the extent of papillomavirus infection in the United States and other
countries, and to present some of the problems associated with the infection, I
have summarized information from epidemiological reports on the virus infections from national survey data and population-based studies in the United States,
and from STD clinics and cytological screening programmes in several countries.

Extent of the problem

National survey and population-based data on genital warts
In the United States, the most widely quoted surveillance mechanism for sexually
transmitted diseases is the National Disease and Therapeutic Index (IMS
American Ltd, 1983). This survey is based upon a random sample of
patient–physician interactions from the private medical sector. In a review of
these survey data, Becker et al (1987) observed that consultations for external
genital warts increased approximately seven-fold between 1966 and 1984, from
169,000 to 1,150,000. Private patient consultations for genital warts increased
among both men and women. The greatest proportion of consultations occurred
in the 20–29 year age range; for most years of the study, consultations for women
at all ages outnumbered those for men. Since only about one-half of all people
with STD in the United States are treated in the private sector (Weisner, 1981),
these survey data considerably underestimate the total numbers of patient visits
for genital warts throughout the country.

Supporting the data from the national survey, a population-based study of genital wart infections by Chuang and co-workers in Rochester, Minnesota, also indicated increasing numbers of cases of external genital warts (Chuang et al, 1984). This study showed an increase in the numbers of cases during the decades of the 1960s and 1970s. The Rochester study also showed that the greatest proportion of persons presenting with genital warts were young adults in their twenties. Unfortunately, neither the Rochester study nor the national survey included racial data, information which could identify groups that may be at high risk to acquire genital warts.

STD clinic data
Reports from STD clinics in several countries show that cases of external genital warts are common, and account for a significant proportion of patient visits for STD-related complaints (Chief Medical Officer's report United Kingdom, 1983; Centers for Disease Control Report, 1979; Environmental Health Branch Report, 1984; Short et al, 1984; Stone et al, 1986). In the United States, STD clinics have witnessed a recent rise in clinically apparent genital wart infections. In an Ohio STD clinic, the frequency of patients initially presenting for genital warts increased from 1980 to 1985 by 138% in white women, and 225% in black women (Table 1). Rates for both heterosexual and homosexual men during the same period, 1980 to 1985, also increased (Stone et al, 1986). Despite the greater increase among black women than among white women in the Ohio report, other STD clinic data in the United States still showed greater numbers of cases among whites than among blacks (Becker, 1984; Becker et al, 1984) (Table 2). STD clinic data in the US also indicate that among both blacks and whites, the rates of infections are highest among persons in the second decade of life.

Table 1 Trends in cases of genital warts compared with cases of all other STD in a Colombus STD clinic, 1980–85

Year	Cases of genital warts No. (% of total)		Other STD cases No. (% of total)	
1980	451	(3.0)	14,661	(97.0)
1981	549	(3.6)	14,872	(96.4)
1982	582	(3.8)	14,648	(96.2)
1983	476	(3.6)	13,376	(96.4)
1984	628	(5.0)	11,994	(95.0)
1985	686	(6.3)*	10,808	(93.7)

* $p < 0.001$, Mantel extension test

Subclinical HPV infections
Advances in diagnostic methods and increasing physician awareness of papillomavirus infections have resulted in growing numbers of reports of asymptomatic, subclinical genital HPV infections. Subclinical infections may be diagnosed by the presence of koilocytes on a cytological smear or biopsy specimen, by DNA hybridization studies, by immunoperoxidase stains, or by colposcopic features. Relying on cytological features of HPV infections, several researchers have reported frequent findings of HPV-infected cells in Pap smears. Evidence of cervical HPV infection was observed in 1–3% of all Pap smears sent

to a Quebec City pathology laboratory during the years 1974 to 1979 (Meisels & Morin, 1982; Meisels et al, 1982), and in 1.7% of cervical specimens from Planned Parenthood clinics throughout the United States during 1984 and 1985 (n=629,000) (Becker et al, 1987). In Texas, Planned Parenthood clinics showed koilocytotic evidence of cervical HPV infection in 1% of 120,000 smears in 1985 (Becker et al, 1987). In Victoria, Australia, Drake et al (1984) found that 2.6% of Pap smears taken in 1984 revealed evidence of cervical HPV infection (n=275,975).

Table 2 Demographics of an Ohio STD population with first diagnosed genital HPV infection, 1983

	HPV patients		Total STD patients	
Sex				
Male	416	(73%)	13,557	(67%)
Female	151	(27%)	6,580	(33%)
Total	567	(100%)	20,137	(100%)
Race				
White	415	(73%)	11,139	(55%)
Non-white	152	(27%)	8,998	(45%)
Marital status				
Single	445	(78%)	4,831	(74%)
All other	122	(22%)	5,306	(26%)
Sex preference				
Heterosexual	509	(90%)	17,679	(88%)
Homosexual	45	(8%)	1,842	(9%)
Bisexual	5	(1%)	207	(1%)
Unknown	8	(1%)	409	(2%)

Cytological evidence alone, however, is not sufficiently sensitive for diagnosis of cervical HPV infection. Among patients attending an STD clinic in London, HPV DNA sequences were identified in 10% of women with normal cytological and colposcopic studies (Wickenden et al 1985). In Seattle, Washington, 5% of women attending an STD clinic who had normal Pap smears also have evidence of cervical HPV DNA (Kiviat, 1986). In Germany, HPV DNA was identified in approximately 10% of women aged 15–50 years with normal cervical cytological smears (De Villiers et al, 1987). Using the combined diagnostic techniques of cervicography, cytology, and DNA hybridization (Reid, 1986) found that over 5% of STD clinic attendees and 20% of gynaecology clinic attendees in Detroit had evidence of cervical HPV infection.

Asymptomatic HPV infection has also been reported among men; these reports are based on koilocytotic changes in penile skin cells and upon colposcopic findings of acetowhitening of penile skin. HPV has also been detected in males from semen and urine specimens (Ostrow et al, 1986). Several researchers have described the high prevalence of HPV-associated penile lesions in men who are the sex partners of women with histological evidence of condylomata (Derkson, 1987; Sedlacek et al, 1986) and of cervical intraepithelial neoplasia (Campion, 1986; Levine et al, 1984). Many of these male partners were unaware of any signs or symptoms of HPV infection at the time of clinical evaluation. Such data suggest that clinically inapparent infections in men, as in women, are probably more common than clinically apparent HPV lesions.

HPV and genital cancers

A growing body of laboratory and epidemiological evidence suggests that genital HPV infection is associated with cervical and other lower genital tract malignancies. Published data show that cervical HPV infection is associated with a high proportion of cervical dysplasia cases, and that a relationship exists between HPV-induced cellular changes and pre-invasive carcinomas of the cervix (Kaufman & Adam, 1986; Fujii et al, 1984). Laboratory studies have demonstrated HPV genome in malignant cervical tissue and in lymph nodes from patients with metastatic cervical cancer (Lancaster et al, 1986). HPV can also induce dysplastic lesions in human cervical tissue in an experimental animal model (Kreider et al, 1986). In addition, associations have been made between HPV infection and dysplastic or neoplastic lesions in vulvar, penile, and anal lesions (Gross et al, 1985; Beckman et al, 1986b; Barrasso et al, 1987; Pfister, 1987).

Epidemiologists in both North and Central America have observed strong links between HPV lesions and development of genital tract cancers. A population-based study from the Mayo Clinic in Rochester, Minnesota, determined that women with prior histories of genital warts were 3.8 times more likely to develop cervical carcinoma *in situ* than women without a history of genital tract warts (Chuang et al, 1984). Several case-control studies have also shown an increased risk of development of cervical carcinoma among subjects reporting histories of genital warts (Peters et al, 1986; Reeves et al, 1986). In Seattle, Washington, a study of randomly selected women attending an STD clinic showed the risk of developing cervical neoplasia was increased 18-fold in association with cervical HPV infection (Kiviat, 1986). These studies strongly suggest that HPV should be viewed as a potential oncogene in the genital tract. Further investigation is warranted, however, to determine the precise role and importance of HPV as an aetiological agent in the development of genital cancers.

The widespread distribution of genital HPV infection, the increasing frequency of diagnosis of both clinically apparent and asymptomatic lesions, and the potential oncogenic effect of this virus are causes for growing alarm. In addition, many currently used forms of therapy for external warts and for internal genital HPV infection are inadequate to achieve cure. Further laboratory and epidemiological studies are clearly needed to examine more closely the role of HPV in the development of genital tract malignancies, and to develop more adequate diagnostic tools and treatments for genital HPV infections.

REFERENCES

Barrasso R, De Brux J, Croissant O, Orth G 1987 High prevalence of papillomavirus-associated penile intraepithelial neoplasia in sexual partners of women with cervical intraepithelia neoplasia. New England Journal of Medicine 15: 916–923
Becker T M 1984 Genital warts—a sexually transmitted disease epidemic? Colposcopy and Gynecologic Laser Surgery 1: 193–199

Becker T M, Hadgu A, Nahmias A J 1984 Genital warts: The most neglected sexually transmitted disease. Epidemic Intelligence Atlanta, Georgia (Abstract) 1984

Becker T M, Blount J F, Guinan M E 1985 Trends in genital herpes infections among private practitioners in the United States, 1966–1981. Journal of American Medical Association 253: 1601–1603

Becker T M, Blount J F, Douglas J et al 1986a Trends in molluscum contagiosum infections in the United States, 1966–1983. Sexually Transmitted Disease 13: 88–92

Becker T M, Stone K M, Coates W 1986b Epidemiology of genital herpes infections in the United States: The current situation. Journal of Reproductive Medicine 31: 359–364

Becker T M, Stone K M, Alexander E R 1987 Genital human papillomavirus infection: A growing concern. Obstetrics and Gynecology Clinics of North America 14: 389–396

Beckman A, Darling J R, Coates R et al 1986 Human papillomavirus in anal cancers. Second International Conference in Human Papillomaviruses and Squamous Cancer. Rush-Presbyterian, St Luke's Medical Center and Sinai Hospital of Detroit (Abstract)

Campion M 1986 Subclinical penile human papillomavirus infection: The clue to the high risk male. Second International Conference on Human Papillomavirus and Squamous Carcinoma. Rush-Presbyterial, St Luke's Medical Center and Sinai Hospital of Detroit (Abstract)

Centers for Disease Control 1979 Non-reported sexually transmissable diseases, United States. Morbidity and Mortality, Weekly Reports 28: 61–63

Centers for Disease Control 1987 Morbidity and Mortality Weekly Report. Human Immunodeficiency Virus infection in the United States. A Review of Current Knowledge 1987; 36s: 1–48

Chief Medical Officer, Department of Health and Social Security, United Kingdom. 1983 Sexually transmitted diseases. British Journal of Venereal Disease 59: 134–137

Chuang T, Su W, Ilstrup et al 1983 Incidence and trend of herpes progenitalis: A 15-year population study. Mayo Clinic Proceedings 58: 436–441

Chuang T, Perry H O, Kurland L T et al 1984 Condyloma acuminatun in Rochester, Minnesota, 1950–1978. Archives of Dermatology 120: 469–475

Derkson D 1987 Human papillomavirus infections in male and female sex partners in a family practice clinic. New Mexico Association of Family Practitioners Annual Conference (Abstract)

De Villiers E M, Schneider A, Miklaw H et al 1987 Human papillomavirus infections in women with and without abnormal cervical cytology. Lancet, September 26: 703–706

Drake M, Medley G, Mitchell H 1984 Cytologic detection of human papillomavirus infection. In: Reid R (ed) Obstetrics and Gynecology Clinics of North America. Saunders Company, Philadelphia

Environmental Health Branch, Department of Health, Australia: Communicable Disease Intelligence 1984, Bulletin No. 84/24

Fujii T, Crum C P, Winkler B et al 1984 Human papillomavirus infection and cervical intraepithelia neoplasia: Histopathology and DNA content. Obstetrics and Gynecology 63(1): 99–104

Gross G, Hagedorn M, Ikenberg H et al 1985 Papillomavirus infection of the anogenital region: correlation between histology, clinical picture and virus type. Journal of Investigations in Dermatology 85: 147–152

IMS America Ltd 1983 Coding Manual and Descriptive Information for the National Disease and Therapeutic Index. Rockville, Maryland

Kaufman R H, Adam E 1986 Herpes simplex virus and human papillomavirus in the development of cerival carcinoma. Clinical Obstetrics and Gynecology 29(3): 678–692

Kiviat N 1986 What is the true prevalence of genital HPV infection: The Seattle experience. Presented at the Second International Conference on Human papillomaviruses and Squamous Carcinoma. Rush-Presbyterian-S Luke's Medical Center and Sinai Hospital of Detroit, Chicago, October 27–29

Kreider J W, Howett M K, Lill N L et al 1986 In vivo transformation of human skin with human papillomavirus type II from condylomata acuminata. Journal of Virology 59: 369–376

Lancaster W D, Castellano C, Santos C et al 1986 Human papillomavirus deoxyribonucleic acid in cervical carcinoma from primary and metastatic sites. American Journal of Obstetrics and Gynecology 154(1): 115–119

Levine R U, Crum C P, Herman E et al 1984 Cervical papillomavirus infection and intraepithelial neoplasia: A study of male sexual partners. Obstetrics and Gynecology 64: 16–20

Meisels A, Morin C 1982 Human papillomavirus and cancer of the uterine cervix. Gynecology and Oncology 12: S111–123

Meisels A, Morin C, Casas-Cordero M 1982 Human papillomavirus and cancer of the uterine cervix. International Journal of Gynecology and Pathology 1: 75–94

Ostrow R S, Zachow K R, Niimura M et al 1986 detection of papillomavirus DNA in human semen. Science 321: 731–733

Peters R K, Thomas D, Hagan D G et al 1986 Risk factors for invasive cervical cancer among Latinas and non-Latinas 77: 1063–107

Pfister H 1987 Relationship of papillomaviruses to anogenital cancer. Obstetrics and Gynecology Clinics of North America 14: 349–36

Reeves W, Causey H, Brinton L et al 1986 Cervical cancer in Latin America. Second International Conference on Human Papillomavirus and Squamous Carcinoma. Rush-Presbyterian-St Luke's Medical Center and Sinai Hospital of Detroit, Chicago, October 27–29, (Abstract)

Reid R 1986 What is the true prevalence of genital HPV infection: The Detroit experience. Presented at the Second International Conference on Human Papillomarvirus and Squamous Carcinoma. Rush-Presbyterian-St Luke's Medical Center and Sinai Hospital of Detroit, Chicago, October 27–29 (Abstract)

Sedlacek T V, Cunnane M, Carpiniello V 1986 Colposcopy in the diagnosis of penile condyloma. American Journal of Obstetrics and Gynecology 154: 494–496

Short D L, Stockman D L, Wolinsky S M et al 1984 Comparative rates of sexually transmitted diseases among heterosexual men, homosexual men, and heterosexual women. Sexually Transmitted Disease 11: 271–274

Stone K M, Lossick J G, Mosure D et al 1986 The epidemiology of genital warts in an STD clinic. Second International Conference on Human Papillomavirus and Squamous Carcinoma. Rush-Presbyterian-St Luke's Medical Center and Sinai Hospital of Detroit. Chicago October 27–29 (Abstract)

Weisner P J 1981 Magnitude of the problem of sexually transmitted diseases in the United States. Sexually Transmitted Diseases 1980 Status Report, NIH Publication No. 82–2213, US Government Printing Office

Wickenden C, Malcolm A D B, Steele A et al 1985 Screening for wart virus infection in normal and abnormal cervices by DNA hybridization of cervical scrapes. Lancet 1: 65–67

World Health Organization 1987 World Health Statistics Annual Report Geneva: World Health Organization, p 15

Discussion: Treatment of human papillomaviruses

Richard Reichman and Thomas Becker

The relationship between immunodeficiency and HPV disease was discussed. Although it is clear that immunosuppression (e.g. from HIV or drugs) increases the expression of HPV, there are no quantitative data. Renal transplant recipients who have HIV-DNA in skin lesions do not typically develop warts; however, large or refractory genital warts are a recognized problem in HIV-infected patients. Some people have observed an apparent increase in the frequency of condyloma in patients with Type I diabetes mellitus or leukaemia. It has been suggested that there is an increased risk of cervical cancer in renal transplant recipients compared with the general population, but systemic studies have not been done. If we can succeed in keeping AIDS patients alive longer, we may see more consequences of papillomavirus infection in that group.

There was some discussion of the relative merits of different techniques for diagnosing HPV infection. For grossly visible warts (e.g. condyloma), the diagnosis is wrong about 10% of the time if gross morphology alone is used. Histopathological examination will clarify the diagnosis in virtually every case. For clinically silent infections, e.g. the cervix, *in situ* hybridization is 2–5 times more sensitive than cytopathology.

One participant questioned the evidence documenting transmission of HPV from mothers with cervical infection to the newborn. There are two observations supporting transmission from mother to child at birth. One is that the HPV types causing laryngeal papillomatosis are the same as those causing cervical infection (namely 6 and 11), and the other is that in studies of children with laryngeal papillomatosis retrospective histories have shown a history of genital warts in about 50% of their mothers. But prospective longitudinal studies have not been done.

There are two large prospective studies on treatment of laryngeal papillomatosis that are now nearing completion, one sponsored by the Burroughs Wellcome Company and one by the NIH. The data have not been published but they are thought to show that patients get better when treated with systemic alpha interferon but regress when it is stopped. The interferon therapy has the clear advantage that the treated children require fewer surgical procedures.

The role of co-factors (e.g. herpes simplex virus) in production of cancers by HPV requires further clarification. The data still support a role for herpes simplex virus as a co-factor; however, some epidemiological data show that smoking may be a greater risk factor for HPV-induced cervical neoplasia than herpes simplex virus infection. Studies showing the presence of nicotine metabolites in cervical mucus support this epidemiological association.

4. Management of chronic hepatitis virus infection

Howard C. Thomas

INTRODUCTION

With the availability of synthetic nucleoside analogues, lymphoblastoid and recombinant alpha interferons and of molecular probes to monitor viral replication, progress in the treatment of chronic hepatitis B (HBV), delta virus (HDV) and non-A, non-B hepatitis has been rapid.

HBV INFECTION

Recovery from HBV infection is dependent on the integrated activity of the patient's immune system. Chronic HBV infections arise because of defects in these defences. These must be understood before logical therapies can be developed.

Acute hepatitis B infection

HBV is not cytopathic and the liver damage is caused by immune lysis of infected hepatocytes. Analysis of the inflammatory infiltrate demonstrates the presence of NK and cytotoxic T-cells (Eggink et al, 1982). Viral antigens are seen on the surface of the hepatocyte (Gudat et al, 1975) and these, in association with the class I MHC proteins, make the cell a target for cytotoxic T-cell lysis (Doherty & Zinkernagel, 1975). Studies in patients with chronic HBV infection suggest that HBc and HBe antigens are an important target (Eddleston et al, 1982; Pignatelli et al, 1987). Hepatocytes usually express very little MHC class I glycoprotein (Thomas et al, 1982) but, in the early stage of acute HBV infection, following the production of alpha interferon, MHC expression on hepatocytes increases and co-incidentally transaminases rise (Fig. 4.1). Interferon also activates a series of enzymes, including the 2-5A synthetase system, which leads to inhibition of viral protein synthesis (Fig. 4.2). These changes would be expected to produce an antiviral state in uninfected, regenerating liver cells, preventing re-infection. This, along with development of virus neutralizing antibodies, should prevent short and long term relapse or re-infection.

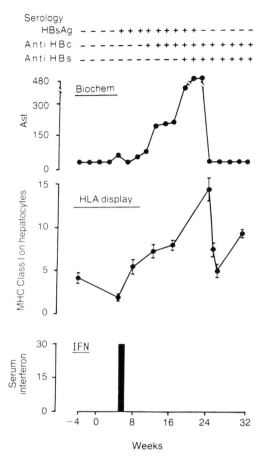

Fig. 4.1 Acute HBV infection in the chimpanzee. Markers of virus infection appear early, coinciding with a detectable pulse of circulating IFN. This is followed by enhanced MHC display on hepatocytes. Liver damage (rising AST) coincides with the appearance of host immunity to HBV (anti-HBc). AST: aspartate aminotransferase (SGOT)

Chronic hepatitis B infection

It is likely that there are many different reasons why patients develop the chronic carrier state.

Chronic HBV infection following exposure in neonatal life
Ninety per cent of babies born to HBV 'e' antigen positive mothers become infected, and over 90% of these develop a chronic carrier state (Beasley et al, 1981). These infants probably receive a large inoculum of virus from maternal blood before or during birth, and by close contact with secretions soon after birth. The reason for these infants failing to clear the virus is unknown but likely relate to the immaturity of the neonatal immune system (Nash, 1985). HBe antigen, a low molecular weight soluble protein, passes across the placenta and may

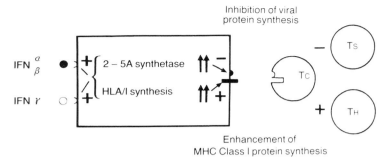

Fig. 4.2 Effect of IFN on virus-infected cell. Alpha and beta IFN acting through a common receptor and gamma IFN acting through a separate receptor activate several enzyme systems, including a 2-5A synthetase. This catalyses production of oligo-adenylates that activate an endogenous ribonuclease leading to cleavage of viral RNA. IFN also causes enhanced expression of MHC Class I proteins on the hepatocyte surface, facilitating recognition of virus-infected cells by the cellular immune mechanisms of the host. HBe and HBc antigens are the target of this component of the hose immune response. Tc, Ts, Th: cytotoxic, suppressor and helper T cells (+) and (-) denote enhancement and suppression, respectively

suppress the development of the cellular immune response to the nucleocapsid proteins which are the target during immune clearance of infected hepatocytes (Fig. 4.3). Other factors such as the immaturity of the neonatal immune system (Nash, 1985), the presence of immunosuppressive factors such as alpha fetoprotein and the large inoculum of the virus, may also contribute to the high incidence of chronic infection resulting from exposure at or before birth.

Fulminant hepatitis following exposure in neonatal life
Rarely, children born to HBs antigen anti-HBe positive mothers develop fulminant hepatitis. The mechanism is once again unknown. One hypothesis is that maternal anti-HBe and anti-HBc pass across the placenta and initially modulate the lysis of infected hepatocytes by cell-mediated immune responses (Pignatelli et al, 1987). The virus spreads throughout the liver and as the maternal antibodies disappear at three to six months, cytotoxic T-cells sensitized to HBe and HBc rapidly destroy the infected cells.

Chronic HBV infection following exposure after the neonatal period
In marked contrast to the situation at birth, only 5–10% of subjects infected after this period develop chronic infection. There are probably several different causes for the development of chronic infection at this stage of life. One defect, which has recently been documented, is the production of sub-normal quantities of alpha interferon by peripheral blood mononuclear cells (Ikeda et al, 1986a). These individuals also have evidence of abnormal activation of their hepatocytes by interferon. Levels of hepatic 2–5A synthetase (an enzyme induced by IFN) are only minimally elevated (Ikeda et al, 1986b), and MHC Class I proteins, which are known to be induced by interferon, are present in very low density on infected hepatocytes (Montano et al, 1982). This appears to be due to the ability of HBV within the hepatocyte to selectively 'switch off' the responsiveness of the cell to interferons. *In vitro* transfection of HBV into cells in tissue culture,

makes them partially non-responsive to interferon: they remain susceptible to lysis by Sindbis virus and HLA induction does not occur (Onji et al, 1988).

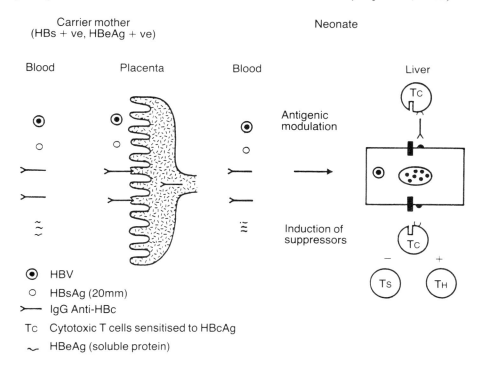

Carrier mother
(HBs + ve, HBeAg + ve)

Neonate

Blood Placenta Blood Liver

Antigenic modulation

Induction of suppressors

⊙ HBV
○ HBsAg (20mm)
>— IgG Anti-HBc
Tc Cytotoxic T cells sensitised to HBcAg
∽ HBeAg (soluble protein)

Fig. 4.3 Neonatal HBV infection: postulated mechanism of viral persistence. It is proposed that HBe antigen crosses the placenta from the maternal blood and, in neonates, induces tolerance to HBe antigen which is one of the targets of the cellular immune response. Maternal IgG anti-HBc also crosses the placenta into the foetal circulation. HBV infection of the neonatal liver is thus facilitated as maternal IgG blocks recognition of virus-infected cells by cytotoxic T cells. Early exposure to soluble virus protein (HBe) may induce a state of antigenic tolerance to the virus with specific suppressor cells inhibiting the host defence mechanism

Management of chronic HBV
There is no established place in the treatment of chronic HBV infection for regimens involving solely anti-inflammatory or immunosuppressive drugs (Scullard et al, 1981; Weller et al, 1982b).

A variety of synthetic and natural antiviral compounds have been developed and are being evaluated in clinical trials.

Indications for therapy (not definitively identified)

(1) Infectivity—HBe antigen and HBV-DNA positivity.
(2) Evidence of progressive liver disease—histological evidence of chronic active or lobular hepatitis.

Contra-indication for therapy

(1)   Evidence of decompensated cirrhosis.

Goals of therapy

(1)   Inhibition of HBV replication (by direct effect or by stimulation of the host antiviral response).
(2)   Long term control of inflammatory necrosis of hepatocytes.
(3)   Prevention of malignant transformation of hepatocytes.

Types of response
There are three types of response (Fig. 4.4)

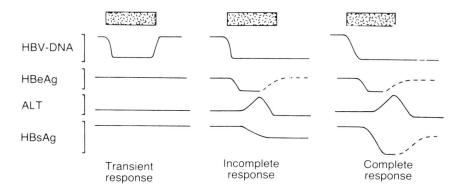

Fig. 4.4 Pattern of response to antiviral treatment

(1)   Transient response: inhibition of HBV replication—loss of HBV-DNA and DNA polymerase but not HBeAg or HBsAg—during therapy but return of these markers on cessation of therapy.
(2)   Incomplete response: sustained inhibition of HBV replication—loss of HBV-DNA and DNA polymerase continuing after cessation of therapy, conversion from HBeAg to anti-HBe but continued HBs antigenaemia due to translation of integrated HBV-DNA.
(3)   Complete response: sustained inhibition of HBV replication—loss of HBV-DNA and DNA polymerase continuing after cessation of therapy, with permanent seroconversion from HBeAg and HBsAg to anti-HBe and anti-HBs.

Active drugs

(1)   Adenine arabinoside: potent inhibitor of HBV replication but clinical usefulness limited by poor aqueous solubility and relatively low therapeutic ratio. In one small, randomized, controlled study a ten day course produced sustained or temporary HBe antigen/antibody seroconversion in 40% of cases (Bassendine et al, 1981).

56

(2)   Adenine arabinoside monophosphate: equally effective inhibitor of HBV replication which can be given by i.m. bolus injection (Scullard et al, 1982; Weller et al, 1982a). A course of 10 mg/kg/24 hours for four days followed by 5 mg/kg/24 hours for a further 23 days has been evaluated in four controlled studies (Hoofnagle et al, 1984; Trepo et al, 1984; Weller et al, 1985; Perillo et al, 1985). Variability of response may be related to heterogeneity of patient population being studied. In one study none of 24 homosexual HBV carriers responded whereas 10 of 22 heterosexual (predominantly Southern European) carriers did (Thomas & Scully, 1986) (Fig. 4.5).

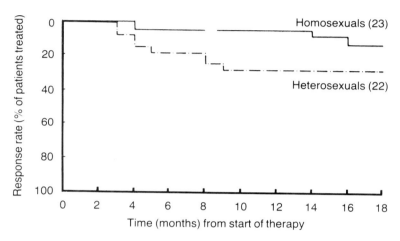

Fig. 4.5 Response to ARA-AMP in homosexual and heterosexual men

(3)   Acycloguanosine (Acyclovir) is active against herpes simplex in low concentrations because of phosphorylation to active metabolites by virus encoded thymidine kinase. This enzyme is not present in HBV infected cells so that this mode of action does not operate. Higher concentrations (near the maximum tolerated level) do partially inhibit HBV replication (Sidwell et al, 1982; Weller et al, 1983) but this has not been shown to be clinically useful.

(4)   Type I interferon (alpha and beta): both natural and recombinant DNA produced preparations have been examined.

(a)   Leucocyte alpha IFN: has been shown to inhibit HBV replication when given daily in moderate doses (5–10 megaunits/m^2/day over three to six months (Greenberg et al, 1976). A randomized controlled study showed that low doses for four to six weeks produced no long term responses (Schalm & Heijtink, 1982).

(b)   Lymphoblastoid alpha IFN: given thrice weekly for three months in moderate doses has been shown in a randomized controlled study to produce HBe antigen clearance in 45% of cases, significantly more often than occurred spontaneously in the control group (Brook et al, submitted[a]). This response rate is similar to that seen with ARA-MP (Lok et al, 1986) but in homosexual patients IFN is significantly better than ARA-MP. Further analysis of these studies show that Chinese carriers (presumably infected from birth) show no response whereas European carriers exhibit a 55% conversion rate (Thomas & Scully, 1986) (Fig. 4.6). Further studies reveal that six months of therapy is no better than three (Fig. 4.7) (Scully et al, 1987).

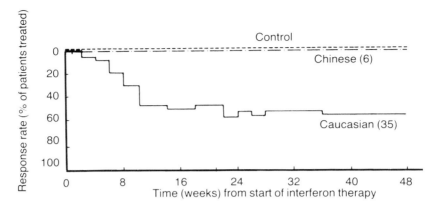

Fig. 4.6 Response to alpha interferon in Chinese and Caucasian carriers (Thomas & Scully, 1986)

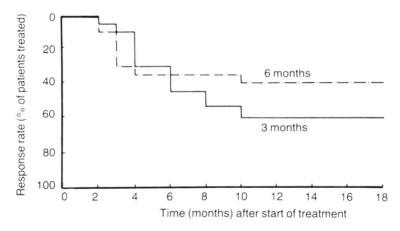

Fig. 4.7 Response to alpha interferon: comparison of 3 and 6 months' therapy (Scully et al, 1987)

(c) Recombinant alpha IFN: given daily in high doses inhibits HBV replication but is toxic (Smith et al, 1983). Moderate doses (10 megaunits/m^2 daily or thrice weekly) are better tolerated and can be given for three to six months (McDonald et al 1987). Preliminary analysis of one randomized controlled study showed 45% of patients clearing HBe antigen (McDonald et al, 1987; Brook et al, submitted[b]).

(d) Beta IFNs: of natural and recombinant types have been used and shown to have similar activity to alpha IFN. No controlled studies are reported.

(5) Type II interferon (gamma): both natural and recombinant gamma interferon are available. These are predominantly immunostimulant with less

direct antiviral activity. Inhibition of HBV replication does occur after several months' therapy. Optimal dosaging has not been established.

(6) Interleukin II: this is a lymphokine which amplifies immune function. It has been tried safely in individual patients but its place has not been established.

(7) Combination therapy:

(a) Short course prednisolone plus antiviral therapy (ARA-MP or IFN): withdrawal of protracted immunosuppressant therapy may result in HBeAg seroconversion (Scullard et al, 1981; Weller et al, 1982b). However short courses of prednisolone do not precipitate seroconversion (Hoofnagle et al, 1982). When followed by ARA-MP or alpha IFN, 60–70% seroconversion rates have been reported in small controlled studies (Perrillo et al, 1985). Care must be taken when withdrawing steroids particularly in patients with severe liver disease: fatalities have been recorded.

(b) Acyclovir and alpha interferon: preliminary studies did not include appropriate controls treated with interferon alone and therefore summative or synergistic effects could not be conclusively identified (Schalm et al, 1985).

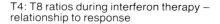

T4: T8 ratios during interferon therapy –
relationship to response

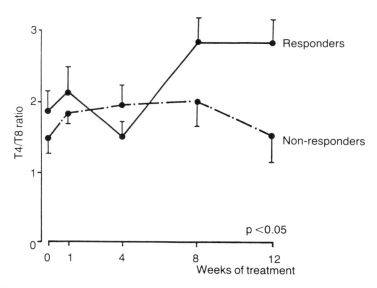

Fig. 4.8 Changes occurring during interferon therapy

General comment
The mechanism of action of interferon in inducing seroconversion hepatitis is unknown. Several changes have been noted both in the immune system and in the infected hepatocyte (Fig. 4.8). An increase in MHC Class I protein display (Pignatelli et al, 1986) and alteration in viral protein expression on the hepatocyte (Thomas et al, 1987) occur within 24 hours after the start of therapy. An increase in the helper/cytotoxic suppressor cell ratio occurs at six to eight weeks when the

seroconversion hepatitis starts and is not seen in those that do not respond.

Changes in humoral immunity also occur. Patients who respond to therapy either have IgM anti-HBc present before treatment or develop it during the course of therapy (Chen et al, submitted). Changes in cell-mediated immunity may also occur but have not yet been documented.

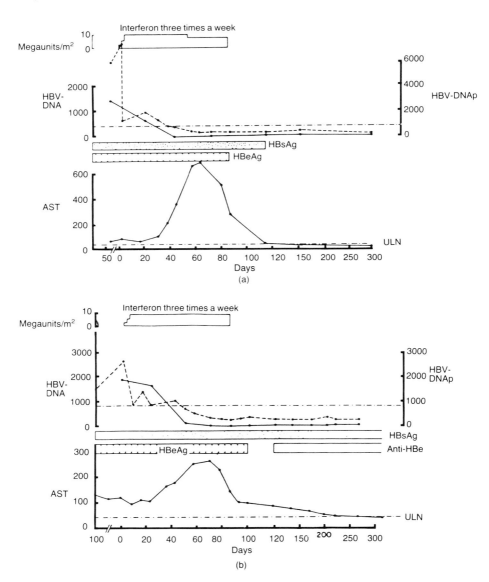

Fig. 4.9 (*a*) Complete response: inhibition of HBV replication and clearance of HBs antigen. (*b*) Incomplete response: inhibition of HBV replication associated with a transient exacerbation and then normalization of the liver function tests. Note the patient remains HBsAg positive, presumably because of the presence of integrated HBV sequences. Benefits to the patient include reduced infectivity and cessation of inflammatory liver disease

Inhibition of viral replication associated with HBe antigen/antibody seroconversion, is usually long lasting and accompanied, after a transient exacerbation, by amelioration of the inflammatory liver disease (Fig. 4.9). Reactivation may occur, particularly in homosexual patients with or without HIV infection (Davis & Hoofnagle, 1985).

Patients treated early in the course of the disease will lose HBs antigen from their serum if cessation of HBV replication is achieved (Fig. 4.9a).

If integration of HBV sequences into the host cell genome has occurred before starting treatment, HBs antigenaemia will continue after cessation of detectable HBV replication (Fig. 4.9b). However, inflammatory liver disease will ameliorate in those patients if long term inhibition of HBV replication is achieved.

Evidence that successful antiviral therapy improves hepatic histology

Several investigations have shown improvement in alanine aminotransferase levels following clearance of HBe Ag and HBV-DNA from the serum. A review of 50 treated and 25 untreated control patients has conclusively shown a reduction in inflammatory necrosis of liver cells and probably a diminished rate of development of cirrhosis, in patients responding to therapy with loss of markers of HBV replication (Brook et al, submitted[a]).

The need to select patients for treatment

Infectivity and progressive liver disease are the major reasons for attempting therapy with either adenine arabinoside monophosphate or the alpha interferons. Currently interferons are the most satisfactory therapy, but less than 50% of patients respond and the side effects of interferon are substantial. For this reason, both clinical and serological features, which predict a greater chance of response have been sought. The clinical features include marked inflammatory activity, high transaminases and more recently the presence of IgM anti HBc (Chen et al, submitted) and low serum HBV-DNA (McDonald et al, 1987).

HDV INFECTION

HDV carriers superinfected with HDV show a marked exacerbation of their disease. Many progress from minimal liver disease to established cirrhosis within a few years. HDV infection is common in Central Africa and the Mediterranean Basin. In the Western World it is seen virtually exclusively in haemophiliacs and drug addicts, although a few cases have been reported in homosexual men.

The cloning of HDV has provided molecular probes capable of detecting delta virus RNA both in serum and liver tissues. Preliminary studies by three groups have shown that delta virus replication can be inhibited by moderate doses of alpha interferon given thrice weekly for several weeks (Rosina et al, 1987; Hoofnagle et al, 1986; Thomas et al, 1987).

The liver function tests and liver histology show a more variable response to interferon therapy. In patients treated early on in the course of the disease, before the development of cirrhosis, when the hepatitis delta virus RNA falls in the serum, the liver transaminases fall. However, in patients treated later in the course of the disease and in those with established cirrhosis the improvement in liver function is more variable in spite of the reproducible fall in HDV-RNA in serum.

The duration of therapy required to produce long-term control of this agent is currently unknown. Even after three months of interferon therapy, delta virus replication resumes in the majority of cases when the treatment is stopped.

NON-A, NON-B VIRUS INFECTION

There are at least two parenterally transmitted non-A, non-B hepatitis viruses. These can be differentiated by different incubation periods.

Short incubation non-a, non-b
This virus has not been isolated and characterized. Preliminary studies in haemophiliac and agammaglobulinaemic (Thompson et al, 1987) patients, and in carriers of the haemophilia gene, have shown a marked improvement in transaminases after several weeks' interferon therapy. Both lymphoblastoid and recombinant alpha interferon are active against this agent and the dosage required to maintain control of the inflammatory activity is between 2 and 3 million units/m^2 given thrice weekly. When treatment is withdrawn after three months of therapy in approximately 50% of cases the transaminases become abnormal again. Long-term therapy may, therefore, be required in some cases. Side effects have been minimal and this therapy has now been continued for at least one year in a small number of cases.

Long incubation non-a, non-b
These patients have an incubation period of six to seven weeks. The virus has once again not been isolated or characterized. Preliminary data show that the virus may be sensitive to lipid solvents thereby indicating that it is probably enveloped.

Recombinant (Hoofnagle et al, 1987) and lymphoblastoid (Jacyna et al, 1988) interferon have been given to small numbers of patients and once again a rapid improvement in liver function tests has been observed. The minimum dose required to maintain this improvement is 1.5 to 2 million units/m^2 thrice weekly. In one randomized controlled trial liver function tests returned to normal by five weeks after the commencement of interferon (Jacyna et al, 1988). Relapse may be seen with withdrawal of interferon and long term maintenance therapy may be required in some cases. Randomized controlled trials are continuing to determine the practicality of this long term therapy.

CONCLUSIONS

It is now clear that both synthetic and natural antiviral compounds, including lymphoblastoid and recombinant alpha interferons, have a place in the management of chronic viral hepatitis. The optimal regimens and duration of treatment remain to be determined.

REFERENCES

Bassendine M F, Chadwick R G, Saberon J, Thomas H C, Sherlock S 1981 Adenine arabinoside therapy in HBsAg positive chronic liver disease: a controlled study. Gastroenterology 80: 1016–1022

Beasley R P, Hwang L-Y, Lin C-C et al 1981 Hepatitis B immune globulin (HBIG) efficacy in the interruption of perinatal transmission of hepatitis B carrier state. Lancet: 388–393

Brook M G, Petrovic L, McDonald J A, Scheuer P J, Thomas H C Evidence of histological improvement following anti-viral treatment in chronic hepatitis B virus carriers and identification of histological features that predict response. Journal of Hepatology (submitted[a])

Brook G, McDonald J A, Caruso L, Karayiannis P, Foster G, Harris J R W, Thomas H C A controlled randomised trial of interferon alpha 2a (Roferon-A) for the treatment of chronic hepatitis B virus (HBV) infection in patients attending a sexually transmitted disease clinic. Gut (submitted[b])

Chen G, Karayiannis P, McGarvey M J, Thomas H C Subclasses of anti HBc in chronic HBV carriers: changes during treatment with interferon and predictions of response. Gut (submitted)

Davis G L, Hoofnagle J H 1985 Reactivation of chronic type B presenting as acute hepatitis. Annals In Medicine 102: 762–765

Doherty PC, Zinkernagel RM 1975 A biological role for the major histocompatibility antigen. Lancet 1: 1405–1409

Eddleston A W L F, Mondelli M, Mieli-Vergani G, Williams R 1982 Lymphocyte cytotoxicity to autologous hepatocytes in chronic hepatitis B virus infection. Hepatology 2: 122S–127S

Eggink H F, Houthoff H J, Huitema S, Gips C H, Poppema S 1982 Cellular and humoral immune reactions in chronic active liver disease. Lymphocyte subsets in liver biopsies of patients with untreated idiopathic auto-immune, chronic active hepatitis B and primary biliary cirrhosis. Clinical Experimental Immunology 50: 17–24

Greenberg H B, Pollard R B, Lutwick L I, Gregory P B, Robinson W S, Merigan T C 1976 Effect of human leukocyte interferon on hepatitis B virus infection in patients with chronic active hepatitis. New England Journal Medicine 295: 517–522

Gudat F, Bianchi L, Sonnabend W, Thiel G, Aenishaenslin W, Stadler C A 1975 Pattern of core and surface expression in liver tissue reflects state of immune response in hepatitis British Journal of Laboratory Investigations 32: 1–9

Hoofnagle J H, Davis G L, Pappas S C et al 1982 A short course of prednisolone/azathioprine in chronic B viral hepatitis. Gut 23: 650–655

Hoofnagle J H, Hansor R G, Minuk G Y et al 1984 Randomised controlled trial of adenine arabinoside monophosphate for chronic type B hepatitis. Gastroenterology 86: 150–157

Hoofnagle J H, Mullen K D, Jones B et al 1986 Treatment of chronic non-A, non-B hepatitis with recombinant human alpha interferon. New England Journal Medicine 315: 1575–1578

Hoofnagle J, Mullen K D, Peters M et al 1987 Treatment of chronic delta hepatitis with recombinant human alpha interferon. In: Liss A R (eds) The hepatitis delta virus Alan R Liss Inc 291–298

Ikeda T, Lever A M L, Thomas H C 1986a Evidence for a deficiency of IFN production in patients with chronic HBV infection acquired in adult life. Hepatology 5: 962–965

Ikeda T, Pignatelli M, Lever A M L, Thomas H C 1986[b] Relationship of HLA protein display to activation of 2–5A synthetase in HBe antigen or anti-HBe positive chronic HBV infection. Gut 27 (12): 1498–1501

Jacyna M, Brook G, Loke R H T, Crossey M, Murray-Lyon I M, Thomas H C 1988 A controlled trial of lymphoblastoid interferon in chronic non-A, non-B hepatitis. British Medical Journal (in press)

Lok A S F, Karayiannis P, Brown D et al 1986 A randomised study of the effect of adenine arabinoside monophosphate (four or eight week courses) versus lymphoblastoid interferon or hepatitis B virus (HBV) replication. Hepatology 3: 865–871

McDonald J A, Caruso L, Karayiannis P, Scully L J, Harris J R W, Forster G, Thomas H C 1987 Diminished responsiveness of male homosexual chronic HBV carriers with HIV antibodies to recombinant alpha interferon. Hepatology 7: 719–723

Montano L, Miescher G C, Goodhall A H, Wiedmann K H, Janossy G, Thomas H C 1982 Hepatitis B virus and HLA display in the liver during chronic hepatitis B virus infection. Hepatology 2: 557–561

Nash A A 1985 Tolerance and suppression in virus diseases. British Medical Bulletin: 41–45

Onji M, Lever A, Thomas H C 1988 Hepatitis B virus reduces the sensitivity of cells to interferon. Hepatology (in press)

Perrillo R P, Regerstein F G, Bodicky C J, Campbell C, Sanders G E, Sunwoo Y C 1985 Comparative efficacy of ARA-MP in prednisolone withdrawal followed by ARA-MP in treatment of HBV induced CAH. Gastroenterology 780–786

Pignatelli M, Waters J, Lever A M L, Brown D, Iwarson S, Schaff Z, Gerety R, Thomas H C 1986 HLA Class I antigens on hepatocyte membrane: Increased expression during interferon therapy of chronic hepatitis B. Hepatology 6 (3): 349–353

Pignatelli M, Waters J, Lever A M L, Iwarson S, Gerety R, Thomas H C 1987 Cytotoxic T-cell responses to the nucleocapsid proteins of HBV in chronic hepatitis. Journal of Hepatology 4: 15–21

Rosina F, Saracco G, Lattore V, Quartarone V, Rizzetto M, Verme G, Trinchero P, Sansalvadore F, Smedile A 1987 In: The hepatitis delta virus Alan R Liss Inc 299–303

Schalm S W, Heijtink R A 1982 Spontaneous disappearance viral replication and liver cell inflammation in HBs-Ag positive chronic active hepatitis: results of placebo vs. interferon trial. Hepatology 2: 791–794

Schalm S W, Heijtink R A, Van Buuren H R, de Man R A 1985 Acyclovir enhances the antiviral effect of interferon in chronic hepatitis B. Lancet 1: 358–360

Scullard G H, Smith C I, Merigan T C, Robinson W S, Gregory P B 1981 Effects of immunosuppressive therapy on viral markers in chronic active hepatitis B. Gastroenterology 81: 987–991

Scullard G H, Andres L L, Greenberg H B et al 1982 Antiviral treatment of HBs and HBeAg positive chronic liver disease: prolonged inhibition of viral replication by highly soluble adenine arabinoside 5'-monophosphate (ARA-MP). Gut 23: 717–723

Scully L J, Shein R, Karayiannis P, McDonald J A, Thomas H C 1987 Lymphoblastoid interferon therapy of chronic HBV infection: a comparison of 12 v 24 weeks of thrice weekly treatment. Journal of Hepatology 5: 51–58

Sidwell R W, Huffman J H, Khare G P et al 1982 Broad spectrum antiviral activity of virazole : 1–β–D ribofuranosyl –1, 2, 4–triazole 3–carboxamide. Science 177: 705–706

Smith C I, Weissberg J, Bernhardt L, Gregory P B, Robinson W S, Merigan T C 1983 Acute Dane particke supression with leukocyte recombinant interferon in chronic HBV infection. Journal of Infectious Diseases 148: 907–913

Thomas H C, Shipton U, Montano L 1982 The HLA system: its relevance to the pathogenesis of liver disease. Grune & Stratton (eds) In: Progress in Liver Disease 16: 517–527

Thomas H C, Scully L J 1986 Antiviral therapy in chronic hepatitis B virus infection. British Medical Bulletin 41: 374–380

Thomas H C, Farci P, Shein R, Karayiannis P, Smedile A, Caruso L, Gerlin L 1987 Inhibition of hepatitis delta virus (HDV) replication by lymphoblastoid human interferon. In: The hepatitis delta virus Alan R Liss. Inc. 277–290

Thompson B J, Doran M, Lever A M L, Webster A D B 1987 Alpha interferon therapy for non-A, non-B hepatitis transmitted by glammaglobulin replacement therapy. Lancet 1: 539:541

Trepo C, Hantz O, Ouzan D et al 1984 Therapeutic efficacy of ARA-MP in symptomatic HBe Ag positive CAH: a randomised, placebo control study. (Abstract 193) Hepatology 4: 1055

Weller I V D, Bassendine M F, Craxi et al 1982a Successful treatment of HBs and HBeAg positive chronic liver disease: prolonged inhibition of viral replication by highly soluble adenine arabinoside 5'-monophosphate (ARA-MP) Gut 23: 717–723

Weller I V D, Bassendine M F, Murray A K, Croxi A, Thomas H C, Sherlock S 1982b The effects of prednisolone/azathioprine in chronic hepatitis B viral infection. Gut 23: 650–655

Weller I V D, Carreno V, Fowler M J F et al 1983 Acyclovir in hepatitis B antigen-positive chronic liver disease: inhibition of viral replication and transient renal impairment with iv bolus administration. Journal of Antimicrobial Chemotherapy 11: 223–231

Weller I V D, Lok A S F, Minel A et al 1985 A randomised controlled trial of adenine arabinoside 5'-monophosphate (ARA-AMP) in chronic hepatitis B virus infection. Gut 26: 745–751

Discussion of paper presented by Howard Thomas

Discussant: Robert Perrillo

A COMMENTARY ON ANTIVIRAL THERAPY OF CHRONIC
HEPATITIS VIRUS INFECTION

The past decade has witnessed relatively slow progress in the development of effective drug regimens for chronic viral hepatitis. The majority of trials have focused on chronic type B hepatitis where the effects on viral proliferation are easily measurable. Most studies have been small, poorly controlled trials involving a number of different treatment regimens, and there has often been marked disparity in patient characteristics between centres. The latter feature is particularly important because it has become increasingly evident that certain patient-related variables, such as sexual lifestyle (Novick et al, 1985; Perrillo et al, 1988) and pretherapy aminotransferase and HBV DNA levels (Perrillo et al, 1988) may have a substantial bearing on response rates. The end result of these clinical studies has been imprecise estimates of treatment-induced HBeAg seroconversions and a large probability that a beneficial effect of treatment has been missed (type II error) (Perrillo, 1988).

Of the current antiviral agents under study, alpha interferon appears to be the most promising. Relatively low doses of interferon inhibit viral replication and are generally well tolerated. Moreover, interferon has immunomodulatory effects that are helpful in the clearance of hepatitis B virus (Peters et al, 1986). Thomas and associates have previously observed that responders to interferon express significantly higher serum levels of B_2 microglobulin than do non-responders (which is assumed to reflect HLA I antigen display on hepatocytes) (Pignatelli et al, 1986). Moreover, an increase in the peripheral CD4 to CD8 lymphocyte ratio occurs at the time of interferon-induced HBeAg sero-conversion. Interesting as these data are, experiments in our laboratory employing a monoclonal antibody (W6/32) to HLA I group antigen have failed to demonstrate a convincing difference in class 1 antigen density on the peripheral blood mononuclear cells of responders and non-responders (Fig. 1). While the reason for this discrepancy is not clear, it should be remembered that immunological studies of the peripheral blood and peripheral blood lymphocytes do not necessarily reflect events within hepatic tissue (Table 1) (Ikeda et al, 1986; Jilbert et al, 1986; Pirovino et al, 1986; Paul & Perrillo, 1987) nor does evaluation of the peripheral blood necessarily lead to greater understanding of the important effector mechanisms involved in this viral clearance. Thus, in the author's opinion, critical information is needed on the state of interferon activation in hepatocytes (Pignatelli et al, 1986; Ikeda et al, 1986) and infiltrating mononuclear cells during treatment.

The suggestion by Dr Thomas to limit treatment to patients with HBeAg-positive chronic active hepatitis and to exclude patients with decompensated cirrhosis appears to be restrictive. In making a decision on the appropriateness of treatment with interferon, several factors need to be considered: first, interferon can induce a marked improvement in the patient's liver disease (Perrillo et al, 1988), and this has critical importance in patients with advanced liver disease in whom the only other option may be future hepatic transplantation; second, there is no alternative medical therapy that is proven to be effective;

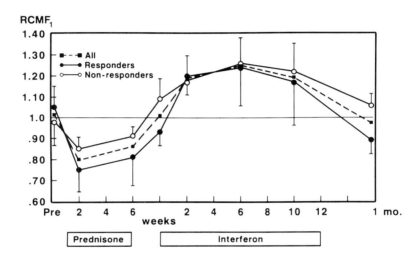

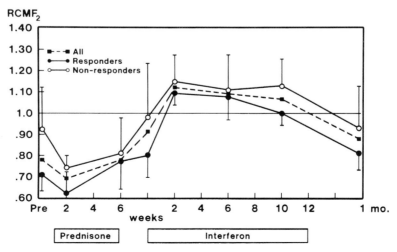

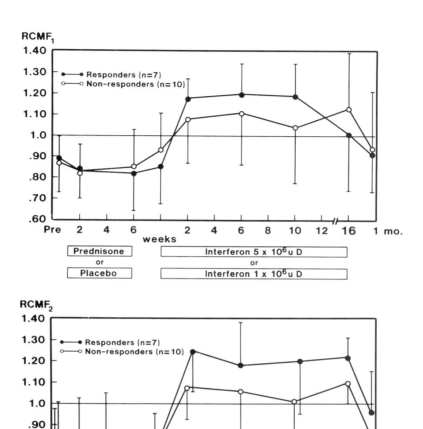

Fig. 1 HLA 1 antigen density expressed as relative mean channel fluorescence (RMCF) in the following groups: (a) peripheral lymphocytes of responders and non-responders treated with a combination of short term prednisone followed by recombinant alpha interferon; (b) peripheral monocytes of the same patients in (a); (c) peripheral lymphocytes of responders and non-responders treated with either placebo or prednisone followed by recombinant alpha interferon; (d) peripheral monocytes of the same patients in (c)

third, therapy may be justified to limit the infectivity of highly promiscuous patients with active viral replication; and fourth, it has become less certain that chronic persistent hepatitis invariably implies a benign prognosis. Thus, in the author's opinion, treatment is also indicated for the following groups: (1) individuals with mildly to moderately decompensated cirrhosis who also have evidence of viral proliferation; (2) HBeAg negative patients with active liver disease in whom HBV DNA can be detected intermittently; and (3) HBeAg/HBV-DNA-positive patients whose initial evaluation reveals mild histological disease such as chronic persistent hepatitis. The first and second groups not uncommonly express low levels of HBV-DNA in serum and may respond quite readily; moreover, experience at our medical centre indicates that patients with clinically advanced liver disease may tolerate low doses of interferon given two to three times weekly (Fig. 2). A combination of immunostimulation (short-term corticosteroids) and antiviral therapy may prove to be a particularly effective strategy for the treatment of selected patients with chronic type B hepatitis. As Dr Thomas advises, combination therapy should not be utilized in individuals with decompensated liver disease because steroid withdrawal is likely to induce a flare of their disease and further decompensation. In clinically stable patients, on the other hand, such therapy is usually very well tolerated (Perrillo & Regenstein, 1986). At our medical centre we have treated more than 40 such patients with a combination of short-term steroids and an antiviral agent without serious adverse effects.

Table 1 HLA 1 antigen density on PBMCs (mean channel fluorescence) and hepatocyte membranes (staining grade) in chronic hepatitis B virus carriers

			Mean channel fluorescence		Liver biopsy†
Subject	HBeAg	ALT	Lymphs	Monos	Grade
1*	−	14	49	104	0
2*†	−	17	52	98	+ +
3	−	33	38	87	0
4	+	73	40	73	0
5	+	235	43	103	0
6	+	140	44	96	0
7	+	74	44	83	0
8	+	49	44	95	0
9	+	320	46	79	0
10†	+	66	71	130	+
11	+	172	40	79	+ +
12	+	284	41	79	+ +
13	+	253	43	83	+ +
14	+	120	44	74	+ +
Mean ± SD of 5 normals:			44 ± 5	87 ± 12	

* Patients 1 and 2 became HBsAg negative < 6 months earlier.
† HIV antibody-positive
  0 = no staining
  + = focal, non-generalized staining
  + + = generalized, honeycomb pattern of staining

Substantial progress in the area of antiviral therapy of chronic viral hepatitis will be at hand during the next few years. Recently initiated multicentre trials on the treatment of chronic type B and non-A, non-B hepatitis will each evaluate 150 to 200 patients. The studies on chronic hepatitis B will evaluate the comparative efficacy of six weeks of steroid followed by recombinant alpha interferon to that of interferon alone. Moreover, these investigations will provide important dose–response data on a relatively homogenous population of clinically stable patients (HBeAg and HBV DNA positive, HIV and HDV-negative), as well as permiting a more definite assessment of patient-related features that negatively or positively correlate with response. The multicentre trial on interferon for post-transfusion chronic non-A, non-B hepatitis should not only scientifically validate the efficacy of this agent, but provide dose–response data and a more accurate indication of relapse rates than the small previous trials.

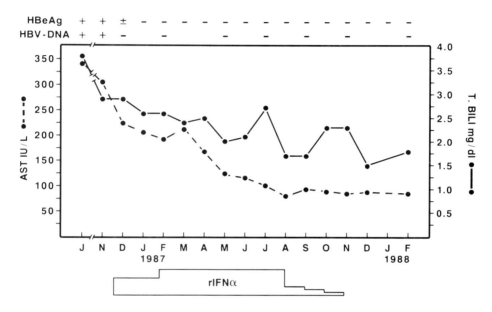

Fig. 2 Biochemical and virological events in a 39-year-old male hepatitis B carrier with decompensated cirrhosis. The patient was treated with 3 x 10^5 units of recombinant alpha interferon two to three times weekly due to a low platelet count (55,000/mm^3). HBeAg and HBV-DNA disappeared within one month of the initiation of therapy accompanied by progressive decline in liver chemistries

As important as these studies will be, they are unlikely to provide uniformly effective ways of managing the vast numbers of patients with chronic viral hepatitis. In many instances therapy appears to be suppressive rather than eradicative, and it appears that high rates of relapse are especially likely after treatment of chronic delta virus and non-A, non-B infections. Long-term suppressive therapy with low dose daily or thrice weekly interferon may eventually be required for individuals who are incapable of sustaining a clinical and virological response off treatment. In these instances, suppressive therapy would have the theoretical advantage of limiting infectivity as well as possibly diminishing the amount of liver injury.

REFERENCES

Ikeda T, Lever A M L, Thomas H C 1986 Evidence for a deficiency of interferon production in patients with chronic hepatitis B virus infection acquired in adult life. Hepatology 6: 962–965

Jilbert A R, Burrell C J, Gowans E J, Hertzog P J, Linnane A W, Marmion B P 1986 Cellular localization of alpha interferon in hepatitis B virus-infected liver tissue. Hepatology 6: 957–961

Novick D M, Lok A S F, Thomas H C 1985 Diminished responsiveness of homosexual men to antiviral therapy for HBeAg-positive chronic liver disease. Journal of Hepatology 1: 29–35

Paul R, Perrillo R 1987 Lack of correlation of HLA 1 antigen expression on hepatocytes and PBMCs in HBV carriers. Hepatology 7: (abstract 396) 1121

Perrillo R P, Regenstein F G, Peters M G, et al 1988 Prednisone withdrawal followed by recombinant alpha interferon in the treatment of chronic type B hepatitis: a randomized, controlled trial. Ann Intern Med 109: 95–100

Perrillo R P 1988 Antiviral therapy of chronic viral hepatitis. Current Opinion in Gastroenterology 4: 420–427

Perrillo R P, Regenstein F G 1986 Corticosteroid therapy for chronic active hepatitis B: is a little too much? Hepatology 6: 1416–1418

Peters M, Davis G L, Dooley J S, Hoofnagle J H 1986 The interferon system in acute and chronic viral hepatitis. In: Progress in Liver Disease. Vol 7 Grune & Stratton, New York pp 453–467

Pignatelli M, Waters J, Brown D et al 1986 HLA class 1 antigens on the hepatocyte membrane during recovery from acute hepatitis B virus infection and during interferon therapy in chronic hepatitis B virus infection. Hepatology 6: 349–355

Pirovino M, Aguet M, Huber M, Altorfer J, Schmid M 1986 Absence of detectable serum interferon in acute and chronic viral hepatitis. Hepatology 6: 645–647

Discussion: Treatment of hepatitis virus

Howard Thomas and Robert Perrillo

The rationale for glucocorticoid pre-treatment of patients with chronic HBV infection was discussed. Their use is based upon the observation that if one treats a patient with a short or long course of steroids and then withdraws therapy, a rise in hepatic transaminases is frequently seen, supporting the notion that there is a renewed immunological recognition of HBV antigens with lysis of liver cells. There is also a fall in serum levels of DNA polymerase but these eventually return to pre-therapy levels. About two thirds of patients develop increases in plasma HBV-DNA levels, particularly at the later phase of the cycle as the dose is reduced. Steroids are therefore thought of as being an adjuvant to therapy. As steroids have the potential to enhance expression of HBV, and this may have adverse effects in an immunosuppressed patient, one must select patients carefully for this regimen. The typical steroid response is not seen in homosexual men, and this may be explained in part by the concurrent immunosuppression which is seen in this group. There is also a steroid responsive element in the HBV genome so there may be a direct effect operating as well.

There are still unresolved areas in the immune response to HBV. For example, cytotoxic T-cells to HBsAg have not been detected, and the explanation for this is unknown. There are some data to suggest that HBsAg will induce suppressor cells, and this may be one explanation. On the other hand, HBcAg is highly immunogenic, and is partially T-independent as well as T-dependent; and there is a very marked humoral and cell mediated immune response to it. There are no sequential studies of cytolytic T-cell activity during acute hepatitis or during seroconversion hepatitis. When those are done we will have a much better idea of exactly what is happening, as we can only piece things together by very indirect routes at the present time.

5. Herpes group viruses

Paul Fiddian

INTRODUCTION

If the 1960s are remembered as the decade when the first tentative steps towards chemotherapy of herpesvirus infections were taken, the 1970s saw the identification of more selective and effective agents, and the 1980s witnessed the wider acceptance and recognition of antiviral therapy, what will the 1990s bring? In order to attempt to answer that question it will be necessary to review the current situation with respect to each of the herpesviruses; but before doing that it may be useful to consider a number of general factors which appear to have a bearing on research in this field.

Although the earliest antiherpes agents play a very limited role in the current management of herpes infections we should not forget the lessons they have taught us in their development. For instance *in vitro* and animal models have been improved, we know more about the epidemiology and natural history of many herpes infections, diagnostic tools have been refined and above all clinical trial methodology has been markedly advanced. Perhaps more than anything else the development of acyclovir over the last ten years has spawned a growth industry in such aspects related to antiviral therapy. It is to be hoped that these advances will not be sacrificed in the search for new agents although recent trends in this regard have not been encouraging. Only by use of carefully controlled trials can efficacy be properly determined and the generation of open case series may actually delay the general acceptance of potential new therapies.

Whilst understandable in some regards there is also a tendency for drug developers to focus on areas that have already proved successful. Hence there is a general concentration of effort on the search for a new agent for herpes simplex whilst cytomegalovirus receives much less attention. Likewise there have been numerous attempts to find an analogue to acyclovir with a similar or improved profile rather than an emphasis on alternative approaches. Obviously commercial implications play a significant role in determining such directions but if we are to see a further revolution in antiviral chemotherapy for herpes group viruses then more adventurous steps probably need to be taken. Otherwise the future is more likely to hold a series of relatively minor victories against these viruses as we have seen of late with antibacterial therapy.

The recent emergence of the acquired immunodeficiency syndrome (AIDS), and the encouraging preliminary attempts to develop antiviral therapy for human immunodeficiency virus infection, may also serve to direct research away from the herpesviruses. There will thus need to be a determined effort by those interested in further advances in the field of herpes group viruses to keep this area active. Even without the discovery of new chemical entities there is still a considerable amount of work to be done in fully exploiting the existing agents and further improving our understanding of herpes infections so that therapeutic intervention can be optimized. Whilst such clinical research may not appear to be as exciting as that offered by the new pandemic the author hopes that this will not deter too many from pursuing it.

HERPES SIMPLEX VIRUS

Although some antiviral agents have markedly different activity against herpes simplex types 1 and 2 *in vitro*, it is difficult to see an advantage in developing agents with selective activity against only one type. Furthermore, it is now accepted that the site of infection is not clearly diagnostic of one type or the other (Corey & Spear, 1986). Therefore this section will not draw specific distinction between the virus types but will consider the various infections according to body site, with additional reference to the immune status of the host or other special situations.

Ocular herpes simplex infections
The greatest range of antiviral therapies is available for the treatment of herpes keratitis (Wood & Geddes, 1987). In different parts of the world this includes idoxuridine, vidarabine, trifluorothymidine, acyclovir and interferon. Where a choice is offered the preference lies between trifluorothymidine and acyclovir (Nicholson, 1984a), the former having the advantage of greater solubility (allowing formulation as drops) whilst the latter is less toxic and so can also be given systemically (Hung et al, 1984). The interferons are capable of enhancing the efficacy of the other antiviral agents, although the real value of this is uncertain, but are not accepted as sole therapies for herpes keratitis (Nicholson, 1984a).

For the management of uncomplicated corneal epithelial herpes infection topical application of the preferred antiviral is very satisfactory and further significant advances are unlikely to be made unless latency could be prevented. Nevertheless any new agents developed for other herpes simplex infections are likely to be tried in the eye because of the relative ease of evaluation. Complicated and/or deeper infections of the eye may also respond to trifluorothymidine or acyclovir (Fiddian & Grant, 1985), aided by the ability of both drugs to penetrate the cornea and the fact that they can be given over longer periods. In some situations the equivalent efficacy of orally administered acyclovir (Collum et al, 1986) may offer an advantage over local applications and so deserves further study. The wide usage of these agents has not been associated to date with the development of clinically significant viral resistance so that earlier concerns appear to have been unfounded and do not justify restriction of their use for ocular infections.

Mucocutaneous herpes simplex in the normal host

Before the advent of acyclovir most attempts to treat labial or genital herpes had concentrated on topical application of antiviral agents (Corey & Holmes, 1983). This unfortunately led to an initial focusing of efforts with acyclovir in the same direction (Spruance et al, 1982; Corey et al, 1982a). Perhaps at last it has been recognized that such agents are not ideally suited for penetration of intact skin. Whilst methods of improving penetration can be devised they by and large rely on disruption of the integument (Kingsley & Fiddian, 1985). Where the infection itself leads to significant cutaneous damage, as with the more serious initial episodes of genital herpes for instance, then the efficacy of topical acyclovir can be readily demonstrated (Corey et al, 1982b; Fiddian et al, 1983a). For milder infections, such as recurrent genital herpes or herpes labialis, it has, however, proved to be impossible to consistently demonstrate efficacy (Corey et al, 1982a; Fiddian et al, 1983a; Yeo & Fiddian, 1983; Shaw et al, 1985).

When attention was directed towards systemically administered acyclovir it was easier to show statistically significant benefits in a reproducible manner. Both intravenous (Mindel et al, 1982; Corey et al, 1983) and oral (Nilsen et al, 1982; Bryson et al, 1983) therapy were shown to be highly effective for the treatment of initial genital herpes. Oral acyclovir was also more reliably demonstrated to be effective in recurrent episodes of genital herpes but the clinical benefit was still not great (Nilsen et al, 1982; Salo et al, 1983). Since viral shedding in typical recurrences only lasts about three days (Corey et al, 1981) it seems unlikely that antiviral therapy could reduce the duration of such episodes by more than a day or two at most if treatment were started after the onset of lesions. Therefore subsequent studies were set up to look at either oral or topical therapy initiated at the earliest possible time after the onset of prodromal symptoms (Kinghorn et al, 1983; Reichman et al, 1984).

If such early intervention could reliably alter the natural history of recurrent episodes rather than merely shortening it, then greater benefits would ensue. Although abortive episodes seemed to be increased by therapy in some studies (Fiddian et al, 1983a; Ruhnek-Forsbeck et al, 1985; Goldberg et al, 1986) this issue remains somewhat controversial (Corey & Gold, 1987). Otherwise the clinical benefits of both topically applied acyclovir (in an improved formulation of modified aqueous cream) and oral acyclovir are generally marginal (Nicholson, 1984a; Raborn et al, 1988). This is often exaggerated by the tendency of such trial designs to include many mild recurrences, thus limiting the opportunity to demonstrate an effect (Kingsley & Fiddian, 1985). Nevertheless there are some patients with more severe recurrences for whom episodic therapy may be warranted (Fiddian et al, 1982; Leigh, 1988; Thin, 1988). The need to take acyclovir five times daily makes this form of treatment somewhat cumbersome but recent data (Goldberg et al, 1986) suggest that twice daily administration of higher doses may be at least as effective and warrants further evaluation. Unless alternative drugs could somehow consistently abort episodes it seems unlikely that they could produce markedly greater benefit overall. It is regrettable that some regulatory authorities have already permitted marketing of certain agents which, whilst largely innocuous have not been clearly proven to be effective (Mindel et al, 1987).

As shown in Table 5.1, the most dramatic demonstration of antiviral efficacy has been the use of suppressive therapy to prevent recurrences of herpes simplex (Straus et al, 1984; Mindel et al, 1984). For patients with frequent reactivations of disease (Mattison et al, 1988; Kinghorn, 1988) or those at specific risk over an identifiable period (Spruance, 1988; Schadelin et al, 1988) this form of treatment reduces the number of recurrences by 70–90% and is very well tolerated even over prolonged periods (Mertz et al, 1988; Mostow et al, 1988). Using this approach it is clearly possible to alter the natural history of recurrent disease whilst therapy continues (Guinan, 1986; Sacks, 1987). Unfortunately when acyclovir is discontinued it does not appear that there is any lasting effect on recurrences (Douglas et al, 1984; Thin et al, 1985). This is consistent with a general lack of demonstrable effect on latency following treatment of primary infections (Bryson et al, 1985; Corey et al, 1985; Mindel et al, 1986). However, it is hard to believe from current understanding that any virustatic agent could influence latent virus and so this should not be viewed as a specific deficiency of acyclovir. The future hope for such ultimate control of the disease by prevention of latency, if it is possible, is more likely to lie with vaccination.

Table 5.1 Long term, placebo (PCB) controlled studies of suppression of recurrent HSV with oral acyclovir (ACV)

Author	Number of patients	Dose	Duration	Recurrence rates/year ACV	PCB*
Mertz et al, 1988	348	400 mg × 2	2 years	1.6	(12.7)
	300	400 mg × 2	1 year	1.9	12.2
Kinghorn, 1988	196	200 mg × 4 ⎱ 400 mg × 2 ⎰	1 year	0.8	(13.1)
Mattison et al, 1988	47	400 mg × 2	1 year	1.0	8.0
Mostow et al, 1988	22	800 mg × 1	2 years	2.2	11.7

* or (historical controls)

Other aspects that are receiving attention include evaluation of the role of antiviral therapy in the treatment of primary gingivostomatitis (Leigh, 1988), eczema herpeticum (Niimura & Nishikawa, 1988) or herpetic whitlow (Gill et al, 1988) and the prevention of erythema multiforme associated with reactivation of herpes simplex (Leigh, 1988). Whilst attempts have been made to use topical applications in the management of at least some of these conditions (Fawcett et al, 1983; Gibson et al, 1986) it seems likely that orally administered acyclovir will offer the best prospects for the foreseeable future. It is too early to predict whether one or more of the various alternatives undergoing development, such as the analogues to acyclovir (Fiddian, 1988), will offer any significant advantages in the clinical situation to current therapy.

Mucocutaneous herpes simplex in the immunocompromised host
As in the normal host early studies of acyclovir also involved topical application

and, as might be expected, it was possible to demonstrate some benefit in these generally more serious infections (Whitley et al, 1984a). Nevertheless it is because of the risk of a worse outcome that systemic therapy is more likely to be considered for routine usage in such patients. Intravenous acyclovir has been clearly shown to be effective in the treatment of established mucocutaneous infection (Meyers et al, 1982). Not surprisingly the greatest benefit can be demonstrated in those patients, such as bone marrow-transplant recipients (Wade et al, 1982), who on average experience the most severe infections. In a single study in this group of patients oral acyclovir, at a dose of 400 mg five times daily, was also reported to be effective (Shepp et al, 1985a). Unfortunately because of wide availability and usage of acyclovir in these patient populations confirmatory studies have not been carried out with oral therapy. For example, it is not possible at present to identify the optimum dosage for the managment of AIDS patients who have perianal ulceration caused by herpes simplex (Thin, 1988).

At the same time intravenous vidarabine was also reported to be effective in immunocompromised patients (Whitley et al, 1984b). No direct comparison between acyclovir and vidarabine has been made for this indication so the clinician must make up his own mind which to opt for. However, on the basis of overall available data for each agent the consensus appears to favour acyclovir as the treatment of first choice (Wood & Geddes, 1987; Saral, 1988). Future candidates will almost certainly have to be compared with acyclovir, therefore, since placebo-controlled trials would no longer be accepted for this indication. The design, conduct and interpretation of such studies requires particularly careful attention since it is likely to be harder to distinguish between two seemingly effective therapies.

As in the normal host the most impressive results have come from studies designed to look at the prevention of reactivation of herpes simplex in at-risk patients. Initially intravenous (Saral et al, 1981) and then oral acyclovir (Gluckman et al, 1983; Wade et al, 1984) were shown to be effective when given prophylactically to bone marrow-transplant recipients or other im-munocompromised patients (Saral et al, 1983; Anderson et al, 1984) during the period of greatest risk of reactivation. In addition to almost completely abolishing clinical disease in such patients there are those that advocate this form of management as a means of minimising the possibility of emergence of drug resistance (Ambinder et al, 1984). With the increasing demands placed on infectious disease specialists and others by both iatrogenic and naturally occurring immune impairment these issues are likely to receive further attention. As possible insurance for the future these clinicians would undoubtedly like to see the development of additional anti-herpes simplex agents, but for this to be a rational goal then particular emphasis should be placed on compounds with an entirely different mechanism of action from acyclovir.

Herpes simplex encephalitis
Developments in chemotherapy for herpesviruses, including many of the controversies, are amply illustrated by consideration of this particular infection and the progress made since the early 1970s. Issues covered by a careful review

of clinical research into this disease reveal the whole gamut of scientific endeavours, both good and bad (Longson, 1977; Longson et al, 1980; Whitley, 1988). Succinctly early enthusiastic anecdotes concerning idoxuridine and cytarabine were quelled by the application of modern controlled clinical trial methodology (Boston IVSG NIAID Study, 1975; Longson et al, 1980). The initial development of vidarabine in a placebo-controlled trial was unfortunately brought to a somewhat premature termination because of ethical concerns (Whitley et al, 1977). Although the drug appeared to be effective (Whitley et al, 1981) there were certainly those who considered the issue unresolved (Campbell et al, 1982). Further argument has also raged regarding the correct diagnosis of this disease and in particular the place of brain biopsy in clinical management (Klapper et al, 1981; Alford et al, 1982).

In some respects the advent of acyclovir has helped resolve these issues or at least led to some sort of truce (Editorial, 1986; Whitley et al, 1987). In two controlled trials, acyclovir has been shown to be clearly more effective than vidarabine regardless of the method of diagnosis (Skoldenberg et al, 1984; Whitley et al, 1986). In addition to a reduction in mortality the surviving patients were shown to have a significantly better outcome. Whilst brain biopsy is not essential to make a clinical diagnosis of herpes encephalitis and should not be allowed to delay initiation of treatment (Nicholson, 1984b; Jeffries, 1986) it may offer the only means of diagnosing the cause of the infection in those presumptive cases not due to herpes (Whitley et al, 1987; Dorsky & Crumpacker, 1987). Since early therapy is so critical to outcome, current efforts should be directed towards improving the recognition and diagnosis of this disease (Whitley, 1988).

It remains to be seen whether newer agents will be able to improve the results even further, but it needs to be recognized that it will become increasingly difficult to demonstrate what are likely to be smaller improvements in efficacy, given the relative sparsity of patients.

Neonatal herpes simplex infections
In contrast to the previous disease category vidarabine was convincingly demonstrated to be effective in reducing mortality compared with placebo (Whitley et al, 1980). Unfortunately because of the low incidence of such infections progress has been rather slow. Following completion of the placebo-controlled trial which employed a dose of vidarabine of 15 mg/kg/day, this dose was compared with a higher one of 30 mg/kg/day (Whitley et al, 1983). Although no difference in mortality or morbidity was apparent this higher dose was then selected for comparison with acyclovir (Whitley, 1988). There have been several reports which have alluded to the data but the definitive results of this study remain to be published. Nevertheless it appears that there were no differences in efficacy between vidarabine and acyclovir at equivalent daily doses.

As with encephalitis there are a number of important factors which may determine outcome, including prevention, prompt diagnosis, early treatment and, in some cases, the need for prolonged therapy. In addition since it is the children with CNS or disseminated disease who do the worst it may be worth exploring higher doses of acyclovir in those groups. Because any new drugs are unlikely to be developed first in children, especially neonates, it is unlikely that the existing drugs will be superseded in the next decade and so their use must be optimized. Of particular interest is the managment of babies who may be prone to develop recurrent infections (Dankner & Spector, 1986) and for whom prophylactic therapy might be indicated.

VARICELLA-ZOSTER VIRUS

Since the most significant infections occur in the immunocompromised host more emphasis has tended to be placed on this area. In addition, before acyclovir, there were no systemic agents that could be considered routinely for use in the normal host. Furthermore, because the activity of acyclovir against varicella-zoster is less than it is against herpes simplex, and because oral bioavailability of higher doses was initially uncertain, clinical development has lagged behind that seen with herpes simplex. However, major advances have been made in recent years.

Varicella in the immunocompromised host

Interferon (Arvin et al, 1982), vidarabine (Whitley et al, 1982a) and acyclovir (Nyerges et al, 1988) have all been shown in placebo controlled trials to be effective in the treatment of this infection in children (Table 5.2). Interferon appears to be less beneficial and is not generally considered to be an acceptable mode of treatment for this indication compared with the specific antiviral drugs (Meyers, 1985). Recently comparative studies have indicated that acyclovir is the treatment of choice over vidarabine (Feldman et al, 1986; Vilde et al, 1986). Used early in the course of the infection such therapy will prevent visceral dissemination, especially to the lungs (Prober et al, 1982), and markedly reduce the impact of the disease.

Table 5.2 Antiviral therapy of chickenpox in immunocompromised children

	Treatment			
Outcome	Acyclovir ($n=53$)	Vidarabine ($n=39$)	Interferon ($n=23$)	Placebo ($n=73$)
Visceral dissemination, number (%)	0	6 (15)	2 (9)	20 (27)
Deaths, number (%)	0	1 (3)	2 (9)	6 (8)

Only the intravenous route of administration of acyclovir has so far been proven to be effective. However, since children at risk of infection can often be identified, current studies are addressing the possible role of high dose oral acyclovir (Novelli et al, 1985) for either prevention or early treatment of chicken-pox. Whilst this may prove to be successful the development of a more potent therapy that would allow less frequent dosing would be an advantage (Fiddian, 1988). Despite enthusiastic preliminary reports surrounding a number of potential candidates, which have been made over the past few years, none has yet emerged as clearly effective or safe for use in this particular patient population (Balfour, 1988). The ultimate role of varicella vaccination in immunocompromised children may also affect the direction of future research in this area (Balfour, 1988). Another issue that warrants further attention is the recurrence of infection (van Weel-Sipman et al, 1981) seen in a minority of children, usually associated with a failure to develop antibodies (Nyerges & Meszner, 1988).

Herpes zoster in the immunocompromised host

Again interferon (Merigan et al, 1978), vidarabine (Whitley et al 1982b) and acyclovir (Balfour et al 1983) have all been demonstrated to be effective in the treatment of herpes zoster infection in susceptible patients (Table 5.3) (Meyers, 1985). As for varicella the choice seems to lie between vidarabine and acyclovir. A small but seemingly definitive study comparing these two therapies concluded that acyclovir should be considered the current treatment of choice (Shepp et al, 1986). Whilst fluoroiodoarabinosylcytosine (FIAC), a nucleoside analogue active against herpes viruses *in vitro*, also appeared to be better than vidarabine in one controlled trial (Leyland-Jones et al, 1986), these findings remain to be substantiated. Despite numerous anecdotal reports of another antiviral drug with good *in vitro* activity, bromovinyldeoxyuridine (Wildiers & de Clercq, 1984), no controlled trials have been documented to enable assessment of its efficacy. Future comparative studies should presumably take acyclovir as the baseline for comparison and be suitably large to avoid large type I and type II errors.

Table 5.3 Antiviral therapy of herpes zoster in immunocompromised patients

Outcome	Treatment			
	Acyclovir ($n = 80$)	Vidarabine ($n = 95$)	Interferon ($n = 45$)	Placebo ($n = 145$)
Cutaneous dissemination, number (%)	2 (4)	11 (13)	9 (20)	40 (31)
Visceral dissemination, number (%)	0	3 (3)	0	12 (8)
Deaths, number (%)	0	1 (1)	0	3 (2)

The usual dose of intravenous acyclovir is 10 mg/kg or 500 mg/m^2 every eight hours for seven days. Although such therapy would be appropriate for patients with severe infections requiring hospitalization some patients might preferably be managed at home. Whilst topically applied acyclovir has been shown to be of some benefit in the treatment of herpes zoster (Levin et al, 1985) it is unlikely that this would be a generally accepted form of therapy. What is required, therefore, is an orally administered treatment. High-dose oral acyclovir has been suggested to be of value in children with varicella-zoster infections (Novelli et al, 1984) but controlled trials remain to be reported. Certainly oral acyclovir has been proven to be effective in preventing reactivation of varicella-zoster virus in patients at risk following transplantation (Lundgren et al, 1985; Perren et al, 1988). It remains to be determined if sufficient plasma levels can be achieved to treat active infection reliably in severely immunocompromised patients, such as those with AIDS.

Varicella in the normal host

Since the infection is usually relatively mild and because the early antivirals were considered too toxic, little work has been conducted in this area. Even with acyclovir there have been only limited studies reported to date in adults reputed to have more severe disease (Straus et al, 1988). Ironically the patients enrolled in a placebo-controlled trial of intravenous acyclovir were subsequently found to have only mild infections and, as patients were enrolled in the trial up to 72 hours after onset of the rash, many were probably treated too late. Nevertheless marginal benefits on rash and fever were reported (Al-Nakib et al, 1983). Similar results were obtained in another study employing high-dose oral acyclovir (Fiddian, unpublished data). Routine therapy is probably not called for but certain patients, for instance smokers, may be at greater risk of developing complications such as pneumonia (Chitkara et al, 1987) and so warrant early intervention in their disease.

Otherwise, the major issue remains the question of whether children should be treated (Balfour, 1988). Placebo-controlled trials are currently in progress to determine the role, if any, of oral acyclovir in the treatment of childhood chicken-pox. Certainly of primary importance is the need for early initiation of therapy, probably within 24 hours of the rash developing. The wide application of a varicella vaccine to normal children is also likely to be the subject of future debate (Heath, 1986).

Herpes zoster in the normal host

Although topically applied idoxuridine (in dimethyl sulphoxide) was shown to have some benefit in localized disease (Wildenhoff et al, 1981), it was considered desirable to have a systemic form of therapy (Juel-Jensen et al, 1983). Several controlled trials of intravenous acyclovir were conducted shortly after it became available (Peterslund et al, 1981; Bean et al, 1982; McGill et al, 1983a). These authors demonstrated the efficacy of the drug in reducing both the duration of the rash and the acute pain of an attack of herpes zoster (Bean et al, 1983). There remained two major issues for future study: the development of oral medication to allow out-patient management of the disease, and a means of reducing the incidence of post-herpetic neuralgia. Following preliminary studies with moderate doses of oral acyclovir (McKendrick et al, 1984; Cobo et al, 1986) it was determined that high doses of 800 mg every four hours could be safely given and were required to affect this disease reliably (McKendrick et al, 1986). Two large-scale trials have now been completed which confirm the benefits of this dose in the acute manifestations of shingles (Wood et al, 1988; Huff et al, 1988). As with the other self-limiting herpes infections the importance of early initiation of therapy was noted.

Unfortunately the issue of post-herpetic neuralgia remains unresolved. One of the above studies did show a significant reduction in the incidence of chronic pain after the episode of herpes zoster (Huff et al, 1988) but the other one (Wood et al, 1988) failed to show any differences between acyclovir and the controls. The reasons for the apparent discrepancies are unclear but may be due to subtle differences in trial methodologies. What is clear from both studies is that the incidence of post-herpetic neuralgia by six months is actually quite low and therefore very large numbers of patients are required for proper evaluation. It is also apparent that since it is not possible to predict which patients will suffer from this complication and because all those with acute pain may benefit in the short term, oral acyclovir still offers an important advance. Current work includes the potential use of steroids in combination with acyclovir to further elucidate this aspect (Esmann et al, 1987).

Another complication that causes concern is where involvement of the face may lead to spread to the eye. Since early use of systemic acyclovir can prevent many such ocular complications (Cobo et al, 1986) it is likely that it will be used in most cases of trigeminal zoster even though the rash itself may be quite mild. Nevertheless, some patients may still present with ocular manifestations and these will require management by the specialist. Some controversy surrounds the use of steroids as primary treatment for such complications but it is generally accepted that topical acyclovir should be applied as soon as possible (McGill et al, 1983b).

Of the newer agents in pre-clinical or early clinical development there are none that may be currently considered as appropriate for use in the normal host because of uncertainties about their safety. Future developments, however, are likely to occur since, even if vaccination for chicken-pox becomes widely accepted and practiced, it will not affect the incidence of herpes zoster for several decades—if at all.

CYTOMEGALOVIRUS

Until a decade or so ago the major interest in this virus related to the problems of congenital infection. More recently the emphasis has switched to an urgent search for an effective antiviral agent for use in immunocompromised patients. This has arisen because of the increase in iatrogenic immunosuppression for bone marrow transplantation and of late the devastating effects of AIDS. Severe sight- and life-threatening infections caused by cytomegalovirus play a significant role in both these clinical situations. Unfortunately the haste in which active drugs have been sought may actually have delayed their expeditious development and licensure.

Cytomegalovirus infection in the immunocompromised host
Vidarabine, acyclovir and interferon, or a combination of the latter with one of the antiviral drugs, have all been tried for the treatment of established infections (Meyers, 1985) (Table 5.4). Generally they failed to show clinical efficacy when used to treat cytomegalovirus pneumonia occurring after marrow transplantation. Whilst none of these agents has very great *in vitro* activity against this virus it may be incorrect to conclude that they have no possible *in vivo* role to play. Certainly even the acyclovir analogue, ganciclovir, which is very active *in vitro*, does not appear to affect the mortality of cytomegalovirus pneumonia in marrow transplant recipients (Shepp et al, 1985b).

Recently it has been reported that high doses of intravenous acyclovir may reduce the incidence of cytomegalovirus infections, including pneumonia, and consequent deaths, when given prophylactically in such patients (Meyers et al, 1988). Given the place of this drug in the management of other herpes infections in this patient population, it would seem to be worthwhile to attempt to confirm these findings. Otherwise there has been a dearth of good controlled trials in this indication despite the availability of several potential candidate drugs, including ganciclovir (Cheng et al, 1983) and the less active foscarnet (Akesson-Johansson et al, 1986). Clearly it is necessary to establish a baseline with one of these agents so that future therapies can be compared with it. The potential role of immunoglobulins, in particular in combination with antiviral therapy (Meyers, 1988), also needs to be evaluated further.

Table 5.4 Intravenous acyclovir for prevention of CMV infection and disease after bone marrow transplantation (from Meyers et al, 1988)

% Probability**	Acyclovir* ($n = 86$)	Control ($n = 65$)	p value
CMV excretion—all sites	70	87	< 0.001
—oropharynx	44	77	< 0.001
CMV disease—all	19	38	< 0.01
—pneumonia	19	31	< 0.05
Survival	71	46	< 0.01

* 500 mg/m^2 8-hourly from day -5 to day $+30$
** in first 100 days after transplantation

Regarding the management of AIDS patients the situation is also complicated by an abundance of anecdotal reporting as opposed to controlled trial data. Whilst ganciclovir seems to have good clinical benefit in cytomegalovirus retinitis (Henderly et al, 1987) the use of this drug, or others, in the treatment of other manifestations of the virus is less clear cut. There are also a number of apparent limitations of ganciclovir which should encourage development of alternative therapies (Collaborative DHPG Treatment Study Group, 1986; Masur et al, 1986). These would include concerns about safety of the drug over long periods (Holland et al, 1986), acceptability for use in other lower risk groups (King & Fiddian, 1986) and in particular poor oral bioavailability which may preclude oral therapy (Jacobson et al, 1987). Since HIV infections in AIDS patients usually recur if therapy if stopped, most patients are given maintenance therapy. However, long-term intravenous dosing is less than completely satisfactory. Whilst a number of potential candidates have been suggested, based on *in vitro* data, it is not possible to predict their ultimate clinical utility. The search for an orally bioavailable agent that can interfere with the replication of cytomegalovirus, without significantly affecting cellular processes, remains the most urgent challenge in antiviral chemotherapy of the herpes group viruses.

EPSTEIN-BARR VIRUS

This virus has had rather less therapeutic attention directed towards it in the past than the other herpes group viruses. Yet it can be a cause of significant morbidity in young adults experiencing the primary infection and more rarely in immunocompromised patients with chronic infection. It has also been associated with malignant transformation causing several types of tumour, including nasopharyngeal carcinoma, Burkitt's lymphoma and EBV-associated lymphomas in transplant recipients. Recently it has been linked to a benign lesion, hairy leukoplakia (Greenspan et al, 1985), seen on the tongue in many AIDS patients, and it seems likely that increasing interest in the virus will unearth other possible associations.

Infectious mononucleosis

Several studies have now reported that acyclovir given intravenously (Pagano et al, 1983; Ernberg & Andersson, 1986) or in high oral doses (Andersson & Ernberg, 1988) can affect virus excretion in the throats of infected patients during treatment. Once therapy is stopped viral shedding resumes as before. Clinical benefits, however, could not be demonstrated (Andersson et al, 1986, 1987) suggesting either that therapy was initiated too late or that antiviral efficacy alone is not sufficient to reduce the symptoms of the disease. To address this latter point the use of a combination of acyclovir plus steroids is currently being evaluated (Andersson & Ernberg, 1988). It should be recognized though that several days and even weeks have usually elapsed before a patient seeks treatment and so any active intervention may be ineffective. Any further advances in this area in the near future are likely to be empirical since this virus is not generally seen as a viable target for drug development.

Chronic infection in the immunocompromised host

Although occasionally patients with apparently normal immune functions develop persistent or relapsing symptoms of Epstein-Barr virus infection, it is more often seen in those with congenital or acquired immune deficiency (Andersson & Ernberg, 1988). Generally it is not possible to gather sufficient numbers of homogenous cases to conduct controlled trials and so only anecdotal reports are available (Hanto et al, 1985). As with infectious mononucleosis it is possible to demonstrate an antiviral effect but clinical benefit may be less clearly definable. The most visible effects have been the responses seen in AIDS patients with hairy leukoplakia treated with acyclovir in various forms (Friedman-Kein, 1986; Schofer et al, 1987; Resnick et al, 1988), but even here real benefit is uncertain (Table 5.5). It remains to be seen whether future clinical demands will be sufficient to stimulate a more positive approach to therapy of this virus.

Table 5.5 Oral acyclovir for hairy cell leukoplakia

Author	Dose	Number of patients	Response*
Resnick et al, 1988	800 mg × 4	6	3CR, 2PR, 1NR
Schofer et al, 1987	400 mg × 5	2	2CR
Freidman-Kein, 1986	800 mg × 4	9	9CR

*CR = cure
 PR = partial response
 NR = no response

HUMAN B-CELL LYMPHOTROPIC VIRUS (HERPES VIRUS TYPE 6)

It may be a little premature to introduce such a newly identified herpes group virus (Salahuddin et al, 1986) into a discussion of antiviral chemotherapy, but if one is expected to crystal-ball gaze into the future then it is surely appropriate to mention this as a possible direction for research interests. Of particular relevance is the need to determine whether this, or one of the established herpesviruses, plays a role in progression of human immunodeficiency virus infection to its end-stage sequelae (Mosca et al, 1987; Rando et al, 1987). If such were the case then anti-herpes agents could yet find a role in the management of an even wider range of infections.

CONCLUSION

Significant progress has been made in the past decade in the development of effective and well-tolerated therapy for use in the management of both herpes simplex and varicella-zoster virus infections. In particular it is the impact of acyclovir, in both its intravenous and oral formulations, that has done most of late to stimulate research in this field of antiviral chemotherapy. Such progress was facilitated by the earlier work done by the pioneers of anti-herpes therapy. It is important that we continue to build on the experience that has been gained to date. For both herpes simplex and varicella-zoster viruses future developments may be less dramatic than we have seen in the past decade, but there are still advances to be made. We must fully exploit the agents that are available to us and optimize their usage. Although we know for instance that acyclovir is effective in a given situation we may not be so sure that the dose or frequency of dosing is optimum. Equally we need to select the most appropriate approach to a given situation, which might involve either treatment or prevention, as the case may be.

The most active area in the next decade may involve one or more of the other herpesviruses. Undoubtedly there is likely to remain a significant demand for an alternative approach to cytomegalovirus infections. Whilst the existing agents are a step in the right direction there is also considerable scope for improvement. For Epstein-Barr virus infections modest academic interest and limited clinical need may well only keep the field ticking over until greater demands occur. We may even see the emergence of a new and valid target amongst the herpesviruses if recent events are anything to go by. Overall, therefore, it seems reasonable to predict that the 1990s will continue to be an exciting and productive area of research for those with an interest in the antiviral chemotherapy of herpes group viruses.

REFERENCES

Akesson-Johansson A, Lernestedt J-O, Ringden O, Lonnqvist B, Wahren B 1986 Sensitivity of cytomegalovirus to intravenousfoscarnet treatment. Bone Marrow Transplantation 1: 215–220
Alford Jr C A, Dolin R, Hirsch M S, Karchmer A W, Whitley R J 1982 Herpes simplex encephalitis and clinical trials design. Lancet 1: 1013

Al-Nakib W, Al-Kandari S, El-Khalik D M A, El-Shirbiny A M 1983 A randomised controlled study of intravenous acyclovir (Zovirax) against placebo in adults with chickenpox. Journal of Infection 6, supplement 1: 49–56

Ambinder R F, Burns W H, Lietman P S, Saral R 1984 Prophylaxis: a strategy to minimise antiviral resistance. Lancet 1: 1154–1155

Anderson H, Scarffe J H, Sutton R N P, Hickmott E, Brigden D, Burke C 1984 Oral acyclovir prophylaxis against herpes simplex virus in non-Hodgkin lymphoma and acute lymphoblastic leukaemia patients receiving remission induction chemotherapy: a randomised double-blind, placebo controlled trial. British Journal of Cancer 50: 45–49

Andersson J, Ernberg I 1988 Management of Epstein-Barr virus infections. American Journal of Medicine 85, supplement 2A:107–115

Andersson J, Britton S, Ernberg I et al 1986 Effect of acyclovir on infectious mononucleosis: a double-bind, placebo controlled study. Journal of Infectious Disease 153: 283–290

Andersson J, Skoldenberg B, Henle W et al 1987 Acyclovir treatment in infectious mononucleosis: a clinical and virological study. Infection 15, supplement 1: S14–S20

Arvin A M, Kushner J H, Feldman S, Baehner R L, Hammond D, Merigan T C 1982 Human leucocyte interferon for the treatment of varicella in children with cancer. New England Journal of Medicine 306: 761–765

Balfour Jr H H 1988 Varicella zoster virus infections in immunocompromised hosts: a review of the natural history and management. American Journal of Medicine 85, supplement 2A:68–73

Balfour Jr H H, Bean B, Laskin O L et al 1983 Acyclovir halts progression of herpes zoster in immunocompromised patients. New England Journal of Medicine 308: 1448–1453

Bean B, Braun C, Balfour Jr H H 1982 Acyclovir therapy for herpes zoster. Lancet 2: 118–121

Bean B, Aeppli D, Balfour Jr H H 1983 Acyclovir in shingles. Journal of Antimicrobial Chemotherapy 12, supplement B: 123–127

Boston Intergroup Virus Study Group and the NIAID-sponsored Cooperative Antiviral Clinical Study 1975 Failure of high dose 5-iodo-2'-deoxyuridine in the therapy of herpes simplex virus encephalitis: evidence of unacceptable toxicity. New England Journal of Medicine 292: 599–603

Bryson Y J, Dillon M, Lovett M et al 1983 Treatment of first episodes of genital herpes simplex virus infection with oral acyclovir: a randomised, double-blind, controlled trial in normal subjects. New England Journal of Medicine 308: 916–921

Bryson Y, Dillon M, Lovett M, Bernstein D, Garratty E, Sayre J 1985 Treatment of first episode genital herpes with oral acyclovir: long-term follow-up of recurrences. Scandinavian Journal of Infectious Diseases, supplement 47: 70–75

Campbell M, Klapper P E, Longson M 1982 Acyclovir in herpes encephalitis. Lancet 1: 38

Cheng Y-C, Huang E-S, Lin J-C et al 1983 Unique spectrum of activity of 9--guanine against herpes viruses in vitro and its mode of action against herpes simples virus type 1. Proceedings of the National Academy of Sciences USA 80: 2767–2770

Chitkara R, Gordon R E, Khan F A 1987 Acyclovir in the treatment of primary varicella pneumonia in non-immunocompromised adults. New York State Journal of Medicine April: 237–238

Cobo L M, Foulks G N, Liesegang T et al 1986 Oral acyclovir in the treatment of acute herpes zoster ophthalmicus. Ophthalmology 93: 763–770

Collaborative DHPG Treatment Study Group 1986 Treatment of serious cytomegalovirus infections with 9-(1,3-dihydroxy-2-propoxymethyl) guanine in patients with AIDS and other immunodeficiences. New England Journal of Medicine 314: 801–805

Collum L M T, McGettrick P, Akhtar J, Lavin J, Rees PJ 1986 Oral acyclovir (Zovirax) in herpes simplex dendritic corneal ulceration. British Journal of Ophthalmology 70: 435–438

Corey L, Gold D 1987 Acyclovir prophylaxis for herpes simplex virus infection. Antimicrobial Agents and Chemotherapy 31: 1865

Corey L, Holmes K K 1983 Genital herpes simplex virus infections: current concepts in diagnosis, therapy, and prevention. Annals of Internal Medicine 98: 973–983

Corey L, Spear P G 1986 Infections with herpes simplex viruses (second of two parts). New England Journal of Medicine 314: 749–757

Corey L, Homes K K, Benedetti J, Critchlow C 1981 Clinical course of genital herpes: implications for clinical trials. In: Nahmias A J, Dowdle W R, Schinazi R F (eds.). The human herpes viruses: an interdisciplinary perspective. Elsevier New York pp 496–502

Corey L, Benedetti J K, Critchlow C W et al 1982a Double-blind controlled trial of topical acyclovir in genital herpes simplex virus infections. American Journal of Medicine 73, supplement 1A: 326–334

Corey L, Nahmias A J, Guinan M E et al 1982b A trial of topical acyclovir in genital herpes simplex virus infections. New England Journal of Medicine 306: 1313–1319

Corey L, Fife K H, Benedetti J K et al 1983 Intravenous acyclovir for the treatment of primary genital herpes. Annals of Internal Medicine 98: 914–921

Corey L, Mindel A, Fife K H, Sutherland S, Benedetti J, Adler M W 1985 Risk of recurrence after treatment of first-epidose genital herpes with intravenous acyclovir. Sexually Transmitted Diseases 12: 215–218

Dankner W M, Spector S A 1986 Recurrent herpes simplex in a neonate. Paediatric Infectious Disease 5: 582–586

Dorsky D I, Crumpacker C S 1987 Drugs five years later: acyclovir. Annals of Internal Medicine 107: 859–874

Douglas J M, Critchlow C, Benedetti J et al 1984 A double-blind study of oral acyclovir for suppression of recurrences of genital herpes simplex virus infection. New England Journal of Medicine 310: 1551–1556

Editorial 1986 Herpes simplex encephalitis. Lancet 1: 535–536

Ernberg I, Andersson J 1986 Acyclovir efficiently inhibits oropharyngeal excretion of Epstein-Barr virus in patients with acute infectious mononucleosis. Journal of General Virology 67: 2267–2272

Esmann V, Geil J P, Kroon S et al 1987 Prednisolone does not prevent post-herpetic neuralgia. Lancet 2: 126–129

Fawcett H A, Wansborough-Jones M H, Clark A E, Leigh I M 1983 Prophylactic topical acyclovir for frequent herpes simplex infection with and without erythema multifiorme. British Medical Journal 287: 789–799

Feldman S, Robertson P K, Lott L, Thornton D 1986 Neurotoxicity due to adenine arabinoside therapy during varicella zoster virus infections in immunocompromised children. Journal of Infectious Diseases 154: 889:893

Fiddian A P 1988 New analogues to acyclovir with increased potency to herpes viruses. In: Kurstak E, Marusyk R G, Murphy F A, van Regenmortel M H V (eds) New vaccines and chemotherapy. Applied Virology Research 1. Plenum Medical. New York. p 223–240

Fiddian A P, Grant D M 1985. Developments in anti-herpes agents: progress and prospects. Abstracts on Hygiene and Communicable Diseases 60: R1–R22

Fiddian A P, Halsos A M, Kinge B R, Nilsen A E, Wikstrom K 1982 Oral acyclovir in the treatment of genital herpes: preliminary report of a multicenter trial. American Journal of Medicine 73, supplement 1A: 335–337

Fiddian A P, Kinghorn G R, Goldmeier D et al 1983a Topical acyclovir in the treatment of genital herpes: a comparison with systemic therapy. Journal of Antimicrobial Chemotherapy 12, supplement B: 67–77

Freidman-Kein A E 1986 Viral origin of hairy leukoplakia. Lancet 2: 694–695

Gibson J R, Klaber M R, Harvey S G, Tosti A, Jones D, Yeo J M 1986 Prophylaxis against herpes liabiais with acyclovir cream—a placebo controlled study. Dermatologica 172: 104–107

Gill M J, Arlete J, Tyrrell D L, Buchan K A 1988 Herpes simplex virus infection of the hand: clinical features and management. American Journal of Medicine 85, supplement 2A: 53–56

Gluckman E, Lotsberg J, Devergie A et al 1983 Prophylaxis of herpes infections after bone marrow transplantation by oral acyclovir. Lancet 2: 706–708

Goldberg L H, Kaufman R, Conant M A et al 1986 Oral acyclovir for episodic treatment of recurrent genital herpes. Journal of the American Academy of Dermatology 15: 256–264

Greenspan J S, Greenspan D, Lennette E T et al 1985 Replication of oral 'hairy' leukoplakia, an AIDS-associated lesion. New England Journal of Medicine 313: 1564–1571

Guinan M E 1986 Oral acyclovir treatment and suppression of genital herpes simplex virus infection: a review. Journal of the American Medical Association 255: 1747–1749

Hanto D W, Frizzera G, Gajl-Peczalaska K J, Balfour Jr H H, Simmons R L, Najarian J S 1985 Acyclovir therapy of Epstein-Barr virus-induced post transplant lymphoproliferative diseases. Transplantation Proceedings 17: 89–92

Heath R B 1986 Varicella: clinical manifestations and prevention. Research and Clinical Forums 8, supplement 6: 27–35

Henderly D E, Freeman W R, Causey D M, Rao N A 1987 Cytomegalovirus retinitis and response to therapy with ganciclovir. Ophthalmology 94: 425–434

Holland G N, Sakamoto M J, Hardy D et al 1986 Treatment of cytomegalovirus retinopathy in patients with acquired immunodeficiency syndrome: use of the experimental drug 9- guanine. Archives of Ophthalmology 104: 1794–1800

Huff J C, Bean B, Laskin O et al 1988 Therapy of herpes zoster with oral acyclovir (Zovirax) in the eye. British Journal of Ophthalmology 68: 192–195

Hung S O, Patterson A, Rees P J, 1984 Pharmacokinetics or oral acyclovir (Zovirax) in the eye. British Journal of Ophthalmology 68: 192–195

Jacobson M A, de Miranda P, Cederberg D M et al 1987 Human pharmacokinetics and tolerance of oral ganciclovir. Antimicrobial Agents and Chemotherapy 31: 1251–1254

Jeffries D J 1986 Acyclovir update. British Medical Journal 293: 1523

Juel-Jensen B E, Khan J A, Pasvol G 1983 High dose intravenous acyclovir in the treatment of zoster: a double-blind, placebo controlled trial. Journal of Infection 6, supplement 1: 31–36

King D H, Fiddian A P 1986 New antiviral agents. In: Lietman P, Ohtani S, Fiddian A P (eds) Clinical Advances in Antiviral Therapy, University Press, Tokyo. p 65–71

Kinghorn G R 1988 Long-term suppression with oral acyclovir of recurrent herpes simplex virus infections in otherwise healthy patients: A European multicenter study. American Journal of Medicine 85, supplement 2A: 26–29

Kinghorn G R, Turner E B, Barton I G, Potter C W, Burke C A, Fiddian A P 1983 Efficacy of topical acyclovir cream in first and recurrent episodes of genital herpes. Antiviral Research 3: 291–301

Kingsley S R, Fiddian A P 1985 Acyclovir cream—an effective therapy for cutaneous herpes simplex infections. In: Kono R, Nakajima A (eds) Herpes Viruses and Virus Chemotherapy. Excerpta Medica, Amsterdam. p 133–137

Klapper P E, Laing I, Longson M 1981 Rapid non-invasive diagnosis of herpes encephalitis. Lancet 2: 607–609

Leigh I M 1988 Management of non-genital herpes simplex virus infections in immunocompetent patients. American Journal of Medicine 85, supplement 2A: 34–38

Levin M J, Zaia J A, Hershey B J, Davis L G, Robinson G V, Segretti A C 1985 Topical acyclovir treatment of herpes zoster in immunocompromised patients. Journal of the American Academy of Dermatology 13: 590–596

Leyland-Jones B, Donnelly H, Groshen S et al 1986 2'-fluoro-5-iodoarabinosylcytosine, a new potent antiviral agent: efficacy in immunocompromised individuals with herpes zoster. Journal of Infectious Diseases 154: 430–436

Longson M 1977 The treatment of herpes encephalitis. In: Oxford J S, Drasar F A, Williams J D (eds) Chemotherapy of Herpes Simple Virus Infections. Academic Press. London. p 115–123

Longson M, Bailey A S, Klapper P 1980 Herpes encephalitis. Recent Advances in Clinical Virology 2: 147–157

Lundgren G, Wilczek H, Lonnqvist B, Lindholm A, Wahren B, Ringden O 1985 Acyclovir prophylaxis in bone marrow transplant recipients. Scandinavian Journal of Infectious Diseases, supplement 47: 137–144

McGill J, MacDonald D R, Fall C, McKendrick G D W, Copplestone A 1983a Intravenous acyclovir in acute herpes zoster infection. Journal of Infection 6: 157–161

McGill J, Chapman C, Mahakasingham M 1983b Acyclovir therapy in herpes zoster infection: a practical guide. Transations of the Ophthalmological Society of the United Kingdom 103: 111–114

McKendrick M W, Care C, Burke C, Hickmott E, McKendrick G D W 1984 Oral acyclovir in herpes zoster. Journal of Antimicrobial Chemotherapy 14: 661–665

McKendrick M W, McGill J I, White J E, Wood M J 1986 Oral acyclovir in acute herpes zoster. British Medical Journal 293: 1529–1532

Masur H, Lane C, Palestine A et al 1986 Effect of 9-(1,3-dihyrdroxy-2-propoxymethyl) guanine on serious cytomegalovirus diease in eight immunosuprressed homosexual men. Annals of Internal Medicine 104: 41–44

Mattison H R, Reichman R C, Benedetti J et al 1988 Double-blind, placebo-controlled trial comparing long–term suppressive with short–term oral acyclovir therapy for management of recurrent genital herpes. American Journal of Medicine 85, supplement 2A: 20–25

Merigan T C, Rand K H, Pollard R B, Abdullah P S, Jordan G W, Fried R P 1978 Human leucocyte interferon for the treatment of herpes zoster in patients with cancer. New England Journal of Medicine 298: 981–987

Mertz G J, Eron L, Kaufman R et al 1988 Prolonged continuous versus intermittent oral acyclovir treatment in normal adults with frequently recurring genital herpes simplex virus infection. American Journal of Medicine 85, supplement 2A: 14–19

Meyers J D 1985 Treatment of herpes virus infections in the immunocompromised host. Scandinavian Journal of Infectious Diseases, supplement 47: 128–136

Meyers J D 1988 Management of cytomegalovirus infection. American Journal of Medicine 85, supplement 2A: 102–106

Meyers J D, Wade J C, Mitchell C D et al 1982 Multicentre collaborative trial of intravenous acyclovir for treatment of mucocutaneous herpes simplex virus infection in the immunocompromised host. American Journal of Medicine 73, supplement 1A: 229–235

Meyers J D, Reed E C, Shepp D H et al 1988 Acyclovir for prevention of cytomegalovirus infection and disease after allogeneic marrow transplantation. New England Journal of Medicine 318: 70–75

Mindel A, Adler M W, Sutherland S, Fiddian A P 1982 Intravenous acyclovir treatment for primary genital herpes. Lancet 1: 697–700

Mindel A, Weller I V D, Faherty A, Sutherland S, Hindley D, Fiddian A P 1984 Prophylactic oral acyclovir in recurrent genital herpes. Lancet 2: 57–59

Mindel A, Weller I V D, Faherty A, Sutherland S, Fiddian A P, Adler M W 1986 Acyclovir in first attacks of genital herpes and prevention of recurrences. Genitourinary Medicine 62: 28–32

Mindel A, Kinghorn G, Allason-Jones E et al 1987 Treatment of first-attack genital herpes—acyclovir versus inosine pranobex. Lancet 1: 1171–1173

Mosca J D, Bednarik D P, Raj N B K 1987 Herpes simplex virus type -1 can reactive transcription of latent human immunodeficiency virus. Nature 325: 67–70

Mostow S R, Mayfield J L, Marr J J, Drucker J L 1988 Suppression of recurrent genital herpes by single daily dosages of acyclovir. American Journal of Medicine 85, supplement 2A: 30–33

Nicholson K G 1984a Antiviral therapy: respiratory infections, genital herpes, and herpes keratitis. Lancet 2: 617–621

Nicholson K G 1984b Antiviral therapy: herpes simplex encephalitis, neonatal herpes infections, and chronic hepatitis B. Lancet 2: 736–739

Niimura M, Nishikawa T 1988 Treatment of eczema herpeticum with oral acyclovir. American Journal of Medicine 85, supplement 2A: 49–52

Nilsen A E, Assen T, Halsos A M et al 1982 Efficacy of oral acyclovir in the treatment of initial and recurrent genital herpes. Lancet 2: 571–573

Novelli V M, Marshall W C, Yeo J, McKendrick G D 1984 Acyclovir administered perorally in immunocompromised children with varicella-zoster infections. Journal of Infectious Diseases 149: 478

Novelli V M, Marshall W C, Yeo J, McKendrick G D 1985 High-dose oral acyclovir for children at risk of disseminated herpes virus infections. Journal of Infectious Dieases 151: 372

Nyerges G, Meszner Z 1988 Treatment of chickenpox in immunocompromised children. American Journal of Medicine 85, supplement 2A: 94–95

Nyerges G, Meszner Z, Gyarmati E, Kerpel-Fronius S 1988 Acyclovir prevents dissemination of varicella in immunocompromised children. Journal of Infectious Disease 157: 309–313

Pagano J S, Sixbey J W, Lin J-C 1983 Acyclovir and Epstein-Barr virus infections. Journal of Antimicrobial Chemotherapy 12, supplement B: 113–121

Perren T J, Powles R L, Easton D, Stolle K, Selby P J 1988 Prevention of herpes zoster in patients by long-term oral acyclovir after allogeneic bone marrow transplantation. American Journal of Medicine 85, supplement 2A: 99–101

Peterslund N A, Seyer-Hansen K, Ipsen J, Esmann V, Schonheyder H, Juhl H 1981 Acyclovir in herpes zoster. Lancet 2: 827–830

Prober C G, Kirk L E, Keeney R E 1982 Acyclovir therapy of chickenpox in immunosuppressed children—a collaborative study. Journal of Paediatrics 101: 622–625

Raborn G W, McGaw W T, Grace M, Percy J 1988 Treatment of herpes labialis with acyclovir: review of three clinical trials. American Journal of Medicine 85, supplement 2A: 39–42

Rando R F, Pellett P E, Luciw P A, Bohan C A, Srinivasan A 1987 Transactivation of human immunodeficiency virus by herpes viruses. Oncogene 1: 13–18

Reichman R C, Badger G J, Mertz G J et al 1984 Treatment of recurrent genital herpes simplex infections with oral acyclovir: a controlled trial. Journal of the American Medical Association 251: 2103–2107

Resnick L, Herbst J S, Ablashi D V et al 1988 Regression of oral hairy leukoplakia after orally administered acyclovir therapy. Journal of the American Medical Association 259: 384–388

Ruhnek-Forsbeck M, Sandstrom E, Andersson B et al 1985 Treatment of recurrent genital herpes simplex infections with oral acyclovir. Journal of Antimicrobial Chemotherapy 16: 621–628

Sacks S L 1987 The role of oral acyclovir in the management of genital herpes simplex. Canadian Medical Association Journal 136: 701–707

Salahuddin S Z, Ablashi D V, Markham P D et al 1986 Isolation of a new virus, HBLV, in patients with lymphoproliferative disorders. Science 234: 596–601

Salo O P, Lassus A, Hovi T, Fiddian A P 1983 Double-blind placebo-controlled trial of oral acyclovir in recurrent genital herpes. European Journal of Sexually Transmitted Diseases 1: 95–98

Saral R 1988 Management of mucocutaneous herpes simplex virus infections in immunocompromised patients. American Journal of Medicine 85, supplement 2A: 57–60

Saral R, Burns W H, Laskin O L, Santos G W, Lietman P S 1981 Acyclovir prophylaxis of herpes simplex virus infections: a randomised, double-blind, controlled trial in bone marrow transplant recipients. New England Journal of Medicine 305: 63–67

Saral R, Ambinder R F, Burns W H et al 1983 Acyclovir prophylaxis against herpes simplex virus infection in patients with leukaemia: a randomised, double-blind controlled study. Annals of Internal Medicine 99: 773–776

Schadelin J, Schilt H U, Rohner M 1988 Preventative therapy of herpes labialis associated with trigeminal surgery. American Journal of Medicine 85, supplement 2A: 46–48

Schofer H, Ochsendorf F R, Helm E B, Milbradt R 1987 Treatment of oral 'hairy' leukoplakia in AIDS patients with vitamin A acid (topically) or acyclovir (systemically). Dermatologica 174: 150–151

Shaw M, King M, Best J M, Banatvala J E, Gibson J R, Klaber M R 1985 Failure of acyclovir cream in treatment of recurrent herpes labialis. British Medical Journal 291: 7–9

Shepp D H, Newton B A, Dandliker P S, Flournoy N, Meyers J D 1985a Oral acyclovir therapy for mucocutaneous herpes simplex virus infections in immunocompromised marrow transplant recipients. Annals of Internal Medicine 102: 783–785

Shepp D H, Dandliker P S, de Miranda P 1985b Activity of 9-[2-hydroxy-1-(hydroxymethyl) ethoxymethyl] guanine in the treatment of cytomegalovirus pneumonia. Annals of Internal Medicine 103: 368:373

Shepp D H, Dandliker P S, Meyers J D 1986 Treatment of varicella-zoster virus infection in severely immunocompromised patients: a randomized comparison of acyclovir and vidarabine. New England Journal of Medicine 314: 208–212

Skoldenberg B, Forsgren M, Alestig K et al 1984 Acyclovir versus vidarabine in herpes simplex encephalitis: randomized multicentre study in consecutive Swedish patients. Lancet 2: 707–711

Spruance S L 1988 Cutaneous herpes simplex virus lesions induced by ultraviolet radiation: a review of model systems and prophylactic therapy with oral acyclovir. American Journal of Medicine 85, supplement 2A: 43–45

Spruance S L, Schnipper L E, Overall J C et al 1982 Treatment of herpes simplex labialis with topical acyclovir in polyethylene glycol. Journal of Infectious Diseases 146: 85–90

Straus S E, Takiff H E, Seidlin M et al 1984 Suppression of frequently recurring genital herpes. New England Journal of Medicine 310: 1545–1550

Straus S E, Ostrove J M, Inchauspe G et al 1988 Varicella-zoster virus infections: biology, natural history, treatment, and prevention. Annals of Internal Medicine 108: 221–237

Thin R N 1988 Management of genital herpes simplex infections. American Journal of Medicine 85, supplement 2A: 3–6

Thin R N, Jeffries D J, Taylor P K et al 1985 Recurrent genital herpes suppressed by oral acyclovir: a multicentre double blind trial. Journal of Antimicrobial Chemotherapy 16: 219–226

van Weel-Sipman M H, van der Meer J W M, de Koning J, Versteeg J 1981 Severe atypical recurrent varicella in childhood leukaemia. Lancet 1: 147–148

Vilde J L, Bricaire F, Leport C, Renaudie M, Brun-Vezinet F 1986 Comparative trial of acyclovir and vidarbine in disseminated varicella-zoster infections in immunocompromised patients. Journal of Medical Virology 20: 127–134

Wade J C, Newton B, McLaren C, Flournoy N, Kleeney R E, Meyers J D 1982 Intravenous acyclovir to treat mucocutaneous herpes simplex virus infection after marrow transplantation. Annals of Internal Medicine 96: 265–269

Wade J C, Newton B, Flournoy N, Meyers J D 1984 Oral acyclovir for prevention of herpes simplex virus reactivation after marrow transplantation. Annals of Internal Medicine 100: 823–828

Whitley R J 1988 Herpes simplex virus infections of the central nervous system: a review. American Journal of Medicine 85, supplement 2A: 61–67

Whitley R J, Soong S J, Dolin R et al 1977 Adenine arabinoside therapy of biopsy-proved herpes simplex encephalitis. New England Journal of Medicine 297: 289–294

Whitley R J, Nahmias A J, Soong S J, Galasso G G, Fleming C L, Alford C A 1980 Vidarabine therapy of neonatal herpes simplex virus infection. Paediatrics 66: 495–501

Whitley R J, Soong S J, Hirsch M et al 1981 Herpes simplex encephalitis: vidarabine therapy and diagnostic problems. New England Journal of Medicine 304: 313–318

Whitley R, Hilty M, Haynes R et al 1982a Vidarabine therapy of varicella in immunosuppressed patients. Journal of Paediatrics 101: 125–131

Whitley R J, Soong S J, Dolin et al 1982b Early vidarabine therapy to control the complications of herpes zoster in immunosuppressed patients. New England Journal of Medicine 307: 971–975

Whitley R J, Yeagar A, Kartus P L et al 1983 Neonatal herpes simplex virus infection: follow-up evaluation of vidarabine therapy. Paediatrics 72: 778–785

Whitley R J, Levin M, Barton N et al 1984a Infections caused by herpes simplex virus in the immunocompromised host: natural history and topical acyclovir therapy. Journal of Infectious Diseases 150: 323–329

Whitley R J, Spruance S, Hayden F G et al 1984b Vidarabine therapy for mucocutaneous herpes simplex infections in the immunocompromised host. Journal of Infectious Diseases 149: 1–8

Whitley R J, Alford C A, Hirsch M S et al 1986 Vidarabine versus acyclovir therapy in herpes simplex encephalitis. New England Journal of Medicine 314: 144–149

Whitley R J, Alford C A, Hirsch M S et al 1987 Factors indicative of outcome in a comparative trial of acyclovir and vidarabine for biopsy-proven herpes simplex encephalitis. Infection 15, supplement 1: S3–S8

Wildenhoff K E, Esmann V, Ipsen J, Harving H, Peterslund N A, Schonheyder H 1981 Treatment of trigemenial and thoracic zoster with IDU. Scandinavian Journal of Infectious Diseases 13: 257–262

Wildiers J, de Clercq E 1984 Oral (E)-5-(2-bromovinyl)-2'-deoxyuridine treatment of severe herpes zoster in cancer patients. European Journal of Cancer and Clinical Oncology 20: 471–476

Wood M J, Geddes A M 1987 Antiviral therapy. Lancet 2: 1189–1193

Wood M J, Ogan P H, McKendrick M W, Care C D, McGill J I, Webb E M 1988 Efficacy of oral acyclovir treatment of acute herpes zoster. American Journal of Medicine 85, supplement 2A: 79–83

Yeo J M, Fiddian A P 1983 Acyclovir in the management of herpes labialis. Journal of Antimicrobial Chemotherapy 12, supplement B: 95–103

Discussion of paper presented by Paul Fiddian

Discussant: Richard Whitley

LESSONS LEARNED FROM THERAPY OF HUMAN HERPESVIRUS
INFECTIONS: A DISCUSSION

Introduction
The past 25 years have witnessed significant progress in the development of
antiviral therapies for human viral infections. Much of the research and
development effort has been focused on inhibitors of herpesvirus replication with
particular emphasis on herpes simplex and varicella-zoster viruses. Epstein-Barr
virus and cytomegaloviruses have been less amenable to drug development,
although certainly these are viruses whose resulting infections are in need of
therapies. A first step in the development of parenteral antiviral therapy was the
demonstration of efficacy for vidarabine therapy of herpes simplex encephalitis,
neonatal herpes simplex and varicella-zoster virus infections in immunocompromised hosts in the late 1970s and early 1980s. In the early 1980s, a landmark
advance was the definition of the value of acyclovir in carefully controlled clinical
trials, as cited by Dr Fiddian. Of special importance, acyclovir was shown to be
a selective and specific inhibitor of herpes simplex replication in contrast to the
prior non-specific inhibitor of herpesvirus replication. This discussion will amplify
comments from the preceding paper with particular reference to the shortcomings
of existing antiviral therapy, rapidity of diagnosis, and targeted areas for future
advances.

Overview of the problems
Of all indications, therapy of mucocutaneous herpes simplex virus infections has
led to the most clinically useful and safest modality of therapy. Similarly,
decreased mortality and improved morbidity can be achieved with therapy of
herpes simplex encephalitis and neonatal herpes simplex infection. Nevertheless,
in spite of these advances, shortcomings in existing therapies of herpesvirus
infections can be identified as shown in Table 1.

Each of these shortcomings involves multiple factors which will continue to
influence the success of any form of antiviral therapy. Such factors include:
(1) the immune status of the host, namely the ability to elicit a purportedly
normal immunological response; (2) rapiditiy and specificity of diagnosis;

(3) drug delivery to a targeted tissue (e.g. drug lipophilicity for delivery across the blood–brain barrier); and (4) the selectivity and specificity of inhibitors of replication for those viral infections for which there is no currently available therapy. The development of compounds which: (1) have a physiological pH, (2) are readily absorbed after oral administration, (3) cross the blood–brain barrier and penetrate infected tissues, (4) are easy to manufacture, and (5) relatively inexpensive to produce, are all of relevance for antiviral drug development. These issues will be considered for selected herpesvirus infections.

Table 1 Problems of antiviral therapy for future attention

Virus	Clinical condition	Problem/potential problem	Future need
HSV[1]	Mucutaneous infection:		Drugs to prevent latency
	Primary	Latency occurs even with therapy of first episode disease	
	Recurrent	Therapy of little clinical value	Drugs given once to prevent future recurrence
	Herpes encephalitis and neonatal herpes	Morbidity/mortality remain high	Pharmacokinetic disposition Enhanced lipophilicity for drug delivery More active drugs
VZV[2]	Chickenpox (primary)	Latency occurs even with therapy of first episode disease	Drugs to prevent latency
	Shingles (recurrent)	Value of therapy unclear	Improved therapy
CMV[3]	All	No safe and routinely acceptable therapy	Rapid diagnosis Need for safe and specific therapies
EBV[4]	All	No safe and routinely acceptable therapy	Rapid diagnosis Need for safe and specific therapies
ALL[5]	Pesistent/ intermittent treatments	Viral resistance	New approaches and drugs

[1] HSV = Herpes simplex virus infection
[2] VZV = Varicella-zoster virus infection
[3] CMV = Cytomegalovirus infection
[4] EBV = Epstein-Barr virus infection
[5] ALL = All of the aforementioned herpes viruses

Mucocutaneous herpes simplex virus infections

A unique characteristic of all herpesviruses is their ability to become latent and reactivate upon proper provocation. While understood phenomenologically, the molecular basis for reactivation is not well understood at the present time. Each of the herpesviruses is capable of being reactivated. The best studied member of this family is herpes simplex virus for which the clinical course following reactivation (herpes simplex labialis or herpes simplex genitalis) are well described. Individuals with frequently recurrent herpetic infections usually have large quantities of neutralizing antibodies as well as intact cell mediated immune responses which, nevertheless, do not appear to prevent the reactivation of latent virus. Regardless, likely because of host immunity, the clinical course of reactivation disease is far less severe than that which is associated with primary infection. While those factors which influence recurrent infections are not well understood currently, recent data suggest that one of the immediate early genes of herpes simplex has a significant role in containing recurrent infection (an anti-sense message to ICP-0).

As described by Dr Fiddian, acyclovir therapy is of established clinical value for primary genital herpes and both treatment and suppression of recurrent herpes simplex virus infections in immunocompromised patients. In addition, the administration of acyclovir to suppress frequently recurrent genital disease in the normal host is of value. The application of molecular biology to clinical therapeutics may lead to the identification of factors which will prevent the reactivation of herpes simplex virus. Such an interventive approach might avoid, hopefully, the necessity for continually administering a medication. Ideally, the ability to provide a single dose of a medication which would prevent all subsequent recurrences may not be untenable as more is learned about the inter-relationship of ICP-O and latency.

Life-threatening disease
Two life-threatening herpes simplex virus infections have attracted particular attention from a therapeutic standpoint; these are herpes simplex encephalitis and neonatal herpes simplex virus infection. While acyclovir therapy, as documented earlier, has clearly improved the prognosis for herpes simplex encephalitis, similar beenfit has not been achieved when compared to vidarabine in the management of neonatal herpes simplex infection. This latter observation warrants careful consideration as it underscores a need to develop new drugs with enhanced activity as well as to understand drug delivery to infected organs (clinical pharmacokinetics). The ability to deliver safe and selective inhibitors of viral replication to target organs for defined diseases is of increasing importance. For herpes encephalitis or neonatal herpes, the ability to improve delivery of a drug such as acyclovir to the central nervous system or targeted organs will be required to improve outcome. In the former discussion, mortality and severe neurological sequelae still account for approximately 50% of patients with biopsy-proven disease. For encephalitis and disseminated infections of the newborn, mortality and severe neurological impairment account for 50% and 70% of babies with culture proven disease, respectively. Thus, enhancing lipophilicity or derivatizing medications in order to allow drugs to be locked into target organ tissues will be of significance in future therapeutic efforts.

Varicella-zoster virus infections
Therapy of varicella-zoster virus infections in the immunocompromised host was one of the early therapeutic triumphs. Matching the apparent clinical need—namely, oral therapy—with the currently available medications—acyclovir—has not led to studies indicating unequivocal clinical value. Clearly, both vidarabine and acyclovir, especially the latter, are effective parenteral

antiviral therapeutics for both chickenpox and shingles in the immunocompromised host. The need for orally bioavailable medications should be stressed. Hopefully, a prodrug of acyclovir or another compound (e.g. bromovinyl arabinosyluracil) will be available for ambulatory care studies.

Other herpesvirus infections
Disease caused by the remaining three herpesviruses, cytomegalovirus, Epstein-Barr virus, and human herpesvirus VI, are not amenable to drugs which have acceptable therapeutic indicies, namely those which are both clinically efficacious and safe to employ. Studies of 9-hydroxyethoxy-methylguanine, ganciclovir, have been performed in the treatment of sight- and life-threatening cytomegalovirus infections in immunocompromised patients. Data for ganciclovir have been largely acquired from immunocompromised hosts with acquired immunodeficiency syndrome, AIDS, or undergoing organ transplantation who received compassionate plea treatment of cytomegalovirus disease (chorioretinitis, colitis and pneumonitis). The results show that disease can be stabilized in high-risk patients; however, relative therapeutic index (efficacy/toxicity), is high. Thus, the exisiting modalities of therapy for cytomegalovirus infection are less than adequate.

When therapy is targeted for an immunocompromised host, the inability of such a host to prevent reactivation or re-excretion of cytomegalovirus is a necessary component in the evaluation of a treatment regimen. Certainly, ganciclovir cannot be used to treat trivial cytomegalovirus infections because of its toxicity. Future drug developments in this area will lead to selective inhibitors of cytomegalovirus infection which can be administered orally and which are without significant toxicity.

No useful therapy has been defined of value for either Epstein-Barr virus or human herpesvirus VI infections. Issues regarding the rapidity and specificity of diagnosis are essential for both of these infections. Since these infections rarely cause life-threatening disease, therapy unequivocally will have to be safe.

Prospects for the future
The advances in antiviral therapy over the last decade have been striking. Much attention has been devoted to treatment of herpesviruses because, in large part, initial strides were made in this area of evaluation. The availability of compounds with an adequate therapeutic index for the management of mucocutaneous herpes simplex virus infection and herpes simplex encephalitis, particularly the absence of toxicity for acyclovir, is an important advance in the development of antiviral therapy. This recognition paired with efficacy provides a bright picture for the future of the development of antiviral drugs.

While current therapeutic efforts have focused on nucleoside analogues, future advances in molecular biology will change this approach. Interest in an anti-sense message to ICP-O, specifically as it relates to maintenance of herpes simplex virus (in a latent state), cannot be understated. The adaptation of molecular biology, particularly the synthesis of anti-sense messages, will be of relevance in the next several years. These anti-sense messages will require novel drug delivery systems to cells. It is essential that these messages should not be cleaved by host enzymes in the plasma, and, once in the cell, will function in a biologically active fashion. While these problems may seem great at the present time, they are clearly reasonable for future drug development.

Acknowledgement

This work was supported by contract AI-62554 from the Developmental and Applications Branch, the National Institutes of Allergy and Infectious Diseases; by grants from the National Cancer Institute, RR-032 from the Division of Research Resources; and by a grant from the state of Alabama.

Discussion: Treatment of herpes group viruses

Paul Fiddian and Richard Whitley

One participant pointed out that it was shown some time ago that the sensitivity of CMV to acyclovir depends very much on the strain. Some fresh isolates may be much more sensitive to acyclovir than the average values shown by Fiddian. Thus it is possible that acyclovir might have prophylactic value against CMV infections.

There was some discussion on the effect of acyclovir or vidarabine treatment of neonatal herpes on the host immune responses to the virus. Most data show no difference between acyclovir and vidarabine on the development of either humoral or cellular immune responses. Specifically, no changes have been seen in total antiviral antibodies, measured by neutralization of ELISA, or in specific antibodies to p66, gB, or gD by immunoblotting. There was some controversy about interpretation of the unpublished outcome data from the study comparing acyclovir with vidarabine for treatment of neonatal HSV infection. Although the mortality was higher in the acyclovir-treated patients with CNS disease (60% vs 40%), the incidence of severe sequelae was lower; thus, the combined incidence of death and severe sequelae was idential in the two groups.

There was also some discussion on the theoretical and actual benefit of glucocorticoid (e.g. dexamethasone) therapy of patients with viral encephalitis. Although they have the theoretical benefit of decreasing cerebral oedema and increasing the penetration of antiviral drugs (by alteration of the blood–brain barrier), no difference in outcome has been seen in clinical trials to date.

Section II
INTERACTION BETWEEN VIRUS PROTEINS AND THE HOST IMMUNE SYSTEM

Chairman: J. Lindsay Whitton

6. Prions causing slow infections

Stanley Prusiner

INTRODUCTION

Over the last 40 years the structures of most viruses, as well as their roles in the causation of disease, have been elucidated (Watson et al, 1987). During this same period, two new classes of infectious pathogens resembling viruses in many respects, have been recognized. These unusual pathogens have been designated viroids and prions. The viroids are small naked RNAs which infect plants (Diener, 1971, 1987b). To date, no animal viroids have been identified. The properties of viroids and prions are antithetical: procedures that hydrolyse or modify nucleic acid inactivate viroids but do not alter prion infectivity, while procedures that hydrolyse or modify proteins inactivate prions but do not alter viroid infectivity (Diener et al, 1982).

Prions cause Creutzfeldt-Jakob disease (CJD), kuru and Gerstmann-Sträussler syndrome (GSS) which are human neurodegenerative diseases and can be transmitted experimentally to animals. In 1920, Creutzfeldt described a progressive dementing illness in a 22-year-old woman. The following year, Jakob described four older patients with a clinically similar presentation and course (Jakob, 1921). During the ensuing four decades, numerous cases of CJD were described clinically and pathologically. While most cases of CJD present with a progressive dementia characterized initially by loss of memory, diminished intellect and poor judgement, a few cases present as progressive cerebellar syndromes with diminished co-ordination, tremor and ataxia. Patients with the ataxic form of CJD eventually become profoundly demented.

Kuru and GSS present as cerebellar syndromes while the dementing phase of these illnesses is often delayed until quite late in their course. In 1959, Klatzo, Gajdusek and Zigas noted the neuropathological similarities between CJD and kuru, a degenerative cerebellar disorder of New Guinea natives (Klatzo et al, 1959). That same year, Hadlow described the neuropathological similarities between kuru and scrapie and suggested that kuru might be transmissible to laboratory animals after a prolonged incubation period (Hadlow, 1959). During the next decade, both kuru and CJD were transmitted to apes and monkeys (Gajdusek et al, 1966; Gibbs et al, 1968).

Three transmissible neurodegenerative diseases of animals, scrapie of sheep and goats, transmissible mink encephalopathy and chronic wasting disease of mule deer and elk, share many features with kuru, CJD and GSS. Whether or not a recently recognized disorder called bovine spongiform encephalopathy is transmissible remains uncertain (Wells et al, 1987).

Of all these human and animal transmissible degenerative central nervous system (CNS) diseases, scrapie is the most well studied. In 1954, Sigurdsson suggested that scrapie and visna, both CNS diseases of sheep, were caused by slow viruses (Sigurdsson, 1954). Diseases caused by slow viruses are characterized by prolonged latent or incubation periods followed by progressive clinical courses. Both scrapie and visna were known to be caused by transmissible, filterable agents which multiply during infection. Based on these properties, it was reasonable to classify these infectious pathogens as viruses. Over the last two decades, it has become clear that visna is caused by a retrovirus similar to the viruses responsible for acquired immune deficiency syndrome (AIDS) (Barre Sinoussi et al, 1983; Gallo et al, 1984; Gonda et al, 1985; Levy, 1988) and scrapie is caused by infectious pathogens which differ significantly from viruses.

In man, the slow transmissible neurodegenerative diseases with prolonged incubation periods ranging from two months to more than three decades have been observed (Gajdusek, 1977). The clinical course may last for periods ranging from a few weeks to a few years (Brown et al, 1986). Neither computerized axial tomography nor magnetic resonance imaging has been useful in establishing the diagnosis of human transmissible neurodegenerative diseases. Positron emission tomography shows non-specific, widespread diminished glucose metabolism (Friedland et al, 1984). The cerebrospinal fluid (CSF) in CJD, GSS and kuru is normal. One study reports the appearance of two abnormal CSF proteins in CJD (Harrington et al, 1986), but their presence in 50% of herpes simplex encephalitis cases and absence in kuru indicate that this finding is non-specific. In Herdwick sheep with scrapie, elevated IgG levels in serum and CSF were reported, but these observations were not reproducible in Suffolk sheep (Strain et al, 1984). Neither a leukocytosis nor a CSF pleocytosis are observed in these neurodegenerative diseases.

NOVEL INFECTIOUS PATHOGENS

As knowledge was accumulated about the infectious agent causing scrapie, the unusual properties of these particles began to be appreciated. Over the decade from 1965 to 1974, new hypotheses on the structure of the scrapie agent were offered at more than one per year (Prusiner, 1982). Radiobiological studies offered the most provocative data suggesting that the scrapie agent is fundamentally different from viruses (Alper et al, 1966, 1967). The unusual features of the scrapie agent (Alper et al, 1966) have been embodied by terms such as 'unconventional virus' and 'virino'. 'Unconventional virus' has been used to contrast the unusual properties of the scrapie agent with those of conventional viruses (Gajdusek, 1977). 'Virino' was originally defined in 1979: 'If the recent experimental results of Marsh and Malone are correct in implicating DNA as a necessary component of the infective unit of scrapie, then an appropriate name for this class of agent would be 'virinos' which (by analogy with neutrinos) are small, immunologically neutral particles with high penetration properties but needing special criteria to detect their presence' (Dickinson & Outram, 1979). Subsequent studies showed that the work of Marsh et al (1978) and Malone et al (1979) could not be confirmed (Prusiner et al, 1980a). The most recent definition of 'virino' is 'host proteins sequestering the agent genome which may code for no product other than copies of itself' (Dickinson & Outram, 1988).

Once an effective protocol for partial purification of the scrapie agent was developed, convincing data was obtained showing that a protein molecule is necessary for infectivity (Prusiner et al, 1981). With these same preparations, attempts to demonstrate that the scrapie agent contains a nucleic acid were unsuccessful. Five procedures that modify or hydrolyse nucleic acids failed to inactivate the scrapie agent, yet these same procedures were capable of inactivating numerous viruses as well as small infectious nucleic acids called viroids (Diener et al, 1982;, Prusiner 1982). Based on these studies, the term 'prion' was introduced in order to distinguish the class of particles causing scrapie from those responsible for viral illnesses (Prusiner, 1982). Prion was given an operational definition: 'small *pro*teinaceous *in*fectious particles which resist inactivation by procedures that modify nucleic acids' (Prusiner, 1982).

To avoid prejudging the structure of these infectious particles, a family of structural hypotheses for the prion was proposed: (1) proteins surrounding a nucleic acid which encodes them (a virus); (2) proteins surrounding a small non-coding polynucleotide; (3) a proteinaceous particle devoid of nucleic acid. Data from many laboratories have made the possibility that scrapie is caused by virus seem remote. While some investigators have chosen to redefine prions as infectious proteins (Carp et al, 1985; Hope & Kimberlin, 1987), we have resisted this oversimplication in order not to bias our experimental approaches (Chamberlin, 1890).

Over the past five years, a large body of experimental data about the particles causing scrapie has been accumulated. Most of the data has been confirmed and much of it is widely accepted (Diener, 1987a). At times, this confirmed body of information has been overshadowed by what seems to be controversy due to the diverse terminology used by different laboratories. The studies described below have constrained the number of putative structures for prions which can now be seriously considered.

Much evidence argues that these novel pathogens are composed largely of protein. Whether or not they contain a second component such as a small nucleic acid remains uncertain.

While both prions and viruses multiply, their properties, structure and mode of replication seem to exhibit some fundamental differences. Viruses contain a nucleic acid genome which encodes progeny viruses, including most or all of the proteins in their protective shells. In constrast, prions contain little or no nucleic acid and the prion protein (PrP) is encoded by a cellular gene (Oesch et al, 1985). Although viruses evoke an immune response during infection, prions do not (Prusiner, 1982; Oesch et al 1985).

PrP 27–30 IS A COMPONENT OF THE SCRAPIE PRION

Development of a more rapid and economical bioassay (Prusiner et al 1980b) greatly facilitated purification of the hamster scrapie agent and led to the discovery of a unique protein, PrP 27–30 (Table 6.1) (Prusiner et al, 1982). This protein migrates in sodium dodecyl sulphate (SDS) polyacrylamide gels as a broad band of apparent molecular weight 27,000 to 30,000 (Fig. 6.1). Much of the microheterogeneity displayed by PrP 27–30 is presumably due to variation in its sialic acid content (Bolton et al, 1985). PrP 27–30 is generated from a larger protein of apparent molecular weight 33,000 to 35,000, designated PrP^{Sc}, by proteinase K digestion (Barry et al, 1986; Barry & Prusiner, 1986; Meyer et al, 1986; Oesch et al, 1985).

Table 6.1 Terminology

Prion	Small *proteinacous infectious* particle which resists inactivation by procedures that modify nucleic acids. It causes scrapie and CJD. Scrapie agent is a synonym.
PrP 27–30	This protein is the only identifiable macromolecule in purified preparations of hamster scrapie prions. Digestion of PrP^{Sc} with proteinase K generates PrP 27–30.
PrP^{Sc}	Scrapie isoform of the prion protein (PrP 33–35^{Sc}).
PrP^{C}	Cellular isoform of the prion protein (PrP 33–35^{Sc}).
Prion rod	An aggregate of prions composed largely, if not entirely, of PrP 27–30 molecules. Created by detergent extraction of membranes. Morphologically and histochemically indistinguishable from many amyloids.

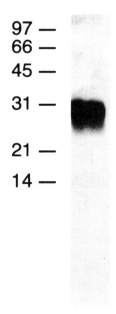

97 —
66 —
45 —
31 —
21 —
14 —

Fig. 6.1 Scrapie prion protein (PrP 27-30). Scrapie-infected golden hamster brains were homogenized and the protease-resistant PrP isoform was purified. The purified scrapie prions were analysed by SDS polyacrylamide gel electrophoresis. The hamster scrapie prion protein (PrP 27-30) was detected by silver staining. Numbers refer to the molecular weights (in kilodaltons) of marker proteins. (Reprinted, by permission of Prusiner, 1987)

Seven lines of evidence argue that PrP 27–30 is a component of the infectious particle:

(1)   PrP 27–30 and the scrapie agent co-purify (Prusiner et al, 1980b, 1983, 1984); PrP 27–30 is the most abundant macromolecule in purified preparations (Prusiner et al, 1983). In fact, PrP 27–30 is the only macromolecule identified to date, which is present in sufficiently high concentrations to be considered a component of the infectious particle. During purification, both the scrapie agent and PrP 27–30 were enriched 3000– to 10,000–fold with respect to cellular proteins. This co-purification indicates that the molecular properties of PrP 27–30 and the infectious particles must be extremely similar.

(2)   PrP 27–30 concentration is proportional to prion titre (McKinley et al, 1983). PrP 27–30 or its precursor PrP^{Sc} is absent in normal, uninfected animals (Barry & Prusiner, 1986; Oesch et al, 1985). The kinetics of PrP 27–30 appearance in scrapie-infected animals coincide with the increase in scrapie prion titre (DeArmond et al, unpublished data).

(3)   Procedures that denature, hydrolyse or selectively modify PrP 27–30 also diminish prion titre (McKinley et al, 1983). The unusual kinetics of PrP 27–30 hydrolysis catalysed by proteases have been shown to correlate with the diminution of scrapie agent titre. Denaturation of PrP 27–30 by boiling in SDS is accompanied by a diminution of prion titre and a change in the protease resistance of PrP 27–30 (Bolton et al, 1982, 1984).

(4)   The PrP gene (*Prn-p*) in mice is linked to a gene controlling scrapie incubation times (*Prn-i*) (Carlson et al, 1986). Prolonged incubation periods are a cardinal feature of both scrapie and CJD. The pre-eminent role of PrP in scrapie pathogenesis has been made all the more compelling by the discovery of a correlation between PrP amino acid sequence and scrapie incubation times (Westaway et al, 1987). Mice with short or intermediate incubation times express prion proteins which are distinct from those found in mice with long incubation times.

(5)   PrP 27–30 and scrapie infectivity partition together into many different forms: membranes, rods, spheres, detergent–lipid–protein complexes (DLPC) and liposomes. These dramatically different physical forms all contain PrP 27–30 and high prion titres (Barry et al, 1985; Gabizon et al, 1987; McKinley & Prusiner, 1986; Meyer et al, 1986; Prusiner et al, 1982, 1983, 1984). To date, all attempts to separate the scrapie PrP isoform (PrP^{Sc}) from infectivity have been unsuccessful.

(6)   Scrapie or CJD PrP proteins have been identified only in tissues of animals with transmissible neurodegenerative diseases and not in other disorders. These proteins have been detected in experimental scrapie of hamsters and mice, experimental CJD of mice as well as CJD, GSS and kuru of humans, but have not been found in control animals, mice with systemic amyloidosis or humans with AD, anoxic encephalopathy or non-neurological disorders (Bockman et al, 1985, 1987; Bolton et al, 1982, 1984; Gibbs et al, 1985; Kitamoto et al, 1986; Prusiner et al, 1982, 1983; Roberts et al, 1986). Thus, protease-resistant PrP molecules are highly specific for prion disease.

(7)   Cultured murine neuroblastoma cells have been infected with both

scrapie and CJD prions (Butler et al, 1988). Clones of the scrapie-infected cells were found to produce PrP^{Sc} while clones exhibiting no infectivity lacked PrP^{Sc}.

In addition to the seven lines of evidence presented above, preliminary studies suggest that PrP 27–30 antisera can neutralize scrapie infectivity in DLPC (Gabizon et al unpublished data). Earlier studies indicated that scrapie infectivity in amyloid rods could not be neutralized by PrP antibodies (Barry & Prusiner, 1987). The neutralization of scrapie infectivity in DLPC directly links PrP 27–30 with the infectious particle.

Investigators from many laboratories have confirmed the presence of PrP 27–30 in scrapie- or CJD-infected brains (Bockman et al, 1987; Diringer et al, 1983; Hope et al, 1986; Manuelidis et al, 1987). Although the amino acid sequence of PrP has been confirmed and there is agreement that PrP is glycosylated, some investigators have suggested that PrP 27–30 may not be a component of the scrapie agent (Braig & Diringer, 1985). One argument revolves around the inability of some investigators to detect PrP mRNA or PrP^{Sc} in spleens of scrapie-infected rodents (Chesebro et al, 1985; Czub et al, 1986). However, investigators in multiple laboratories have clearly shown that both PrP mRNA and PrP^{Sc} are present in spleen (McKinley et al, 1987a; Oesch et al, 1985; Rubenstein et al, 1986; Shinagawa et al, 1986). Another argument centres on experiments which demonstrate the loss of CJD infectivity bound to a lectin column. Neither denaturation of CJD PrP nor neutralization of CJD infectivity by immobilization on the lectin column matrix were considered as explanations (Manuelidis et al, 1987). Denaturation of PrP^{Sc} has been demonstrated to be accompanied by a loss of scrapie infectivity. Indeed, no experimental data have been presented where fractions with high levels of scrapie infectivity contain less than one PrP 27–30 molecule per infectious unit.

PRION PROTEIN ISOFORMS

Once the N-terminal amino acid sequence of PrP 27–30 was determined (Prusiner et al, 1984), oligonucleotides corresponding to a portion of this sequence were synthesized and used to identify a PrP cDNA (Chesebro et al, 1985; Oesch et al, 1985). Southern blotting with PrP cDNA revealed a single gene with the same restriction patterns in normal and scrapie-infected hamster brain DNA. Unexpectedly, PrP mRNA was found at similar levels in both normal and scrapie-infected hamster brain.

Using antisera raised against PrP 27–30, prion proteins of apparent molecular weight of 33,000 to 35,000 were detected in crude extracts of both normal and scrapie-infected brains (Oesch et al, 1985). In healthy cells, the product of the PrP gene is a protein designated PrP^C (Table 6.2) (Barry et al, 1986; Meyer et al, 1986; Oesch et al, 1985), which is susceptible to digestion by proteases (Barry et al, 1986; Barry & Prusiner, 1986; Meyer et al, 1986; Oesch et al, 1985). In contrast, the scrapie isoform PrP^{Sc} is resistant to proteases; proteinase K digestion of PrP^{Sc} yields PrP 27–30. Both PrP^C and PrP^{Sc} are membrane proteins, but upon detergent extraction, PrP^C is solubilized while PrP^{Sc} polymerizes into amyloid rods (Table 6.2). The polymerization of PrP^{Sc} in detergents provided a method to separate the two isoforms and show that scrapie-infected brains contain both PrP^C and PrP^{Sc} (Meyer et al, 1986).

Table 6.2 Prion protein isoforms

Properties	PrP^C	PrP^{Sc}
Normal hamster brain	~1 μg	Absent
Scrapie hamster brain	~1 μg	~10 μg
Protease digestion	Hydrolysed	PrP 27–30 formed
Detergent extraction	Solubilized	Polymerizes into amyloid
Isolated prions	Absent	Copurifies

The discovery of PrP^C may help explain one of the most puzzling questions in scrapie and CJD research. PrP^C may account for the lack of an immune response to a lethal 'slow infection' by rendering the host tolerant to the abnormal PrP isoform (PrP^{Sc}) (Oesch et al, 1985; Prusiner, 1982). The difficulties in raising antibodies to PrP 27–30 may be due, at least in part, to tolerance induced by PrP^C (Barry & Prusiner, 1986).

HAMSTER PRION PROTEIN GENE

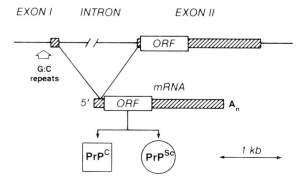

Fig. 6.2 Organization and expression of the hamster PrP gene. The features presented were deduced from the nucleotide sequences of PrP genomic and cDNA clones. Untranslated regions of the mRNA are represented by hatched boxes. An open reading frame or protein coding region is indicated by the open box. The diagonal lines show a splicing event that joins the 5' leader sequences to the remainder of the coding sequences. (Reprinted, by permission of Prusiner, 1987)

PRION PROTEIN GENES

The organization and structure of the hamster PrP gene has been elucidated; the entire open reading frame or protein coding region is contained within a single exon (Fig. 6.2) (Basler et al, 1986). The 5' end of the PrP gene contains multiple initiation sites, located between 82 and 50 nucleotides upstream of a splice donor site. The transcription start sites are preceded by a guanine (G): cytosine (C)-rich region which contains three direct repeats of the nonanucleotide GCCCCGCCC. This promoter structure is reminiscent of several 'housekeeping' genes. A 10,000 base intron follows the splice donor site. A splice acceptor precedes an uninterrupted block of protein coding sequence denoted as the open reading frame. A site which possesses all the features generally needed for initiation of protein synthesis is located 11 nucleotides downstream (or to the right) of the splice junction.

Both normal and scrapie-infected animals (75 days after inoculation) gave the same restriction patterns with these probes corresponding to: (1) the first exon; (2) the intron (Basler et al, 1986); and (3) the second exon (Oesch et al, 1985). From these results, rearrangements of the PrP gene are unlikely to figure in the pathogenesis of scrapie.

Since the entire protein coding region of the PrP gene is contained within exon II (Fig. 6.2), it is unlikely that PrP^C and PrP^{Sc} arise by alternative splicing exons. Thus, the two PrP isoforms appear to have the same amino acid sequence; presumably, the difference in the properties of the two proteins is due to a post-translational event (Basler et al, 1986).

STRUCTURE OF THE PRION PROTEIN

The hamster prion protein is initially synthesized as a polypeptide of 254 amino acids with subsequent cleavage of the first of 22 residues at the N-terminus which comprise a signal peptide (Fig. 6.3) (Basler et al, 1986; Hope et al, 1986). The first 67 amino acids of the mature PrP^{Sc} are not found in PrP 27–30; these amino acids are hydrolysed during purification which utilizes proteinase K digestion (Prusiner et al, 1982, 1983). The digested region of the protein contains an interesting set of repeated glycine-rich sequences. The significance of these repeats is unknown, but it is of interest that they are highly conserved among the hamster, mouse and human proteins (Chesebro et al, 1985; Kretzschmar et al, 1986b; Locht et al, 1986; Oesch et al, 1985). Since these repeats are hydrolysed when PrP 27–30 is generated and there is no loss of scrapie infectivity, they may be important for the cellular function of the prion protein.

Attempts to find meaningful sequence homologies for the PrP cDNA or its translated protein sequence with other macromolecules in computerized data bases have been unsuccessful, to date (Bazan et al, 1987).

Since the entire open reading frame of the PrP gene is found within exon II (Fig. 6.2) it is quite likely that both PrP^C and PrP^{Sc} are translated from the same mRNA and thus have the same amino acid sequence. The profound differences between the molecular properties of PrP^C and those of PrP^{Sc} presumably arise from post-translational events (Basler et al, 1986).

At present, there is evidence for six post-translational modifications of PrP. The first modification to be identified was glycosylation; PrP 27–30 is a sialoglycoprotein (Bolton et al, 1985; Prusiner et al, 1984). Both the cellular and scrapie PrP isoforms possess an intramolecular disulphide bond linking Cys residues 152 and 214 (Turk et al, 1987). Both PrP isoforms have N-linked oligosaccharides which can be removed by digestion with the enzyme peptide:

N-glycosidase F (Haraguchi et al, 1987). Digestion studies with this enzyme suggest that PrP^{Sc} may be glycosylated at two potential sites and the two oligosaccharides differ in their sugar sequences. The PrP amino acid sequence contains two *N*-glycosylation sites of the type Asn-X-Thr at codons 181 to 183 and 197 to 199 (Fig. 6.3) (Basler et al, 1986; Oesch et al, 1985). To date, there is no evidence for *0*-linked sugars. Like the *N*-terminal signal peptide which is cleaved during maturation of the prion protein (Basler et al, 1986; Bazan et al, 1987; Hay et al, 1987a; Hope et al, 1986), the *C*-terminal hydrophobic segment may also be removed (Oesch et al, 1985) and a phosphatidylinositol glycolipid added (Stahl et al, 1987). Both PrP^{Sc} and PrP^{C} possess complex glycolipids. Studies with cultured cells show that PrP^{C} is localized almost exclusively on the external surface of cultured neuronal cells and that it is anchored by the phosphatidylinositol glycolipid. An important avenue of future investigations will be to determine the cellular topology of PrP^{Sc}. Differences in the topology of the PrP isoforms might reflect post-translational modifications which account for their different properties.

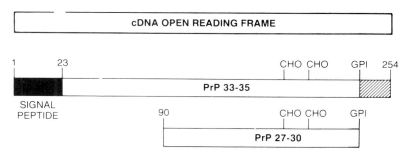

Fig. 6.3 Structure of the hamster prion protein (PrP). The open reading frame encodes a protein of 254 amino acids. The first 22 amino acids comprise a signal peptide which is cleaved during synthesis of PrP 33-35. Asn-linked oligosaccharides (CHO) are probably attached to amino acid residues 181 and 197. A *C*-terminal peptide is removed upon addition of a glycosyl phosphatidylinositol (GPI) moiety. The *C*-terminal amino acid residue remains to be determined. Digestion of the hamster scrapie isoform of PrP 33-35^{Sc} (PrP^{Sc}) with proteinase K generates a smaller protease-resistant polypeptide designated PrP 27-30.

HUMAN PRION PROTEINS

Protease-resistant prion proteins were found in the brains of patients dying of CJD (Bockman et al, 1987). Purified fractions from the brains of two patients with CJD were found to contain protease-resistant proteins ranging in apparent molecular weight from 10,000 to 50,000. These proteins reacted with antibodies raised against hamster scrapie PrP 27–30. Rod-shaped particles were found in sucrose gradient fractions prepared from the brains of these patients that were similar to those isolated from rodents with either scrapie or experimental CJD (Prusiner et al, 1983). After staining with Congo red dye, the protein polymers from patients with CJD exhibited green-gold birefringence when examined under polarized light, suggesting that the amyloid plaques found in the brains of CJD patients might be composed of paracrystalline arrays of prion proteins similar to those in scrapie. Recent studies show that this is the case not only in CJD but also in kuru (Kitamoto et al, 1986; Roberts et al, 1986).

Hybridization studies with human DNA (Oesch et al, 1985) and immunochemical investigations of CJD prion proteins (Bockman et al, 1985) implied that the human genome contains a PrP gene. The amino acid sequence of human PrP was deduced from a sequenced cDNA (Kretzschmar et al, 1986b) and aligned with the hamster sequence (Oesch et al, 1985; Basler et al, 1986). These protein sequences differ in length by one amino acid (253 vs 254) and there are 27 amino acid residues ($\sim 10\%$) which differ between the hamster and human sequences.

Recent studies have shown that CJD prion proteins exhibit species-specific epitopes. Human CJD prions have epitopes distinct from those found in mice. After transmission of human prions to mice, the resulting mouse CJD prion proteins have lost their human-specific epitopes (Bockman et al, 1987). These results are consistent with a cellular gene encoding PrP (Oesch et al, 1985).

HUMAN AND MOUSE PrP GENE CHROMOSOME LOCATIONS

Studies with somatic cell hybrids have localized the human PrP gene (PRNP) to chromosome 20 and the mouse PrP gene (*Prn-p*) to chromosome 2 (Sparkes et al, 1986). These assignments of the human and mouse PrP genes to homologous chromosomes provide additional evidence for the hypothesis that a common ancestor of man and mouse possessed a PrP gene. *In situ* hybridization studies have confirmed the assignment of the human PrP gene (PRNP) to chromosome 20 and have localized it to region 20p12h→pter (Robakis et al, 1986; Sparkes et al, 1986). The mouse PrP gene (*Prn-p*) has been located very near the inosine triphosphatase gene; it is flanked by the β_2 microglobulin gene and the agouti locus as determined by linkage analysis (Carlson et al, 1988). *Prn-p* is also tightly linked to a gene controlling the scrapie incubation time (*Prn-i*) (Carlson et al, 1986).

SCRAPIE AND CJD INCUBATION TIME GENES

A fascinating question in studies on prions concerns the molecular mechanism responsible for the prolonged incubation periods in scrapie and CJD. Early studies with sheep showed that the genetic background of the host could influence both their incubation times and susceptibility to scrapie (Parry, 1983). Dickinson and co-workers, using specific inbred strains of mice and 'strains' of scrapie agent, defined a genetic locus in mice which they labelled *Sinc* (Bruce & Dickinson, 1987; Dickinson & Meikle, 1971).

Two genes, *Pid-1* and *Prn-i*, which influence prion incubation periods in mice have been assigned to chromosomes 17 and 2, respectively. *Pid-1* is located within the D-subregion of the H-2 complex (Kingsbury et al, 1983). Of greater influence than *Pid-1* in both experimental scrapie and CJD is the *Prn-i* gene. The dominant allele of *Prn-i* codes for longer incubation times. Using a restriction fragment length polymorphism, *Prn-i* has been shown to be linked to the gene encoding the prion protein (*Prn-p*) (Carlson et al, 1986). Whether the *Prn-i* and *Prn-p* genes are separate but linked genes or identical genes remains to be determined (Fig. 6.4). To determine if the *Prn-i* and *Prn-p* genes are the same (Fig. 6.4B), the *Prn-p* gene from long incubation time mice must be cloned and injected into the fertilized embryos of short incubation time mice. If the resulting transgenic mice display long instead of short incubation times after inoculation with prions, then the identity of *Prn-i* and *Prn-p* will be established. Studies with congenic mice suggest that *Sinc* is linked to *Prn-p* raising the possibility that *Prn-i* and *Sinc* are the same genetic locus (Carp et al, 1987; Hunter et al, 1987).

PRION GENE COMPLEX *(Prn)*

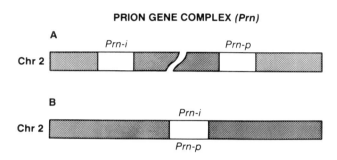

Fig. 6.4 Mouse PrP gene (*Prn-p*) is linked to the scrapie incubation time gene (*Prn-i*). Together *Prn-p* and *Prn-i* form the prion gene complex (*Prn*) on chromosome 2. Whether (A) *Prn-p* and *Prn-i* are different genes separated by as many as 1.4×10^6 base pairs or (B) they are the same gene remains to be established

The most compelling genetic evidence for a central role of PrP in scrapie pathogensis comes from molecular cloning which shows that inbred mice with short and long scrapie incubation times possess distinct prion proteins (Westaway et al, 1987). NZW mice with short incubation times have a PrP gene encoding a leucine at codon 109 and a threonine at 189. I/Ln mice with long incubation times have a phenylalanine codon at 109 and a valine at 190. While codon 109 is not conserved amongst humans, hamsters and most mice, codon 189 is. Using restriction fragment length polymorphism analysis, all mice with short and intermediate incubation times were found to possess a threonine at codon 189 and all three inbred strains of mice known to have long incubation times have a variant amino acid at this codon. The correlation between scrapie incubation times and PrP amino acid sequence emphasizes the pivotal role of PrP^{Sc} in scrapie pathogenesis. Moreover, these findings provide a novel explanation for the instability of scrapie agent 'strains' isolated in long incubation time mice. The change in scrapie agent characteristics upon passage from long to short mice may be a consequence of changing one or both of the above noted amino acids within the PrP molecule; however, not all aspects of scrapie 'strains' can be explained by this mechanism (Dickinson & Outram, 1979). Transgenic mice carrying altered PrP sequences especially at codons 109 and 189 should be useful in deciphering the significance of these amino acid variations in mice with long scrapie incubation periods.

In CJD and Kuru, incubation times of 30 years appear to be common (Alpers, 1979; Gajdusek 1977). Perhaps these studies will help explain why many degenerative diseases manifest themselves late in life. It is tempting to speculate that the prion 'clock' gene (*Prn-i*) might have a more general influence and possibly even play a role in the timing of senescence.

EXPRESSION OF PrP MrNA

In situ hybridization of normal and scrapie-infected hamster brains showed that neurons contain the highest levels of PrP mRNA (~50 copies per cell); glial cells contain less than three mRNA copies per cell (Kretzschmar et al, 1986a). These findings are in accord with the observation suggesting that CNS neurons are probably the only cell type which undergoes degeneration in prion diseases (Zlotnik, 1962).

Although PrP mRNA levels were unchanged throughout the course of scrapie infection (Oesch et al, 1985), we have found that the expression of the PrP gene is developmentally regulated (McKinley et al, 1987b). During the first 20 days after birth, PrP mRNA increases in the neonatal hamster brain at different rates in various regions of the brain. In the septum, the kinetics of the PrP mRNA increase parallel to those for choline acetyltransferase. Both PrP mRNA and choline acetyltransferase were stimulated by intraventricular injections of nerve growth factor (NGF) (Mobley et al, 1987). Stimulation of PrP gene transcription by NGF was unexpected since the G:C-rich promoter of the PrP gene is typical of 'housekeeping' genes (Fig. 6.2) (Basler et al, 1986). Similar promoters for other genes do not generally respond to hormones or trophic factors. By 20 days of age, PrP mRNA levels reach a maximum and apparently remain constant throughout the adult life of the hamster.

Interestingly, neonatal hamsters with low brain PrP mRNA levels exhibit significantly shorter scrapie incubation periods. And this acceleration in scrapie can be diminished by intracellular injections of NGF (McKinley et al, 1987c). Further studies are needed to decipher the role of PrP gene transcription in regulating the length of scrapie incubation times.

SCRAPIE AND CJD PRION PROTEINS FORM AMYLOIDS

Many investigators have used the electron microscope to search for a scrapie-specific particle. Spheres, rods, fibrils and tubules have been described in scrapie, kuru and CJD-infected brain tissue (see McKinley & Prusiner, 1986).

The first scrapie-specific structures to be identified by electron microscopy were spherical particles contained within postsynaptic evaginations of scrapie-infected mouse brains (David-Ferreira et al, 1968). Similar particles were found in scrapie-infected sheep brains (Bignami & Parry, 1971) and human brains from patients dying of CJD (Bots et al, 1971). Some investigators were unable to identify these scrapie-associated particles within infected hamster brains (Baringer et al, 1979), but others have recently reported their presence (Narang et al, 1987).

In crude extracts of scrapie-infected rodent brains, fibrillar structures were found and differentiated from amyloids by their well defined morphology. Two types of fibrils consisting of either two or four helically wound subfilaments were reported and labelled scrapie-associated fibrils (SAF) types I and II, respectively (Merz et al, 1981). The regular periodic crossings of the subfilaments as well as the spaces between them were used to distinguish SAF from both amyloids and other filamentous structures (Merz et al, 1981, 1984). Ignoring the fine structure, some investigators have chosen to assign the term, SAF, to the prion amyloid rods (Diener, 1987a; Diringer et al, 1983) described below. While the prion amyloid rods are composed largely, if not entirely, of scrapie or CJD prion proteins (Prusiner et al, 1982, 1983, 1984), the composition of the SAF types I and II as orginally described remains to be established (Diener, 1987a). One investigator has raised the possibility that SAF are composed of the N-terminal portion of PrP^{Sc} which is digested by proteinase formation of PrP 27–30 (Clawson, 1988).

In purified fractions prepared from scrapie-infected brains, rod-shaped particles were found measuring 10 to 20 nm in diameter and 100 to 200 nm in length (Barry et al, 1985; Prusiner et al, 1982, 1983, 1984). Although no unit morphologic structure could be identified, most of the rods exhibited a relatively uniform diameter and appeared as flattened cylinders (Fig. 6.5A). Some of the rods had a twisted structure suggesting that they might be composed of protofilaments, but no consistent substructure could be discerned. Similar rod-shaped particles were isolated from the brains of humans dying of the CJD (Bockman et al, 1985): one patient presented with a cerebellar syndrome and later exhibited a profound dementia (Fig. 6.5B) while another presented with a typical, rapidly progressive dementing illness (Fig. 6.5C). The heterogenous morphology of the prion rods and the lack of consistent structure distinguishes them from viruses.

The ultrastructure of the prion rods is, on the other hand, indistinguishable from many purified amyloids (Prusiner et al, 1983). Histochemical studies with Congo red dye have extended this analogy to purified preparations of prions (McKinley & Prusiner, 1986) as well as to scrapie-infected brain where amyloid plaques have been shown to stain with antibodies to PrP 27–30 (Bendheim et al, 1984). In addition, PrP 27–30 has been found to stain with periodic acid Schiff reagent (Bolton et al, 1985); amyloid plaques in tissue sections readily bind this reagent.

Immunocytochemical studies with antibodies to PrP 27–30 have shown that filaments measuring approximately 16 nm in diameter and up to 1500 nm in length within amyloid plaques of scrapie-infected hamster brain are composed of prion proteins (De Armond et al, 1985). The prion filments have a relatively uniform diameter, rarely show narrowings and possess all the morphological features of amyloids. Except for their length, the prion filaments appear to be identical ultrastucturally with the rods which are found in purified fractions of prions (Figure 6.5A).

NEUROPATHOLOGY OF PRION DISEASES

A prominent and very characteristic feature of prion diseases is the lack of any inflammatory response. In both the brain and eye, prions replicate to near maximal titres before any neuropathological changes are detected (Hogan et al, 1986).

A reactive astrocytosis is found throughout the CNS in all of these disorders (Beck & Daniel, 1979; McKinley et al, 1987b). The extent of astrocytic hypertrophy is generally out of proportion to the degree of neuronal cell damage. Both increased amounts of glial fibrillary acidic protein (GFAP) polymerised into glial filaments (Fig. 6.6A), as well as increased levels of GFAP mRNA have been observed during prion infections (De Armond et al, 1987a; Zlotnik, 1962).

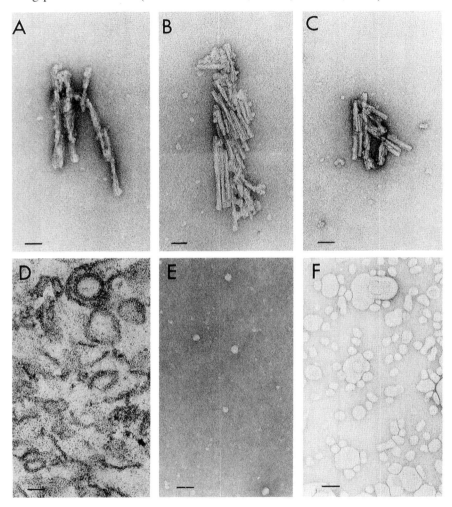

Fig. 6.5 Ultrastructure of the multiple forms of hamster scrapie and human Creutzfeldt-Jakob disease prions. (A) Purified prion amyloid rods which are generated upon detergent extraction of membranes from scrapie-infected brain. (B and C) Human Creutzfeldt-Jakob disease prion rods in purified preparations from a patient who had a cerebellar syndrome on initial evaluation and later had a profound dementia (B) and from a patient who had a typical, rapidly progressive dementing illness on initial evaluation. (D) Microsomal membrane containing prions. (E) Spheres generated from extensive sonication of rods and isolated by sedimentation through a sucrose gradient. (F) Infectious prion liposomes. All structures were negatively strained with uranyl formate and viewed in a JEOL 100B electron microscope at 80 kev. Bar = 50 nm. (Photomicrographs taken by Michael P McKinley). (Reprinted by permission of Prusiner, 1987)

In most cases of prion diseases, neuronal vacuolation is a prominent feature. Usually the grey matter is most affected but vacuolation of the white matter has been reported (Beck & Daniel, 1979; Tateishi et al, 1979; Zlotnik, 1962). Coalescence of intracellular vacuoles into larger ones within the neuropil is called spongiform degeneration (Fig. 6.6B) (Masters & Richardson, 1978). One hypothesis suggests that the abnormal PrP isoform disrupts normal membrane processing which leads to the formation of vacuoles (De Armond et al, 1987a). The prominence of widespread vacuolation in some prion diseases has led some investigators to label these diseases 'transmissible spongiform encephalopathy'. However, spongiform change is rare in natural scrapie of sheep (Kretzschmar et al, 1986a), and some cases of CJD fail to exhibit recognizable vacuolation at the light microscopic level (Prusiner, 1982).

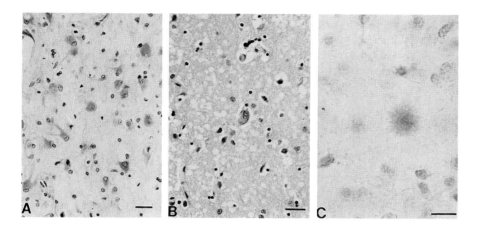

Fig. 6.6 Neuropathological changes in human Creutzfeldt-Jakob disease. (A) Cerebral cortex stained by peroxidase immunohistochemistry for glial fibrillary acid protein (GFAP) with haematoxylin counterstain showing intense reactive astrocytic gliosis, marked nerve cell loss, and status spongiosis. Bar = 100 um. (B) Putamen stained with haematoxylin and eosin showing spongiform degeneration of the neuropil, little nerve cell loss, and little reactive astrocytic gliosis. Bar = 50 um. (C) Prion amyloid plaques in the granular layer of the cerebellar cortex strain intensely with rabbit antiserum raised against purified hamster scrapie PrP 27-30 molecules. The staining employed peroxidase immunohistochemistry with haematoxylin counterstain. Bar = 20 um. (Photomicrographs taken by Stephen J DeArmond). (Reprinted, by permission of Prusiner, 1987)

Neither astrocytosis nor neuronal vacuolation are pathognomonic changes, but their presence in the CNS of hosts with neurological dysfunction is highly suggestive of a prion disease. Until recently, the transmissibility of CNS disease to experimental animals was required to establish with certainty the diagnosis of a prion disorder. The presence of protease-resistant PrP molecules in extracts of infected brain tissue (Bockman et al, 1985, 1987; Gibbs et al, 1985) as well as specific immunostaining of amyloid plaques (Kitamoto et al, 1986; Roberts et al, 1986) has provided a rapid method for establishing the diagnosis of CJD and GSS (Fig. 6.6C).

Using PrP monoclonal antibodies, PrP^C was found confined to cell bodies of neurons (De Armond et al, 1987b). During scrapie infection, PrP immunoreactivity in neuronal cell bodies disappears but becomes very intense within the dendritic trees. How these changes in PrP localization feature in the pathogenesis of scrapie and its attendant neurological dysfunction remains to be established.

PRP 27–30 AND SCRAPIE INFECTIVITY CO-PARTITION INTO LIPOSOMES

Numerous studies emphasized the association of scrapie infectivity with membranes (Hunter, 1979). Detergent extraction of membrane-containing fractions led to the production of infectious particles displaying a continuum of sizes (Prusiner et al, 1978). Only recently has this detergent-induced transition of scrapie infectivity from a membrane form to a rod form been understood (Meyer et al, 1986). The prion rods in purified preparations are created upon detergent extraction of membrane containing PrP^{Sc} (Fig. 6.5D) (Meyer et al, 1986). Detergent extraction of membrane containing only PrP^{c} did not produce rods. These observations support the hypothesis that the rods are aggregates of prions (Prusiner et al, 1982, 1983).

Sonication of the prion rods reduced their mean length to 60 nm and generated many spherical particles without altering infectivity titres (Fig. 6.5E) (McKinley & Prusiner, 1986). The rods were found to be dissociated under non-denaturing conditions with a combination of cholate and phosphatidylcholine (PC). The resulting DLPC as well as liposomes, frequently showed a 10- to 50-fold increase in scrapie infectivity. Electron microscopy showed that the rods (Fig. 6.5A) were completely disrupted upon the formation of lipsomes (Fig. 6.5F).

The increase in infectivity and the decrease in size as measured by sedimentation, electron microscopy and light scattering, all argue for a profound change in the physical state of the scrapie agent upon the incorporation into phospholipid vesicles (Gabizon et al, 1987). We estimate the average number of PrP 27–30 molecules per liposome is between two and four which is in accord with earlier ionizing radiation and size exclusion chromatography studies suggesting that the smallest infectious unit of the scrapie agent has a molecular weight of $< 10^5$ (Alper et al, 1966; Prusiner, 1982). Recent studies show that the ionizing radiation target size is independent of the prion form. Scrapie-infected hamster brain homogenates, microsomal membranes, purified rods and DLPC all exhibited virtually identical ionizing radiation survival curves giving a target size of $55,000 \pm 9000$ daltons (Bellinger-Kawahara et al, 1988).

SEARCH FOR A PRION NUCLEIC ACID

The molecular cloning of a PrP cDNA provided a highly sensitive probe with which to search for PrP-related nucleic acids within the infectious prion. No PrP-related nucleic acids were found in purified preparations of scrapie prions indicating that PrP^{Sc} is not encoded by a nucleic acid carried within the infectious particles (Oesch et al, 1985).

Many attempts to demonstrate the dependence of scrapie agent infectivity upon a nucleic acid have failed over the past two decades (Alper et al, 1967; Bellinger-Kawahara et al, 1987a, 1987b; Diener et al, 1982; Hunter, 1979; Prusiner, 1982). Reports on the identification of scrapie-specific nucleic acids have not been reproducible (Dees et al, 1985; Gilles et al, 1987; Malone et al, 1979; Prusiner et al, 1980a).

The transfer of scrapie infectivity from rods to liposomes provided a new method by which to search for a hidden or cryptic nucleic acid within the prion. Treatment of DLPC as well as liposomes with nucleases, Zn^{++} or psoralens failed to alter scrapie infectivity (Gabizon et al, 1987). While liposomes have been used to protect nucleic acids by entrapping them within vesicles, this is not the case in the presence of detergent where DLPC or fragments of vesicles are formed. The resistance of both purified prion rods and DLPC to ultraviolet irradiation at 254 nm has also been examined (Bellinger-Kawahara et al, 1987a; Gabizon et al, 1988). Both forms of the scrapie agent yielded similar inactivation curves, indicating that if prions possess a nucleic acid, it is likely to be < 5 bases for a single-stranded molecule and 30–45 base pairs for a double-stranded one.

Some investigators continue to argue that the scrapie and CJD agents must possess intrinsic nucleic acids (Braig & Diringer, 1985; Manuelidis et al, 1987; Merz et al, 1984) while others suggest that they may be devoid of nucleic acid but prefer to label them 'viruses' (Gajdusek, 1986). Still other investigators argue that 'strains' of scrapie agent demand a nucleic acid within the infectious particle (Bruce & Dickinson, 1987; Dickinson & Outram, 1988). Changes in properties of scrapie agent 'strains' have been reported, but the evidence that these changes are due to mutations within a scrapie-specific nucleic acid is not convincing. Moreover, studies described above indicate that PrP molecules isolated from short and long incubation period mice have distinct PrP molecules (Westaway et al, 1987). Differences in PrP sequence correlate with the length of the scrapie incubation period and could provide an epigenetic mechanism to explain much of the instability observed with various scrapie agent isolates. Interestingly, some investigators report that different 'strains' of scrapie agent exhibit different PrP immunoblot patterns (Kascsak et al, 1986).

HOW DO PRIONS REPRODUCE?

Compelling evidence presented above argues that the infectious particles causing scrapie are not viruses. Yet these particles clearly multiply. One infectious unit causing scrapie inoculated into a weanling hamster initiates a multiplication process which results in the production of 10^9 infectious units during the ensuing ~130 day period. This increase in the number of prions resembles the replication of viruses and contrasts with protein toxins which do not multiply. Several models for the multiplication of prions can be proposed (Fig. 6.7). If prions contain a small nucleic acid molecule, then this nucleic acid might stimulate the production of PrP^{Sc}. As new copies of the hypothetical small nucleic acid are synthesized, they would combine with PrP^{Sc} to form a highly stable complex which is infectious. Alternatively, prions may be devoid of nucleic acid and PrP^{Sc} stimulates its own synthesis either directly or through a cascade of reactions. If the *Prn-i* and Prp genes are separate (Fig. 6.4A), then one model for prion multiplication might involve PrP^{Sc} forming a complex with the product of the *Prn-i* gene or some other macromolecule. Such a complex would stimulate or catalyse the formation of new PrP^{Sc} molecules. Another possibility is that a PrP^{Sc} oligomer stimulates the biosynthesis of new PrP scrapie molecules, PrP^{C} and PrP^{Sc}, and it will be possible to erect more specific hypotheses. Indeed, if prions are composed only of protein molecules, the term 'amplification' might be more appropriate than replication or infection in describing the multiplication of these novel pathogens.

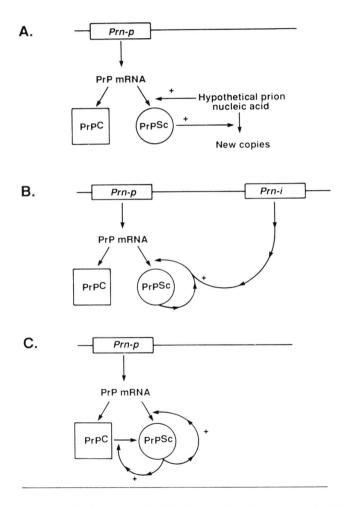

Fig. 6.7 Some possible models for prion multiplication. (A) Small, as yet undetected, prion-specific nucleic acid triggers the synthesis of PrP^{Sc} and together these two molecules form a new prion. (B) PrP^{Sc} combines with the *Prn-i* gene product to stimulate the synthesis of more PrP^{Sc}. (C) PrP^{Sc} by itself triggers a series of reactions which produce more PrP^{Sc} molecules.

Most PrP^{Sc} and prion infectivity is associated with membranes in scrapie-infected tissues, but a fraction of the PrP^{Sc} is polymerized into filaments which coalesce to form amyloid plaques within the extracellular space (Fig. 6.8) (De Armond et al, 1985). Detergent extraction of the membranes isolated from scrapie-infected brains produces rod-shaped polymers composed largely, if not entirely, of PrP^{Sc} or PrP 27–30 (Meyer et al, 1986). Sonication of the rods produces spherical particles composed of PrP 27–30 which retain their infectivity (McKinley & Prusiner, 1986). Boiling the rods in SDS leads to their dissociation, but under these denaturing conditions, PrP 27–30 is rendered protease sensitive and infectivity is diminished (Prusiner et al, 1983, 1984). In contrast, addition of cholate and PC to the rods produces DLPC which retain all of the scrapie infectivity (Gabizon et al, 1987). Removal of the cholate by dialysis leads to the formation of closed liposomes which are also infectious. Extraction of the PC with chloroform: methanol resulted in repolymerization of PrP 27–30 into rods with retention of scrapie infectivity.

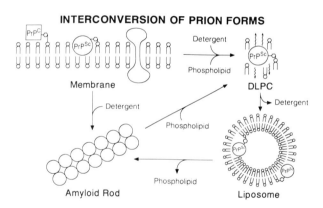

Fig. 6.8 Multiple molecular forms of prions. Scrapie and CJD prions are found associated with membranes. Whether the prion amyloid filaments forming plaques are infectious is unknown. Extraction of membranes from scrapie – or CJD-infected brains – produces prion amyloid rods. Denaturation of PrP 27-30 by boiling in SDS causes dissociation of the amyloid rods. Extensive sonication fragments the rods, and mixing the rods with phospholipid and detergent leads to the formation of DLPC. Removal of detergent produces closed liposomes, and organic solvent extraction of the liposomes recreates the prion amyloid rods.

The existence of multiple forms of prions argues that these particles are likely to be composed of a single type of macromolecule. The membrane, rod and liposome forms of prions favour the macromolecule being a protein. Presumably, hydrophobic interactions are the driving force for the changes in both size and morphology of prions (Fig. 6.8) (Gabizon et al, 1987; Prusiner et al, 1978). Indeed, all the known features of PrP^{Sc} structure are compatible with the hypothesis that PrP^{Sc} is a major, or possibly the only, component of the prion. Despite the profound morphological alterations which prions can undergo during their conversion from one form to another, the dose of ionizing radiation required to inactivate prions remained constant. Exponential survival curves indicate that a single prion is inactivated by one ionization and gives target size of ∼55,000 daltons (Bellinger-Kawahara et al, 1988). This estimate is consistent with the hypothesis that prions may be composed of two PrP^{Sc} molecules. Not only are the multiple forms of scrapie prions uncharacteristic of viruses, but they are incompatible with the structure of viruses which are highly organized entities consisting of water soluble polynucleotides surrounded by a protein lattice or capsid.

The possibility that scrapie is caused by a highly efficient virus (Oesch et al, 1985) has been considered and the ability of prions to exist in multiple forms has been used in searching for this putative 'scrapie virus'. Assuming that the 'scrapie virus' is a filamentous structure, as some investigators have suggested (Merz et al, 1984) and that it is hidden amongst the amyloid rods, then this virus should be detectable among infectious prion liposomes. Using the rod-shaped tobacco mosaic virus as a control, virions could be readily detected by electron microscopy when they were added to the liposomes at a concentration of ‹ 1% of the prion titre; no other elongated particles were discerned demonstrating that a rod-shaped or filamentous 'scrapie virus' does not exist (Gabizon et al, 1987). It is noteworthy that this ultrastructural approach alone could not be used to eliminate the possibility of a spherical 'scrapie virus', but there are no data to support its existence.

PATHOGENIC MECHANISMS IN PRION DISEASES

The three human prion diseases (kuru, CJD and GSS) are probably variants of the same disorder (Alpers, 1987). By analogy with experimental scrapie, it seems likely that all three of these human diseases will require the appearance of an abnormal PrP isoform. Both chromosomal localization (Sparkes et al, 1986) and Southern analyses of human DNA suggest that the human PrP gene is single copy (Hsiao et al, 1987; Oesch et al, 1985; Wu et al, 1987).

The human prion disease illustrates three mechanisms by which CNS degeneration might arise: (1) slow infection; (2) sporadic disease; and (3) genetic disorders (Table 6.3) (Ridley et al, 1986). That these three diseases can be transmitted by inoculation to experimental animals is well documented (Gajdusek et al, 1966; Gibbs et al, 1968; Masters et al, 1981b). Kuru is thought to have been spread exclusively through a slow infectious mechanism by ritualistic cannibalism (Alpers, 1979; Gajdusek, 1977).

Table 6.3 Human prion diseases

Pathogenic mechanism	Disease
Infectious	Kuru (CJD)
Sporadic	CJD
Genetic	GSS (CJD)

While a few CJD cases can be traced to inoculation with prions, i.e. human growth hormone (Gibbs et al, 1985), cornea transplantation and cerebral electrode implantation, the vast majority appear to be sporadic despite considerable effort to implicate scrapie-infected sheep as an exogenous source (Gajdusek, 1977). Though unlikely, it is still possible that sporadic CJD results from prions being ubiquitous in the human chain and having a very low efficiency of infection. Scrapie infection in hamsters by oral route was found to be 10^9 times less efficient than intracerebral inoculation (Prusiner et al, 1985). Whether or not CJD can arise endogenously without any molecules being contributed from an exogenous source remains to be established. If it is then possible for prions to arise endogenously, then it will be important to identify the macromolecule or events which initiate their synthesis.

GSS seems to represent the genetic form of prion disease although 10 to 15% of CJD may also have a genetic basis (Masters et al, 1981b). The genetic mechanism whereby patients develop GSS during their fifth decade of life is unknown. One possibility is that a genetic locus renders these individuals susceptible to infection by exogenous prions. Genetic control of the scrapie and CJD incubation periods in mice after inoculation with prions is well documented (Carlson et al, 1986; Dickinson & Meikle, 1971; Kingsbury et al, 1983). Alternatively, GSS might be due to a gene which activates the synthesis of the abnormal isoform of PrP as well as any other components of the prion, if they exist. Whether or not the PrP gene in GSS patients is different from that in unaffected family members is unknown.

Certainly, all of the considerations raised by these three forms of prion disease are equally compatible with an infectious particle which either possesses a nucleic acid or is devoid of one. However, the former would require that the putative prion-specific nucleic acid be widespread in susceptible mammals all over the planet.

NEURODEGENERATIVE DISEASE

Among the most devastating disorders of older age are neurodegenerative diseases. Such disorders include: Alzheimer's disease (AD), amyotrophic lateral sclerosis (ALS), Parkinson's disease (PD), Huntington's disease, CJD and GSS.

The causes of most neurodegenerative diseases are unknown. Genetic, infectious, metabolic, toxic, immunological and atrophic aetiologies have been proposed for AD, ALS and PD. The lack of animal models, which faithfully reproduce all aspects of most neurodegenerative disorders, is one of the major obstacles impeding investigation.

The lack of AD transmissibility to experimental animals was the first evidence suggesting that the aetiological molecules in AD were not CJD prions even though the two diseases share many clinical and pathological features (Goudsmit et al, 1980). On the other hand, studies on prions have shown that cerebral amyloids may not be inert waste products as many investigators had assumed (Bendheim et al, 1984; De Armond et al, 1985; Prusiner et al, 1983). While this discovery intensified interest in the possible aetiological role of amyloid proteins in AD (Prusiner, 1984), subsequent studies have shown that the major AD protein of vascular amyloid and probably senile plaques is unrelated to PrP based on sequencing (Glenner & Wong, 1984; Masters et al, 1985) as well as immunostaining studies (Bockman et al, 1987; Kitamoto et al, 1986; Roberts et al, 1986). The amyloid proteins comprising neurofibrillary tangles are less well characterized.

Of particular interest is the recent finding that the gene encoding the vascular and plaque AD amyloid β-protein is located on chromosome 21 (Goldgaber et al, 1987; Kang et al, 1987; Robakis et al, 1987; Tanzi et al, 1987). The amyloid β-protein gene as well as a genetic locus for familial AD map to region 21q21; however, this region of chromosome 21 is not required for Down's syndrome (St George-Hyslop et al, 1987).

It is well documented that individuals with Down's syndrome or trisomy 21 who live beyond 40 years of age develop the cerebral amyloid accumulations characteristic of AD. Studies with a mouse model of Down's syndrome (trisomy 16 chimeras) have shown that after inoculation with prions, the onset of clinical scrapie and subsequently death is accelerated compared with that in non-trisomic control chimeras (Epstein et al, 1987). The mechanism by which scrapie is accelerated in these Down's mice is unknown.

It will be important to define the human prion gene complex and learn whether any gene within the complex or nearby plays a role in the pathogenesis of AD. Presumably, a human prion incubation time gene controls the timing of CJD, GSS and kuru. Perhaps this same clock gene regulates the age-dependent susceptibility observed in one or more of some common CNS degenerative diseases such as AD, PD and ALS. Of interest are familial pedigrees which contain multiple cases of both AD and CJD (Masters et al, 1981a).

FRONTIERS OF PRION RESEARCH

While recent research on prions has begun to define the molecular structure of these fascinating pathogens, their complete structure remains to be elucidated. Although the mechanism by which prions replicate is unknown, considerable evidence indicates that replication, at least in part, requires the conversion of a normal cellular protein (PrP^C) or its precursor to an abnormal isoform (PrP^{Sc}). It is likely that the formation of PrP^{Sc} results from a post-translational event (Basler et al, 1986). Defining the chemical and/or conformational differences between PrP^C and PrP^{Sc} is of paramount importance as is learning how to synthesize biologically active prions. Whether prions are composed only of PrP^{Sc} oligomers or contain additional macromolecules such as polynucleotides remains unresolved.

How prions spread from one cell to another is unknown, but secretion must be considered since biogenesis studies have demonstrated a secretory form of PrP (Hay et al, 1987b). Whether prions enter uninfected cells by binding to specific receptors or by partitioning into cell membranes remains to be established. Another major question in prion research concerns the cellular function of PrP^C. Since PrP^C is found almost exclusively on the surface of cells, this observation suggests a cell recognition or adhesion molecule, an enzyme, a receptor or even a hormone-like factor. It will be important to learn about the topology of PrP^{Sc}

relative to PrP^C since this may give new insights into the structural differences between these two isoforms.

The current study of prions may represent a point of departure for future investigations of a whole wastebasket (Krevans, 1963) of degenerative diseases. The cellular origin of prion proteins and the slow amplification mechanisms which account for the replication of prions make these unique macromolecules interesting candidates to explore with respect to many diseases that occur later in life. More important, the study of prion diseases has emphasized the need to learn how normal cellular proteins are converted into abnormal isoforms which polymerize into insoluble filaments (Prusiner, 1984).

Although AD and PD have not been transmitted to experimental animals (Gajdusek, 1977), abnormal protein polymers do accumulate in AD as amyloids and PD as Lewy body filaments; whether these polymers feature in the aetiology of these disorders or they accumulate only as pathological products remains to be determined (Prusiner, 1984). Placed in the most general context, studies on prions raise the possibility that infectious, environmental and genetically programmed events may signal the conversion of normal, necessary proteins into malignant, lethal molecules by modifications which occur after polypeptide chains are assembled. Though seemingly remote, knowledge about prions might also be applicable to studies on some systemic degenerative disorders; for example, amyloids have been found to accumulate in the pancreas of some diabetic patients.

The studies reviewed here demonstrate that the approaches developed first for the investigation of experimental scrapie in rodents are directly applicable to the study of CNS degeneration in humans caused by CJD prions. Because of new knowledge about scrapie and CJD prions, any clinical description of prion diseases in humans must be considered provisional and incomplete. Research on human prions is in its infancy, but the availability of both PrP antibodies and cDNA probes should lead to an explosion of new information about the classification, aetiology, clinical course, pathogenesis and intervention during the next decade.

Acknowledgements
This paper has been adapted from an article published in the New England Journal of Medicine 317: 1517–1518, 1987. Important contributions from Drs R Barry, J Bockman, S DeArmond, R Gabizon, S Kent, V Lingappa, M McKinley, B Oesch, M Scott, N Stahl and D Westaway are gratefully acknowledged. Collaborative studies with Drs G Carlson, J Cleaver, T Diener, W Hadlow, L Hood, E Kempner, D Kingsbury, D Riesner and C Weissmann are greatly appreciated. The author thanks K Bowman, S Coleman, D Groth, M Peterson and M Walchli for technical assistance as well as L Gallagher for manuscript production assistance.

The following abbreviations are used throughout this paper:

AD – Alzheimer's Disease
AIDS – Acquired Immune Deficiency Syndrome
ALS – Amyotrophic Lateral Sclerosis

CJD – Creutzfeldt-Jakob Disease
CNS – Central Nervous System
CSF – Cerebro Spinal Fluid
DLPC – Detergent-Lipid-Protein Complexes
GFAP – Glial Fibrillary Acidic Protein
GSS – Gerstmann-Sträussler Syndrome
PC – Phosphatidylcholine
PD – Parkinson's Disease
PRNP – Human PrP Gene
SAF – Scrapie Associated Fibrils
SDS – Sodium Dodecyl Sulfate.

REFERENCES

Alper T, Haig D A, Clarke M C 1966 The exceptionally small size of the scrapie agent. Biochemical and Biophysical Research Communications 22: 278–284
Alper T, Cramp W A, Haig D A, Clarke M C 1967 Does the agent of scrapie replicate without nucleic acid? Nature 214: 764–766
Alpers M P 1979 Epidemiology and ecology of kuru. In: Prusiner S B, Hadlow W J (eds) Slow transmissible diseases of the nervous system, vol 1. Academic Press, New York, pp 67–92
Alpers M P 1987 Epidemiology and clinical aspects of kuru. In: Prusiner S B, McKinley M P (eds) Prions—novel infectious pathogens causing scrapie and Creutzfeldt-Jakob disease. Academic Press, Orlando, pp 451–465
Baringer J R, Wong J, Klassen T, Prusiner S B 1979 Further observations on the neuropathology of experimental scrapie in mouse and hamster. In: Prusiner S B, Hadlow W J (eds) Slow transmissible diseases of the nervous system, vol 2. Academic Press, New York, pp 111–121
Barre Sinoussi F, Nugeyre M, Dauguet C et al 1983 Isolation of a T-lymphotropic retrovirus from a patient at risk for acquired immune deficiency syndrome. Science 220: 868–871
Barry R A, McKinley M P, Bendheim P E, Lewis G K, DeArmond S J, Prusiner S B 1985 Antibodies to the scrapie protein decorate prion rods. Journal of Immunology 135: 603–613
Barry R A, Kent S B, McKinley M P et al 1986 Scrapie and cellular prion proteins share polypeptide epitopes. Journal of Infectious Diseases 153: 848-854
Barry R A, Prusiner S B 1986 Monoclonal antibodies to the cellular and scrapie prion proteins. Journal of Infectious Diseases 154: 518–521
Barry R A, Prusiner S B Immunology of prions. 1987 In: Prusiner S B, McKinley M P (eds) Prions—novel infectious pathogens causing scrapie and Creutzfeldt-Jakob disease. Academic Press, Orlando, pp 239–275
Basler K, Oesch B, Scott M et al 1986 Scrapie and cellular PrP isoforms are encoded by the same chromosomal gene. Cell 46: 417–428
Bazan J F, Fletterick R J, McKinley M P, Prusiner S M 1987 Predicted secondary structure and membrane topology of the scrapie prion protein. Protein Engineering 1: 125–135
Beck E, Daniel P M 1979 Kuru and Creutzfeldt-Jakob disease; neuropathological lesions and their significance. In: Prusiner S B, Hadlow W J (eds) Slow transmissible diseases of the nervous system, vol 1. Academic Press, New York, pp 253–270
Bellinger-Kawahara C G, Cleaver J E, Diener T O, Prusiner S B 1987a Purified scrapie prions resist inactivation by ultraviolet irradiation. Journal of Virology 61: 159–166
Bellinger-Kawahara C G, Diener T O, McKinley M P, Groth D F, Smith D R, Prusiner S B 1987b Purified scrapie prions resist inactivation by procedures that hydrolyze, modify, or shear nucleic acids. Virology 160: 271–274
Bellinger-Kawahara C G, Kempner E, Groth D, Gabizon R, Prusiner S B 1988 Scrapie prion liposomes and rods exhibit target sizes of 55,000 daltons. Virology 164: 537–541
Bendheim P E, Barry R A, DeArmond S J, Stites D P, Prusiner S B 1984 Antibodies to a scrapie prion protein. Nature 310: 418–421
Bignami A, Parry H B 1971 Aggregation of 35-nanometer particles associated with neuronal cytopathic changes in natural scrapie. Science 171: 389–391
Bockman J M, Kingsbury D T, McKinley M P, Bendheim P E, Prusiner S B 1985 Creutzfeldt-Jakob disease proteins in human brains. New England Journal of Medicine 312: 73–78

Bockman J M, Prusiner S B, Tateishi J, Kingsbury D T 1987 Immunoblotting of Creutzfeldt-Jakob disease prion proteins—host species-specific epitopes. Annals of Neurology 21: 589–595

Bolton D C, McKinley M P, Prusiner S B 1982 Identification of a protein that purifies with the scrapie prion. Science 218: 1309–1311

Bolton D C, McKinley M P, Prusiner S B 1984 Molecular characteristics of the major scrapie prion protein. Biochemistry 23: 5898–5905

Bolton D C, Meyer R K, Prusiner S B 1985 Scrapie PrP 27–30 is a sialoglyco-protein. Journal of Virology 53: 595–606

Bots G, Th A M, DeMan J C H, Verjaal A 1971 Virus-like particles in brain tissue from two patients with Creutzfeldt-Jakob disease. Acta Neuropathologica (Berlin) 18: 267–270

Braig H, Diringer H 1985 Scrapie: a concept of a virus-induced amyloidosis of the brain. EMBO Journal 4: 2309–2312

Brown P, Cathala F, Castaigne P, Gajdusek D C 1986 Creutzfeldt-Jakob disease; clinical analysis of a consecutive series of 230 neuropathologically verified cases. Annals of Neurology 20: 597–602

Bruce M E, Dickinson A G 1987 Biological evidence that scrapie agent has an independent genome. Journal of General Virology 68: 79–89

Butler D A, Scott M R D, Bockman J M et al 1988 Scrapie-infected murine neuroblastoma cells produce protease-resistant prion proteins. Journal of Virology 62: 1558–1564

Carlson G A, Kingsbury D T, Goodman P et al 1986 Prion protein and scrapie incubation time genes are linked. Cell 46: 503–511

Carlson G A, Westaway D, Goodman P A, Peterson M, Marshall S T, Prusiner S B 1988 Genetic control of prion incubation period in mice. In: Marsh J (ed) Novel infectious agents and the central nervous system, Ciba Foundation Symposium No 135 John Wiley and Sons, London 84–94

Carp R I, Merz P A, Kascak R J, Merz G S, Wisinewski H M 1985 Nature of the scrapie agent: current status of facts and hypotheses. Journal of General Virology 66: 1357–1368

Carp R I, Moretz R C, Natelli M, Dickinson A G 1987 Genetic control of scrapie: incubation period and plaque formation in I mice. Journal of General Virology 68: 401–407

Chamberlin T C The method of multiple working hypotheses. 1890 Science 15: 92 (Reprinted in: Science 1965; 148: 754–759)

Chesebro B, Race R, Wehrly K et al 1985 Identification of scrapie prion protein-specific mRNA in scrapie-infected and uninfected brain. Nature 315: 331–333

Clawson G A 1988 Antiheretical speculations on the 'prion' protein and scrapie. Perspectives in Biology and Medicine 31: 212–223

Czub M, Braig H R, Blode H, Diringer H 1986 The major protein of SAF is absent from spleen and thus not an essential part of the scrapie agent. Archives of Virology 91: 383–386

David-Ferreira J F, David-Ferreira K L, Gibbs C J Jr, Morris J A 1968 Scrapie in mice: ultrastructural observations in the cerebral cortex. Proceedings of the Society for Experimental Biology and Medicine 127: 313–320

DeArmond S J, McKinley M P, Barry R A, Braunfeld M B, McColloch J R, Prusiner S B 1985 Identification of prion amyloid filaments in scrapie-infected brain. Cell 41: 221–235

DeArmond S J, Kretzschmar H A, McKinley M P, Prusiner S B 1987a Molecular pathology of prion diseases. In: Prusiner S B, McKinley M P (eds) Prions—novel infectious pathogens causing scrapie and Creutzfeldt-Jakob disease. Academic Press, Orlando, pp 387–414

DeArmond S J, Mobley W C, DeMott D L, Barry R A, Beckstead J H, Prusiner S B 1987b Changes in the localization of brain prion proteins during scrapie infection. Neurology 37: 1271–1280

Dees C, McMillan B C, Wade W F, German T L, Marsh R F 1985 Characterization of nucleic acids in membrane vesicles from scrapie-infected hamster brain. Journal of Virology 55: 126–132

Dickinson A G, Meikle V M 1971 Host-genotype and agent effects in scrapie incubation: change in allelic interaction with different strains of agent. Molecular and General Genetics 112: 73–79

Dickinson A G, Outram G W 1979 The scrapie replication-site hypothesis and its implications for pathogenesis. In: Prusiner S B, Hadlow W J (eds) Slow transmissible diseases of the nervous system, vol 2. Academic Press, New York, pp 13–31

Dickinson A G, Outram G W 1988 Genetic aspects of unconventional virus infections. In: Marsh J (ed) Novel infectious agents and the central nervous system, Ciba Foundation Symposium No 135. John Wiley and Sons, London 63–77

Diener T O 1971 Potato spindle tuber 'virus'. IV. A replicating, low molecular weight RNA. Virology 45: 411–428

Diener T O 1987a PrP and the nature of the scrapie agent. Cell 49: 719–721

Diener T O (ed) 1987b The viroids. Plenum Press, New York, pp 1–344

Diener T O, McKinley M P, Prusiner S B 1982 Viroids and prions. Proceedings of the National Academy of Sciences USA 79: 5220–5224

Diringer H, Gelderblom H, Hilmert H, Ozel M, Edelbluth C, Kimberlin R H 1983 Scrapie infectivity, fibrils and low molecular weight protein. Nature 306: 476–478

Epstein C J, Anneren K G, Foster D, Groner Y, Prusiner S B, Smith S A 1987 Pathogenetic relationships between Down syndrome and Alzheimer disease: studies with animal models. In: Banbury Report 27: Molecular neuropathology of ageing. Cold Spring Harbor Laboratory, Cold Spring Harbor, New York 339–355

Friedland R P, Prusiner S B, Jagust W J, Budinger T F, Davis R L 1984 Bitemporal hypometabolism in Creutzfeldt-Jakob disease measured by positron emission tomography with -2-fluorodeoxyglucose. Journal of Computer Assisted Tomography 8: 978–981

Gabizon R, McKinley M P, Prusiner S B 1987 Purified prion proteins and scrapie infectivity copartition into liposomes. Proceedings of the National Academy of Sciences USA 84: 4017–4021

Gabizon R, McKinley M P, Groth D F, Kenaga L, Prusiner S B 1988 Properties of scrapie prion liposomes. Journal of Biological Chemistry 263: 4950–4955

Gajdusek D C 1977 Unconventional viruses and the origin and disappearance of kuru. Science 197: 943–960

Gajdusek D C 1986 Chronic dementia caused by small unconventional viruses apparently containing no nucleic acid. In: Scheibel A B, Wechsler A F, Brazier M A B (eds). The biological aspects of Alzheimer's disease. Academic Press, Orlando, pp 33–54

Gajdusek D C, Gibbs C J Jr, Alpers M 1966 Experimental transmission of a kuru-like syndrome to chimpanzees. Nature 209: 794–796

Gallo R, Salahuddin S, Popovic M et al 1984 Frequent detection and isolation of cytopathic retroviruses (HTLV-III) from patients with AIDS and at risk for AIDS. Science 224: 500–502

Gibbs C J Jr, Gajdusek D C, Asher D M et al 1968 Creutzfeldt-Jakob disease (spongiform encephalopathy): transmission to the chimpanzee. Science 161: 388–389

Gibbs C J Jr, Joy A, Heffner R et al 1985 Clinical and pathological features and laboratory confirmation of Creutzfeldt-Jakob disease in a recipient of pituitary-derived human growth hormone. New England Journal of Medicine 313: 734–738

Gilles K, Riesner D, Prusiner S B 1987 Search for a nucleic acid in purified scrapie prions. 87th Annual Meeting of American Society for Microbiology, p 313 (Abstract)

Glenner G G, Wong C W 1984 Alzheimer's disease and Down's syndrome: sharing of a unique cerebrovascular amyloid fibril protein. Biochemical and Biophysical Research Communications 122: 1331–1135

Goldgaber D, Lerman M I, McBride O W, Saffiotti U, Gajdusek D C 1987 Characterization and chromosomal localization of a cDNA encoding brain amyloid of Alzheimer's disease. Science 235: 877–880

Gonda M A, Wong-Staal F, Gallo R C, Clements J E, Narayan O, Gilden R V 1985 Sequence homology and morphologic similarity of HTLV-III and visna virus, a pathogenic lentivirus. Science 227: 173–177

Goudsmit J, Morrow C H, Asher D M et al 1980 Evidence for and against the transmissibility of Alzheimer's disease. Neurology 30: 945–950

Hadlow W J 1959 Scrapie and kuru. Lancet 2: 289–290

Haraguchi T, Groth D, Barry R A et al 1987 Deglycosylation demonstrates two forms of the scrapie prion protein. Federation Proceedings 46: 1319 (Abstract)

Harrington M G, Merril C R, Asher D M, Gajdusek D C 1986 Abnormal proteins in the cerebrospinal fluid of patients with Creutzfeldt-Jakob disease. New England Journal of Medicine 315: 279–283

Hay B, Barry R A, Lieberburg I, Prusiner S B, Lingappa V R 1987a Biogenesis and transmembrane orientation of the cellular isoform of the scrapie prion protein. Molecular and Cellular Biology 7: 914–920

Hay B, Prusiner S B, Lingappa V R 1987b Evidence for a secretory form of the cellular prion protein. Biochemistry 26: 8110–8115

Hogan R N, Bowman K A, Baringer J R, Prusiner S B 1986 Replication of scrapie prions in hamster eyes preceeds retinal degeneration. Ophthalmic Research 18: 230–235

Hope J, Kimberlin R H 1987 The molecular biology of scrapie: the last two years. Trends in Neurosciences 10: 149–151

Hope J, Morton L J D, Farquhar C F, Multhaup G, Beyreuther K, Kimberlin R H 1986 The major polypeptide of scrapie-associated fibrils (SAF) has the same size, charge distribution and N-terminal protein sequence as predicted for the normal brain protein (PrP). EMBO Journal 5: 2591–2597

Hsiao K, DeArmond S J, Prusiner S B 1987 Human prion protein gene. Neurology 37 (Suppl): 342 (abstract)

Hunter G D 1979 The enigma of the scrapie agent: biochemical approaches and the involvement of membranes and nucleic acids. In: Prusiner S B, Hadlow W J (eds) Slow transmissible diseases of the nervous system, vol 2. Academic Press, New York, pp 365–385

Hunter N, Hope J, McConnell I, Dickinson A G 1987 Linkage of the scrapie-associated fibril protein (PrP) Gen and *Sinc* using congenic mice and restriction fragment length polymorphism analysis. Journal of General Virology 68: 2711–2716

Jakob A 1921 Uber eigenartige erkrankungen des zentralnervensystems mit bemerkenswertem anatomischen befunde (spatische pseudosclerose-encephalomyelopathic mit disseminierten degenerationsherden). Zeitschrift fur die Gesamte Neurologie und Psychiatrie 64: 147–228

Kang J, Lemaire H-G, Unterbeck A et al 1987 The precursor of Alzheimer's disease amyloid A4 protein resembles a cell-surface receptor. Nature 325: 733–736

Kascsak R J, Rubenstein R, Merz P A et al 1986 Immunological comparison of scrapie-associated fibrils isolated from animals infected with four different scrapie strains. Journal of Virology 59: 676–683

Kingsbury D T, Kasper K G, Stites D P, Watson J C, Hogan R N, Prusiner S B 1983 Genetic control of scrapie and Creutzfeldt-Jakob disease in mice. Journal of Immunology 131: 491–496

Kitamoto T, Tateishi J, Tashima T et al 1986 Amyloid plaques in Creutzfeldt-Jakob disease strain with prion protein antibodies. Annals of Neurology 20: 204–208

Klatzo I, Gajdusek D C, Zigas V 1959 Pathology of kuru. Laboratory Investigation 8: 799–847

Kretzschmar H A, Prusiner S B, Stowring L E, DeArmond S J 1986a Scrapie prion proteins are synthesized in neurons. American Journal of Pathology 122: 1–5

Kretzschmar H A, Stowring L E, Westaway D, Stubblebine W H, Prusiner S B, DeArmond S J 1986b Molecular cloning of a human prion protein cDNA. DNA 5: 315–324

Krevans J R 1963 Out of the wastebasket. Annals of Internal Medicine 58: 701–702

Levy J A 1988 The biology of the human immunodeficiency virus and its role in neurological disease. In: Rosenblum M L, Levy R M, Bredesen D E (eds) AIDS and the nervous system. Raven Press, New York, pp 327–345

Locht C, Chesebro B, Race R, Keith J M 1986 Molecular cloning and complete sequence of prion protein cDNA from mouse brain infected with the scrapie agent. Proceedings of the National Academy of Sciences USA 83: 6372–6376

Malone T G, Marsh R F, Hanson R P, Semancik J S 1979 Evidence for the low molecular weight nature of the scrapie agent. Nature 278: 575–576

Manuelidis L, Sklaviadis T, Manuelidis E E 1987 Evidence suggesting that PrP is not the infectious agent in Creutzfeldt-Jakob disease. EMBO Journal 6: 341–347

Marsh R F, Malone T G, Semancik J S, Lancaster W D, Hanson R P 1978 Evidence for an essential DNA component in the scrapie agent. Nature 275: 146–147

Masters C L, Gajdusek D C, Gibbs C J Jr 1981a The familial occurence of Creutzfeldt-Jakob disease and Alzheimer's disease. Brain 104: 535–558

Masters C L, Gajdusek D C, Gibbs C J Jr 1981b Creutzfeldt-Jakob disease virus isolations from the Gerstmann-Straussler syndrome. Brain 104: 559–588

Masters C L, Simms G, Weinman N A, Multhaup G, McDonald B L, Beyreuther K 1985 Amyloid plaque core protein in Alzheimer disease and Down syndrome. Proceedings of the National Academy of Sciences USA 82: 4245–4249

Masters C L, Richardson E P Jr 1978 Subacute spongiform encephalopathy Creutzfeldt-Jakob disease—the nature and progression of spongiform change. Brain 101: 333–344

McKinley M P, Bolton D C, Prusiner S B 1983 A protase-resistant protein is a standard component of the scrapie prion. Cell 35: 47–62

McKinley M P, Butler D A, Prusiner S B 1987a Prion protein mRNA in hamsters and mice Journal of Cell Biology 105: 317a (Abstract)

McKinley M P, Hay B, Lingappa V R, Lieberburg I, Prusiner S B 1987b Developmental expression of prion protein gene in brain. Developmental Biology 121: 105–110

McKinley M P, Mobley W C, Coleman S, Peterson M, Prusiner S B 1987c Developmental regulation of scrapie incubation times in neonatal Golden hamsters. VIIth International Congress of Virology, Edmonton, Alberta, Canada, p. 147 (Abstract)

McKinley M P, Prusiner S B 1986 Biology and structure of scrapie prions. In: Bradley R J (ed) International review of neurobiology, vol 28. Academic Press, New York, pp 1–57

125

Merz P A, Rohwer R G, Kascsak R et al 1984 Infection-specific particle from the unconventional slow virus diseases. Science 225: 437–440

Merz P A, Somerville R A, Wisniewski H M, Iqbal K 1981 Abnormal fibrils from scrapie-infected brain. Acta Neuropathol (Berl) 54: 63–74

Meyer R K, McKinley M P, Bowman K A, Barry R A, Prusiner S B 1986 Separation and properties of cellular and scrapie prion proteins. Proceedings of the National Academy of Sciences USA 83: 2310–2314

Mobley W C, DeArmond S J, Prusiner S B, Johnston M W, McKinley M P 1987 Nerve growth factor stimulates prion protein gene expression in developing brain. Society for Neuroscience Abstracts 13: 186 (Abstract)

Narang H K, Asher D M, Pomeroy K L, Gajdusek D C 1987 Abnormal tubulovesicular particles in brains of hamsters with scrapie. Proceedings of the Society for Experimental Biology and Medicine 184: 504–509

Oesch B, Westaway D, Walchli M et al 1985 A cellular gene encodes scrapie PrP 27–30 protein. Cell 40: 735–746

Parry H B (ed) 1983 Scrapie Disease in Sheep. Academic Press, New York, pp 1–192

Prusiner S B 1982 Novel proteinaceous infectious particles cause scrapie. Science 216: 136–144

Prusiner S B 1984 Some speculations about prions, amyloid and Alzheimer's disease. New England Journal of Medicine 310: 661–663

Prusiner S B 1987 Prions and neurogenerative diseases. New England Journal of Medicine 317: 1571–1581

Prusiner S B, Bolton D C, Groth D F, Bowman K A, Cochran S P, McKinley M P 1982 Further purification and characterization of scrapie prions. Biochemistry 21: 6942–6950

Prusiner S B, Cochran S P, Alpers M P 1985 Transmission of scrapie in hamsters. Journal of Infectious Diseases 152: 971–978

Prusiner S B, Hadlow W J, Garfin D E et al 1978 Partial purification and evidence for multiple molecular forms of the scrapie agent. Biochemistry 17: 4993–4997

Prusiner S B, Groth D F, Bildstein C, Masiarz F R, McKinley M P, Cochran S P 1980a Electrophoretic properties of the scrapie agent in agarose gels. Proceedings of the National Academy of Sciences USA 77: 2984–2988

Prusiner S B, Groth D F, Cochran S P, Masiarz F R, McKinley M P, Martinez H M 1980b Molecular properties, partial purification and assay by incubation period measurements of the hamster scrapie agent. Biochemistry 19: 4883–4891

Prusiner S B, McKinley M P, Groth D F et al 1981 Scrapie agent contains a hydrophobic protein. Proceedings of the National Academy of Sciences USA 78: 6675–6679

Prusiner S B, McKinley M P, Bowman K A et al 1983 Scrapie prions aggregate to form amyloid-like birefringent rods. Cell 35: 349–358

Prusiner S B, Groth D F, Bolton D C, Kent S B, Hood L E 1984 Purification and structural studies of a major scrapie prion protein. Cell 38: 127–134

Ridley R M, Baker H F, Crow T J 1986 Transmissible and non-transmissible neurodegenerative disease: similarities in age of onset and genetics in relation to etiology. Psychological Medicine 16: 199–207

Robakis N K, Devine-Gage E A, Jenkins E C et al 1986 Localization of a human gene homologons to the PrP gene on the p arm of chromosome 20 and detection of PrP-related antigens in normal human brain. Biochemical and Biophysical Research Communications 140: 758–765

Robakis N K, Wisniewski H M, Jenkins E C et al 1987 Chromosome 21q21 sublocalisation of gene encoding beta-amyloid peptide in cerebral vessels and neuritic (senile) plaques of people with Alzheimer disease and Down syndrome. Lancet 1: 384–385

Roberts G W, Lofthouse R, Brown R, Crow T J, Barry R A, Prusiner S B 1986 Prion protein immunoreactivity in human transmissible dementias. New England Journal of Medicine 315: 1231–1233

Rubenstein R, Kascsak R J, Merz P A et al 1986 Detection of scrapie associated fibril (SAF) proteins using anti-SAF antibody in non-purified tissue preparations. Journal of General Virology 67: 671–681

St George-Hyslop P H, Tanzi R E, Polinsky R J et al 1987 The genetic defect causing familial Alzheimer's disease maps on chromosome 21. Science 235: 885–890

Shinagawa M, Munekata E, Doi S, Takahashi K, Goto H, Sato G 1986 Immunoreactivity of a synthetic pentadecapeptide corresponding to the N-terminal region of the scrapie prion protein. Journal of General Virology 67: 1745–1750

Sigurdsson B 1954 Rida, a chronic encephalitis of sheep with general remarks in infections which develop slowly and some of their special characteristics. British Veterinary Journal 110: 341–354

Sparkes R S, Simon M, Cohn V H et al 1986 Assignment of the human and mouse prion protein genes to homologous chromosomes. Proceedings of the National Academy of Sciences USA 83: 7358–7362

Stahl N, Borchelt D R, Hsiao K K, Prusiner S B 1987 Glycolipid modification of the scrapie prion protein. Cell 51: 229–240

Strain G M, Barta O, Olcott B M, Braun W F 1984 Serum and cerebrospinal fluid concentrations of immunoglobulin G in Suffolk sheep with scrapie. American Journal of Veterinary Research 45: 1812–1813

Tanzi R E, Gusella J F, Watkins P C et al 1987 Amyloid B-protein gene: cDNA, mRNA distribution, and genetic linkage near the Alzheimer locus. Science 235: 880–884

Tateishi J, Ohta M, Koga M, Sato Y, Kuroiwa Y 1979 Transmission of chronic spongiform encephalopathy with kuru plaques from humans to small rodents. Annals of Neurology 5: 581–584

Turk E, Teplow D B, Hood L E, Prusiner S B 1987 Purification of the cellular and scrapie prion protein isoforms. Journal of Cellular Biochemistry 35 (Suppl): 11 (Abstract)

Watson J D, Hopkins N H, Roberts J W, Steitz J A, Weiner A M (eds) 1987 Molecular biology of the gene, 4th ed, vol 2. Benjamin Cummings, Menlo Park, CA, pp 898–959

Wells G A H, Scott A C, Johnson C T et al 1987 A novel progressive spongiform encephalopathy in cattle. Veterinary Record 121: 419–420

Westaway D, Goodman P, Mirenda C, Carlson G, Prusiner S B 1987 Short and long scrapie incubation time mice have distinct prion protein gene alleles. Cell 51: 651–662

Wu Y, Brown W T, Robakis N K et al 1987 A PvuII RFLP detected in the human prion protein (PrP) gene. Nucleic Acids Research 15: 3191

Zlotnik I 1962 The pathology of scrapie: a comparative study of lesions in the brain of sheep and goats. Acta Neuropathologica (Suppl) (Berlin) 1: 61–70

Discussion of paper presented by Stanley Prusiner

Discussant: George A. Carlson

PROGRESS IN TRANSMISSIBLE NEURODEGENERATIVE
DISEASES: PRION PROTEIN AND THE INFECTIOUS AGENT

Introduction

Elucidation of the biochemical nature of the scrapie agent now seems to be a realistic goal. Primarily through the efforts of Stanley Prusiner, his colleagues, students and collaborators, the past ten years have seen an explosion of new knowledge and a resurgence of interest in the transmissible neurodegenerative diseases. It is important to emphasize that although most of the important new discoveries on the nature of the scrapie agent have originated in the Prusiner laboratory, independent confirmation of his results has been repeatedly obtained (Diener 1987). The word 'prion', coined by Prusiner (1982) to distinguish the class of infectious agents responsible for transmissible neurodegenerative diseases from conventional viruses and from viroids, was well chosen. No prion-specific nucleic acid has been detected in infectious preparations. Although conventional viruses also require protein for infectivity, the involvement of prion protein (PrP) in infectivity is fundamentally different—if PrP is indeed a functional component of the infectious prion.

Most current research on scrapie and related diseases now focuses on PrP, the only macromolecule that has been identified in the scrapie prion. Is the consensus that further studies on PrP will lead to the solution of the nature of the scrapie prion warranted? All available evidence, coming from a variety of different approaches, points towards PrP playing a pivotal role in scrapie and related diseases.

PrP 27–30 and infectivity co-purify

Biochemical fractionation of scrapie-infected hamster brains, aimed solely at enriching for infectivity, led to the identification of a 27–30 kD protein, designated PrP 27–30 (Bolton et al, 1982; Prusiner et al, 1982). Although the development and use of a rapid and economical incubation time assay in place of endpoint titration (Prusiner et al, 1980) greatly facilitated purification of scrapie prions, the identification of PrP 27–30 represented a near heroic effort. The minimal conclusion from these and similar co-purification studies is that the molecular properties of PrP 27–30 and infectious prions are extremely similar.

Pathological accumulation of PrP

Accumulation of PrP in the brains of infected animals is diagnostic for prion-induced diseases in all species, including man, that have been tested (Roberts et al, 1986; Bockman et al, 1985; Kitamoto et al, 1986). It is of interest that the findings that PrP 27–30 aggregates to form amyloid (Prusiner et al, 1983) and that the amyloid plaques in the brains of scrapie-infected animals stain with anti-PrP 27–30 (Bendheim et al, 1984), provided impetus for focusing Alzheimer's disease (AD) research on the precursor protein of the amyloid A_4 peptide (Kang et al, 1987). However, the propensity of PrP 27–30 to aggregate led some to argue that the infectious agent was entrapped and that PrP was not a functional component of the agent.

PrP is encoded by a host gene

PrP is encoded by a host gene and not by any cryptic nucleic acid that may be present in the prion (Oesch et al, 1985). The amount of PrP mRNA is not increased above normal levels in infected animals, leading some to conclude that PrP is not a component of the infectious agent (Chesebro et al, 1985). However, this conclusion ignores the finding that there are two isoforms of PrP (Oesch et al, 1985). Limited proteinase K treatment of the scrapie isoform, PrP^{Sc}, yields PrP 27–30, while the same treatment degrades the normal cellular isoform PrP^C. It is most likely that the differences between PrP^C and PrP^{Sc} arise post-translationally (Basler et al, 1986). That PrP is a host protein provides an explanation for the immunological inertness of the prion, one of the peculiar properties of the scrapie agent.

Non-aggregated PrP^{Sc} is infectious

Further compelling evidence that PrP^{Sc} is required for infectivity was provided by the demonstration that solubilized PrP 27–30 incorporated into liposomes was at least as infectious as aggregated prion rods (Gabizon et al, 1987). Tobacco mosaic virus added to the liposomes, at a concentration 100 times lower than the infectious prion titre, were readily seen by electron microscopy, making the hypothesis (Merz et al, 1984) that filamentous virus particles were hidden among prion rods extremely unlikely. Immunoaffinity chromatography using anti-PrP antibodies was made possible by the liposome technology, providing immunological evidence that PrP^{Sc} is a functional component of the infectious particle. If a co-factor, such as a nucleic acid, is a component of the prion it is tightly bound to PrP^{Sc}.

Linkage of prion protein and scrapie incubation time genes

In mice, a single autosomal gene (*Prn-i*) has a profound effect on the scrapie incubation period. This gene was found to be closely linked to the prion protein gene (*Prn-p*), forming a prion gene complex (*Prn*), emphasizing the involvement of PrP in the biology of scrapie (Carlson et al, 1986). Although not formally proven, it is possible that PrP itself may control the incubation period of scrapie because the short and long haplotypes of the prion gene complex encode PrP's that differ from one another at codons 108 and 189 (Westaway et al, 1987).

All available evidence points to PrP^{Sc} as being a functional component, and possibly the only component of prions. The prion protein gene is highly conserved and PrP^C presumably has a normal physiological function. I know of no precedent for an infectious agent comprised of the product of a normal host gene which may also control susceptibility to the disease caused by the agent.

'Strains' of scrapie agent

Much of the criticism levelled against the prion hypothesis was directed against only one of the models for the prion—the 'protein only' model. Extensive work by Dickinson and his colleagues over the past 20 years has led to the identification of a variety of scrapie 'strains' (Bruce & Dickinson, 1987; Dickinson & Fraser, 1977). The differential behaviour of labile scrapie isolates was attributed to host selection and agent mutation, and was based on the assumption that agent-specific nucleic acid was the only possible informational molecule in the prion (Dickinson & Outram, 1988). A prion comprised of a small nucleic acid bound to and protected by PrP is a viable model. However, it may not be necessary to invoke nucleic acid as the informational macromolecule of the prion (Diener, 1987; Westaway et al, 1987; Carlson et al, 1988). For example, the interval between inoculation and the onset of neurological dysfunction (incubation period) in I/LnJ (*Prn-p^b*) inoculated with 30 µg of a 1/10 dilution of the chandler scrapie isolate passaged in NZW/LacJ mice (*Prn-p^a*) was 283 ± 21 days (n=8). Inoculation of I/LnJ mice with I/LnJ-passaged isolate gave an incubation period of 193 ± 6 days (n=16); no further shortening of incubation was seen in second passage I/LnJ scrapie. One obvious difference between NZW-passaged and I/Ln-passaged inocula is that the PrP molecules encoded by the two strains differ in primary amino acid sequence. One interpretation of these and similar results is that interactions between homologous PrP facilitate shorter incubation periods with heterologous molecules being less efficient. Replicating prions would be comprised of host-encoded PrP, compatible with the change in behaviour occurring in a single passage rather than gradually. Experiments are in progress to determine whether or not this hypothesis is correct. Existing biochemical information on the nature of the post-translational modifications responsible for converting PrP^C to PrP^{Sc} is not sufficient to construct a detailed hypothesis to account for 'strains' of protein-only prions, but in many respects a protein-only model is less complicated than one involving a prion-specific nucleic acid that interacts with PrP. A nucleic acid would not only need to utilize host replicative machinery, but also direct the post-translational conversion of PrP^C to PrP^{Sc} and bind to PrP, while remaining under the control of the prion incubation time gene, which may be the prion protein gene itself. To date, the source of variation between different isolates of scrapie prions remains a mystery. This is a central and fascinating issue in scrapie research.

Neurodegenerative disease and biological clocks

Molecular studies of the prion gene complex (*Prn*) and of the post-translational modifications leading to the production of PrP^{Sc} may provide a point of departure for the study of host susceptibility to a variety of neurodegenerative disorders. The human prion diseases kuru, Creutzfeldt-Jakob disease (CJD) and Gerstmann-Straussler syndrome (GSS) appear to occur primarily through three different mechanisms: infectious, sporadic and genetic, respectively (Prusiner, 1987).

Like CJD, the majority of Alzheimer's disease (AD) cases are sporadic, but a significant portion are genetic. Attempts to transmit both sporadic and familial AD to experimental animals have been unsuccessful to date (Goudsmit et al, 1980). While the non-transmissibility of AD is a major feature distinguishing it from CJD, these two neurodegenerative diseases retain a large number of similarities both clinically and pathologically. Familial Alzheimer's disease (FAD) is inherited as an autosomal dominant disorder. Two anonymous RFLP probes and early onset FAD have been linked and mapped to chromosome 21 (Tanzi et al, 1987a; Goldgaber et al, 1987; St George-Hyslop et al, 1987). The B-amyloid gene has also been mapped to chromosome 21 but it is quite distinct from the early onset FAD locus (Tanzi et al, 1987b; Van Broeckhoven et al, 1987). Early onset FAD resembles GSS with respect to the age at which the illness appears. The incidence of sporadic AD begins to rise around age 60, the time at which the incidence of CJD is maximal.

One of the major problems facing investigators studying most neurodegenerative diseases is the lack of animal models that recapitulate all features of these disorders (Glenner, 1988). Although Alzheimer's disease is not transmissible and its amyloid does not contain detectable amounts of PrP, biochemical processes similar to those in prion diseases may be involved. Post-translational modification of a normal cellular protein to an abnormal polymerizing isoform may be a process common to several degenerative diseases, and initiation of the pathological cascade could be caused by defects in the protein gene itself or in 'incubation time' loci, as well as by environmental insults. An exogenous infectious source of initiation of pathology may be restricted to those diseases characterized by accumulation of PrP^{Sc}. Whether studies on *Prn* in mice will lead to the development of more suitable animal models for human neurodegenerative diseases other than those caused by prions remains uncertain. Regardless, it will be of interest to construct transgenic mice with mutant *Prn* genes in order to determine whether such animals spontaneously develop scrapie. If some *Prn* transgenic mice are found to produce prions spontaneously, they will provide an excellent model for elucidating the molecular basis of familial CJD and GSS.

It is intriguing to speculate that prion incubation time genes, and perhaps genes controlling susceptibility to some non-prion genetic diseases, function as biological clocks, eliminating aged individuals from the population. If such deleterious 'incubation time' loci confer a reproductive advantage to young individuals, further selective advantage in the form of reduced competition for limited resources could derive from the death of post-reproductive age parents. Limited evidence for increased fecundity of affected women in GSS families has been presented by Ridley et al (1986).

It is clear that the biochemical nature of the prion is as yet unsolved. However, it is also clear that further research focusing on PrP is likely to be the key. This area of research is one of the most exciting in biology and may have implications far beyond prion diseases. The rapid progress in the field of transmissible neurodegenerative diseases has been largely due to the bold initiative and fertile imagination of Dr Prusiner, and, based on the clear goals and direction of his current research as outlined in his presentation, it is likely that even more excitement is in store.

REFERENCES

Basler K, Oesch B, Scott B, et al 1986 Scrapie and cellular PrP isoforms are encoded by the same chromosomal gene. Cell 46: 417–428
Bendheim P E, Barry R A, DeArmond S J, Stites D P, Prusiner S B 1984 Antibodies to a scrapie prion protein. Nature 310: 418–421
Bockman J M, Kingsbury D T, McKinley M P, Bendheim P E, Prusiner S B 1985 Creutzfeldt-Jakob disease prion proteins in human brains. New England Journal of Medicine 312: 73–78
Bolton D C, McKinley M P, Prusiner S B 1982 Identification of a protein that purifies with the scrapie prion. Science 218: 1309–1311
Bruce M E, Dickinson A G 1987 Biological evidence that scrapie agent has an independent genome. Journal of General Virology 68: 79–89
Carlson G A, Kingsbury D T, Goodman P A et al 1986 Linkage of prion protein and scrapie incubation time genes. Cell 46: 503–511
Carlson G A, Westaway D, Goodman P A, Peterson M, Marshall S T, Prusiner S B 1988 Genetic control of prion incubation period in mice. In: Novel Infectious Agents and the Central Nervous System, Ciba Foundation Symposium 135. John Wiley & Sons, London, pp 84–99
Chesebro B, Race R, Wehrly K et al 1985 Identification of scrapie prion protein-specific mRNA in scrapie-infected and uninfected brain. Nature 315: 331–333
Dickinson A G, Fraser H 1977 The pathogenesis of scrapie in inbred mice: an assessment of host control and response involving many strains of agent. In: V terMulen, M Katz (Eds.) Slow Virus Infections of the Central Nervous System, Springer-Verlag, New York, pp 3–14
Dickinson A G, Outram G W 1988 Genetic aspects of unconventional virus infections: the basis of the virion hypothesis. In: Novel Infectious Agents and the Central Nervous System, Ciba Foundation Symposium 135, John Wiley & Sons, London, pp 63–83
Diener T O 1987 PrP and the nature of the scrapie agent. Cell 49: 719–721
Gabizon R, McKinley M P, Prusiner S P 1987 Purified prion proteins and scrapie infectivity copartition into liposomes. Proceedings of the National Academy of Sciences USA 84: 4017–4021
Glenner G G 1988 Alzheimer's disease: its proteins and genes. Cell 52: 307–308
Goldgaber D, Lerman M J, McBride O W, Saffiotti U, Gajdusek D C 1987 Characterization and chromosomal localization of a cDNA encoding brain amyloid of Alzheimer's disease. Science 235: 877–879
Goudsmit J, Morrow C H, Asher D M et al 1980 Evidence for and against the transmissibility of Alzheimer's disease. Neurology 30, 945–950
Kang J, Lemaire H-G, Unterbeck A et al 1987 The precursor of Alzheimer's disease amyloid A4 protein resembles a cell-surface receptor. Nature 325: 733–736
Kitamoto T, Tateishi J, Tashima T et al 1986 Amyloid plaques of Creutzfeldt-Jakob disease stain with prion protein antibodies. Annals of Neurology 20: 204–208
Merz P A, Rohwer RG, Kascsak R et al 1984 Infection-specific particle from the unconventional slow virus diseases. Science 225: 437–440
Oesch B, Westaway D, Wachli M et al 1985 A cellular gene encodes scrapie PrP 27–30 protein. Cell 40: 735–746
Prusiner S B 1982 Novel proteinaceous infectious particles cause scrapie. Science 216: 136–144
Prusiner S B 1987 Prions and neurodegenerative diseases. New England Journal of Medicine 317: 1571–1581
Prusiner S B, Groth D F, Cochran S P, Masiarz F R, McKinley M P, Martinez H M 1980 Molecular properties, partial purification and assay by incubation period measurements of the hamster scrapie agent. Biochemstry 19: 4883–4891
Prusiner S B, Bolton D C, Groth D F, Bowman K A, Cochran S P , McKinley M P 1982 Further purification and characterization of scrapie prions. Biochemistry 21: 6942–6950

132

Prusiner S B, McKinley M P, Bowman K A et al 1983 Scrapie prions aggregate to form amyloid-like birefringent rods. Cell 35: 349–358

Ridley R M, Baker H F, Crow T J 1986 Transmissible and non-transmissible neurodegenerative disease: similarities in age of onset and genetics in relation to aetiology. Psychological Medicine 16: 199–207

Roberts G W, Lofthouse R, Brown R, Crow T J, Barry R A, Prusiner S B 1986 Prion-protein immunoreactivity in human transmissible dementias. New England Journal of Medicine 315: 1231–1233

St George-Hyslop P H, Tanzi R E, Polinsky R J et al 1987 The genetic defect causing familial Alzheimer's disease maps on Chromosme 21 Science 235: 885–889

Tanzi R E, Gusella J F, Watkins P C et al 1987a Amyloid protein gene: cDNA mRNA distribution and genetic linkage near the Alzheimer locus. Science 235: 880–884

Tanzi R E, St George-Hyslop P H, Haines J L et al 1987b The genetic defect in familial Alzheimer's disease is not tightly lined to the amyloid B-protein gene. Nature 329: 156–157

Van Broeckhoven C, Genthe A M, Bandeberghe A et al 1987 Familial Alzheimer's disease does not segregate with the A_4-amyloid gene in several European families. Nature 329: 153–155

Westaway D, Goodman P A, Mirenda C A, McKinley M P, Carlson G A, Prusiner S B 1987 Distinct prion proteins in short and long scrapie incubation period mice. Cell 51: 651–662.

Discussion: Prion proteins

Stanley Prusiner and George Carlson

The discussion revolved around the cellular protein PrP^C and its scrapie counterpart PrP^{Sc}. In response to a question concerning the possibility that disease was the result of greater accumulation of PrP^{Sc}, rather than greater synthesis *per se*, Dr Prusiner described an *in vitro* model of scrapie-infected neuroblastoma cells. In these cells, PrP^C is synthesized abundantly but is turning over rapidly, while PrP^{Sc} is synthesized much more slowly, but is accumulating. The precise reason for this is unknown. PrP^{Sc} is characterized by relative resistance to protease, while PrP^C is susceptible; possibly a conformational change distinguishes the two forms, since denaturation of PrP^{Sc} renders it susceptible to protease.

Several questions were asked about *in vivo* manipulations of the cellular gene which encodes PrP. Had it been re-introduced into mice? Such experiments have been attempted but to date have borne minimal fruit. Cell-free translation systems, bovine papilloma virus, and baculovirus expression vectors, have been used to try to produce 'infectious PrP'. None of the systems has allowed production of the protease resistant form of PrP, but continued attempts are being made. Also, the hamster PrP gene has been used to generate transgenic mouse lines, but so far expression of the 'exogenous' PrP has not been detected. Again, these experiments continue.

The final series of questions addressed the role of host genes in determining the incubation period of scrapie. The incubation period appears to be determined by a single locus, with at least two allelic forms, which maps close to (and may well be the same as) the gene encoding PrP. Scrapie prions from 'long incubation period' mice will breed true when passed through 'long' mice, but will revert to 'short incubation period' prions after a single passage through 'short' mice, and vice-versa. Prions from long/short F_1 mice (heterozygous at the locus determining scrapie incubation period) behave in a manner consistent with their comprising a mix of 'long' and 'short' incubation prions; however such F_1 preparations have not been purified in large quantities and thus have not been subjected to biochemical analyses.

7. Viral determinants and autoimmunity

Robert S. Fujinami

Virus infection can result in a variety of outcomes. In most instances infection by viruses to which man plays host cause no detectable illness in the majority of individuals, despite cell and tissue invasion (Mims, 1987). In contrast, a virus that cycles through man, to which man is not normally the natural host, can lead to dire consequences. For example, rabies virus infection in humans is often fatal without prompt medical intervention although this virus is maintained in its natural host without serious consequences. There is usually a balanced pathogenesis where virus can replicate and spread to other individuals without a great deal of debilitation to the host species.

Immune responses to virus infections can also vary. Viruses can be readily contained by natural defenses such as phagocytosis by macrophages, or be unable to attach to epithelial cells due to inactivation by glycoprotein inhibitors in the mucus lining the upper respiratory tract (Mims, 1987). Once viruses establish an infection they or their antigens, usually make their way to draining lymph nodes where an immune response is initiated. Both humoral (Sissons, 1984) and cellular (Zinkernagel, 1976) effector mechanisms are brought into play to thwart the invasion. The outcome of the infection is usually determined within the first few days.

Several possible scenarios come to mind. First, an acute infection could occur where virus is rapidly cleared by the mounting immune response and the host completely recovers. Second, the virus could establish a latent infection where the immune response is not able to clear the virus, such as with human cytomegalovirus infection (Rice et al, 1985). Third, the virus can initiate a persistent infection in the host where the agent cannot readily be recovered, yet virus lingers. An example of this would be measles virus infection resulting in subacute sclerosing panencephalitis (ter Meulen et al, 1972). Here, too, the immune response is not able to eliminate the virus, although humoral and cellular responses to virus are intact in these afflicted individuals (Perrin et al, 1977). Lastly, immune responses to viruses can mediate immunopathological disease. A model for this is represented by an acute infection of mice with lymphocytic choriomeningitis virus (Buchmeier et al, 1980). Acutely infected mice die due to T cells reactive for lymphocytic choriomeningitis virus infected cells. These cells are responsible for viral clearance (Oldstone et al, 1986). Immunosuppressed mice do not die but develop a persistent infection thus demonstrating the immunopathological nature of the disease.

Another way the immune system could mediate pathological disease leading to autoimmunity is through molecular mimicry (Fujinami et al, 1983; Fujinami & Oldstone, 1985). Here, immune responses to common antigenic determinants between microbes and host cell proteins could lead to disease induction. In order to test this hypothesis, monoclonal antibodies to various viruses were examined for their ability to bind to host cell proteins. First, a monoclonal antibody to measles virus was found, by immunofluorescent staining experiments, to react with uninfected as well as measles virus infected cells (Fujinami et al, 1983). The staining pattern in mock infected cells had a network-like appearance. In the uninfected cells that were undergoing mitosis, the reactivity was one which gave a speckled veneer which was concentrated between the two dividing cells. This pattern of staining was very suggestive of reactivity with intermediate filament proteins, particularly vimentin or cytokeratin (Franke et al, 1982). In contrast, the monoclonal antibody reacted with viral inclusion bodies in the cytoplasm of measles virus infected cells. In these infected cells no network staining could be detected. To demonstrate specificity, intermediate filament enriched preparations from uninfected cells were obtained and used for absorption studies. When the monoclonal antibody was incubated with the intermediate filament preparation, the reactivity to infected cells could be removed. Next, Western blotting experiments were performed, to determine biochemically what viral and intermediate filament protein the monoclonal antibody reacted with. Here, intermediate filament proteins were separated by electrophoresis on SDS gels and then transferred to nitrocellulose paper. The monclonal antibody was reacted with the proteins bound to the nitrocellulose strip. The antibody bound to a 52–54,000 protein co-migrated with one of the cytokeratin proteins which migrated ahead of vimentin. Similar experiments were performed using cytosol preparations from infected and uninfected cells where the intermediate filament proteins were removed. The antibody bound to the 70,000 molecular weight phosphoprotein of measles virus from infected cells. The monoclonal antibody was also tested for its reactivity to proteins from purified measles virions. Here, viral proteins were separated by electrophoresis on SDS gels and transferred to nitrocellulose strips. Western blotting analysis was performed and again the monoclonal antibody was found to react with the 70,000 molecular weight measles virus phosphoprotein. Thus, the antibody reacted with a 52–54,000 cytokeratin protein and the 70,000 measles virus phosphoprotein found in infected cells and virions.

Similarly, a monoclonal antibody has recently been identified (Fujinami, unpublished) that bound to Theiler's murin encephalomyelitis virus (TMEV). This monoclonal antibody was also found to react with galactocerebroside, a myelin component. Intracerebral TMEV infection of mice produces a chronic demyelinating disease (Lipton, 1975). This is characterized by perivascular cellular infiltrates and demyelination (Dal Canto & Lipton, 1975). Macrophages were observed to be actively stripping myelin lining the axons. In addition vesiculation of the myelin sheath could be found. This TMEV monoclonal antibody had the ability to neutralize the virus and by Western blotting experiments was identified to bind to VP-1. The monoclonal antibody reacted with oligodendrocyte-like cells in newborn mouse brain cultures. The TMEV monclonal antibody reacted with a viral determinant and a component in myelin. In TMEV infected mice antibodies to galactocerebroside were observed (Rosenthal et al, 1986). Some of these antibodies could result in a cross-reacting immune response to TMEV. It is clear that an experimental allergic neuritis-like disease can result in animals immunized with galactocerebroside in adjuvant. Further, antibodies to galactocerebroside, when injected into the sciatic nerve of rats could lead to demyelinating changes in these animals (Saida et al, 1979). Thus, antibodies to galactocerebroside could contribute to the observed pattern of disease, i.e. demyelination.

Monoclonal antibodies are good tools to use to indicate common determinants between viral protein and host cell determinants; however, these reagents cannot precisely define what the cross-reacting elements are, viz. the amino acid sequence. In order to understand this aspect of how viruses could initiate autoimmune events, the model system of experimental allergic encephalomyelitis (EAE) was utilized (Paterson, 1979). This autoimmune disease could be reasonably mimicked by the injection of myelin basic protein and adjuvant into a suitable animal species. Myelin basic protein has been extensively studied and its amino acid sequence is known (Hashim & Schilling, 1973). In addition, the encephalitogenic (disease inducing) regions on the protein have been mapped for a wide variety of species (Spitler, 1972; Martenson, 1975). Therefore, injection of any of these discrete regions with adjuvant into the appropriate animal species leads to the production of EAE. The sequence of the known viral proteins were compared with the encephalitogenic regions on myelin basic protein (Fujinami & Oldstone, 1985). Several common regions were uncovered but one of the better fits was with the encephalitogenic region for the rabbit and a domain from the hepatitis B virus polymerase (HBVP). Six amino acids were found in tandem from each region. The viral stretch was biochemically synthesized and since it shared sequence similarity with one of the rabbit encephalitogenic sites, rabbits were immunized once with the HBVP in adjuvant. The rabbits were then followed for the production of autoantibodies and cellular reactivity to the self antigen, myelin basic protein, and observed for disease induction. The majority of rabbits immunized with the viral peptide were found to have antibodies which reacted with whole myelin basic protein. The binding of these antibodies could be blocked with peptide indicating the specificity of the reaction. In experiments studying cellular reactivity to viral peptide and self protein, all of the rabbits' (eight animals tested) peripheral blood mononuclear cells proliferated in response to HBVP. Peripheral blood mononuclear cells from half of these animals proliferated when cultured in the presence of myelin basic protein. Lastly, when the brains and cervical spinal cords from the rabbits were examined histologically, some of the rabbits (4 out of 11) had inflammatory lesions consistent with EAE. Thus, a viral peptide sharing a common determinant with a self protein could induce autoantibodies, cellular reactivity and disease production.

Recently, by computer analysis, a peptide from the predicted protein sequence from the immediate-early region of human cytomegalovirus was identified to have sequence similarity to the B-chain of the human histocompatibility complex HLA-DR (Fujinami et al, 1988). The homologous region was located in an area that was conserved between the human and mouse histocompatibility antigen. The common stretch between the immediate-early region and DR B-chain had a similar hydrophobility estimate and had predicated B-turn potential, suggesting these areas would be on the surface of the protein. Rabbits were immunized with the viral peptide and the resulting antibodies specifically recognized the human DR B-chain by ELISA and Western blot analysis. Expression of human cytomegalovirus proteins, infection, and reactivation have been associated with graft rejection phenomenon. Immune reactivity to the human cytomegalovirus IE-2 sequences could initiate responses against DR determinants. Patients with rejection events had an increased DR expression (van Es et al, 1984). Human cytomegalovirus infection coincided with an increase in DR appearance. The level of HLA DR subsided to normal after symptoms of cytomegalovirus infection faded. Another study (van Willebrand et al, 1986) suggested that cytomegalovirus infection was associated with the up-regulation of Class II antigen in the parenchymal cells of the graft. The presence of cross-reacting determinants between virus and MHC antigens could explain both of these findings. Another problem for a host is immunosuppression associated with cytomegalovirus infection. Here, cross-reacting antibodies to DR could interfere with effective antigen presentation and may contribute to the immunosuppression observed during active cytomegalovirus infection. Thus, these observations with the sequence similarity in human cytomegalovirus immediate-early region and DR B-chain could explain many of the *in vivo* observations.

In a like manner other microbes having common determinants with self proteins have led to interesting speculations (Dyrberg & Oldstone, 1986). Ankylosing spondylitis and Reiter's syndrome both have an association with the HLA B27 haplotype. Schwimmbeck et al (1987) have found, by computer search, a sequence similarity of six consecutive amino acids between HAL B27.1 and the *Klebsiella pneumoniae* nitrogenase. Both the common regions are hydrophilic which would suggest that these regions were located on the exposed surface of each respective molecule. In analysing sera from patients with ankylosing spondylitis and Reiter's syndrome 29% and 53%, respectively, contained antibodies that reacted with the common peptide region from HLA B27.1 and *Klebsiella pneumoniae*. Only 1 of 22 sera from healthy B27 positive control individuals had antibodies that bound to other peptides. Greater that 40% of the patients with ankylosing spondylitis or Reiter's syndrome had antibodies that reacted with the Klebsiella peptide and none of the normal HLA B27 haplotype controls did. These data suggest that immune responses to *Klebsiella nitrogenase* could cross-react with HLA B27.1 contributing to the disease state in certain individuals. For example, immune attack on HLA determinants located on cells from synovial membranes could initiate pathological changes that result in disease production.

Thus, autoimmunity could arise when microbial determinants reflect those host-protein conformations that are capable of inciting disease, although the viral determinant is required to be different enough from self to provoke an effective immune response. Autoimmune responses probably occur from the breaking of tolerance at either the T or B cell level. Once tolerance is broken and cross-reacting immune responses to self are initiated, exposure of additional self antigen at the site of inflammation could lead to re-stimulation without the original inciting agent being present. This type of outcome may lead to a chronic smoldering type of pathology. Similar events may play a role in autoimmune phenomena linked with myasthenia gravis, arthritis, thyroiditis, diabetes, Guillain-Barre's syndrome and multiple sclerosis.

REFERENCES

Buchmeier M, Welsh R, Dutko F, Oldstone M 1980 The virology and immunobiology of lymphocytic choriomeningitis virus infection. Advances in Immunology 30: 275

Dal Canto M C, Lipton H L 1975 Primary demyelination in Theiler's virus infection. Laboratory Investigations 33: 626

Dyrberg T, Oldstone M B A 1986 Peptides as probes to study molecular mimicry and virus induced autoimmunity. Current Topics in Microbiological Immunology 130: 25

Franke W W, Schmid E, Grund C, Geiger B 1982 Intermediate filament proteins in nonfilamentous structures: Transient disintegration and inclusion of subunit proteins in granular aggregates. Cell 30: 103

Fujinami R S, Nelson J A, Walker L et al 1988[b] Sequence homology and immunologic cross-reactivity of human cytomegalovirus with HLA-DR chain: a means for graft rejection and immunosuppression. Journal of Virology 62: 100

Fujinami R S, Oldstone M B A, Wroblewska Z et al 1983 Molecular mimicry in virus infection: Cross-reaction of measles virus phosphoprotein or of herpes simplex virus protein with human intermediate filaments. Proceedings of the National Academy of Sciences USA 80: 2346

Fujinami R S, Oldstone M B A 1985 Amino acid homology between the encephalitogenic site of myelin basic protein and virus: Mechanism for autoimmunity. Science 230: 1043

Fujinami R S, Zurbriggen A, Powell H C 1988[a] Monoclonal antibody defines determinant between Theiler's virus and lipid-like structures. Journal of Neuroimmunology, in press

Hashim G A, Schilling F J 1973 Allergic encephalomyelitis: Characterization of the determinants for delayed type hypersensitivity. Biochemical Biophysical Research Communications 50: 589

Lipton H L 1975 Theiler's virus infection in mice: An unusual biphasic disease process leading to demyelination. Infection and Immunity, 11: 1147

Martenson R E 1975 The location of regions in guinea pig and bovine myelin basic proteins which induce experimental allergic encephalomyelitis in Lewis rats. Journal of Immunology 114: 592

Mims C A The pathogensis of infectious disease 1987 Academic Press, London p 3.

Oldstone M B A, Blount P, Southern P J et al 1986 Cytoimmunotherapy for persistent virus infection reveals a unique clearance pattern from the central nervous system. Nature (London) 321: 239

Paterson P Y 1979 Neuroimmunologic disease of animals and humans. Reviews of Inflammatory Diseases 1: 468

Perrin L H, Tishon A, Oldstone M B A 1977 Immunologic injury in measles virus infection. III. Presence and characterization of human cytotoxic lymphocytes. Journal of Immunology 118: 282

Rice G P A, Schrier R D, Oldstone M B A 1985 Detection of human cytomegalovirus in peripheral blood lymphocytes in a natural infection. Science 230: 1048

Rosenthal A, Fujinami R S, Lampert P W 1986 Mechanism of Theiler's virus-induced demyelination in nude mice. Laboratory Investigation 54: 515

Saida T, Saida K, Dorfman S H et al 1979 Experimental allergic neuritis induced by sensitization with galactocerebroside. Science 204: 1103

Schwimmbeck P L, Yu D T Y, Oldstone M B A 1987 Autoantibodies to HLA B27 in the sera of HLA B27 patients with ankylosing spondylitis and Reiters syndrome: Molecular mimicry with Klebsiella pneumoniae as potential mechanism of autoimmune disease. Journal of Experimental Medicine 166: 173–181

Sissons J G P 1984 Antibody- and complement-dependent lysis of virus-infected cells. In: Concepts in viral pathogenesis. Springer-Verlag New York, p 40

Spitler L E 1972 Experimental allergic encephalitis dissociation of cellular immunity to brain protein and disease production. Journal of Experimental Medicine 136: 156

ter Meulen V, Katz M, Muller D 1972 Subacute sclerosing panencephalitis: A review. Current Topics in Microbiology 57: 1.

van Es A, Baldwin W M, Oljans P J et al 1984 Expression of HLA-DR on T lymphocytes following renal transplantation, and association with graft-rejection episodes and cytomegalovirus infection. Transplantation 37: 65

van Willebrand E, Pettersson E, Ahonen J et al 1986 CMV infection, class II antigen expression, and human kidney allograft rejection. Transplantation 42: 364

Zinkernagel R M H-2 1976 compatibility requirement for virus-specific T cell mediated cytolysis Journal of Experimental Medicine 143: 437

Discussion of paper presented by Robert Fujinami

Discussant: Thomas Dyrberg

ANTIGEN MIMICKING EPITOPES ON VIRUS AND HOST CELL PROTEINS—IMPLICATIONS FOR DEVELOPMENT OF AUTOIMMUNITY

Autoimmunity appears to be an important component in many diseases. Although in some cases, the pathogenic processes leading to autoimmune disease are known or suspected, the aetiology is only rarely known. Viruses are one of the environmental factors which have been implicated as initiating agents in the development of autoimmunity. Some of the mechanisms whereby virus has been speculated to cause autoimmunity include polyclonal B-cell activation, expression of new antigens or alteration of existing cell antigens, via idiotype mechanism or through cross-reactivity between virus and host cell proteins (Notkins et al, 1984). One variation of the cross-reactivity concept is termed molecular mimicry as presented by Dr Fujinami and by Oldstone (1987).

Molecular mimicry has been defined as the presence of homologous epitopes, either linear or conformational, on virus and host cell proteins. Virus and mammalian cells often share antigen epitopes, demonstrated by the fact that 3.5% of more than 600 monoclonal antibodies to a variety of virus also reacted with uninfected cells from a number of organs (Srinivasappa et al, 1986). One approach to identify the molecular basis of such mimicking epitopes is through computer search analysis for amino acid sequence homologies between host and virus proteins (Dyrberg & Oldstone, 1986). This approach has been made possible through the rapidly growing number of cloned cell and virus proteins from which the predicted amino acid sequence has been established. The limitation of this analysis is, however, that only those proteins for which sequence data are available are compared. Further, at present only linear and not conformational homologies can be investigated. Studies on the pathogenic importance of homologous amino acid sequences between virus and host protein in autoimmune disease can be pursued by generating immune responses in, for example, rabbits or mice to synthetic peptides representing the mimicking epitope and testing the antibodies and immune cells for cross-reactivity to the respective native proteins, as well as by looking for autoantibodies in patient sera reacting with the selected peptides (Dyrberg & Oldstone, 1986).

Along these lines Fujinami and Oldstone (1985) have demonstrated that immunization of rabbits with a viral amino acid sequence mimicking the encephalotigenic epitope of myelin basic protein, not only induced humoral and cellular responses cross-reacting with myelin basic protein but also pathological CNS lesions resembling those seen in experimental allergic encephalitis. Molecular mimicry, as a cause of autoimmunity, has also been shown to be of importance in a number of diseases in man. Well recognized examples are the immunological cross-reactivities between streptococci and cardiac myosin (Dale & Beachey, 1985) associated with rheumatic heart disease, and between *Trypanosoma cruzi* and neuronal cells (Wood et al, 1982) associated with Chagas disease. *Klebsiella pneumoniae* has been implicated in the pathogenesis of ankylosing spondylitis and Reiter's syndrome which predominantly occur in HLA-B27 positive persons. One hypothesis to explain the molecular basis for the association between HLA-B27 and these diseases is described by Schwimmbeck et al (1987). A computer search analysis demonstrated a six amino acid sequence identity between a Klebsiella protein and the first hyper-variable domain of HLA-B27, and it was shown that 29% of sera from patients with ankylosing spondylitis and 53% of patients with Reiter's syndrome contained antibodies specifically reacting with this common sequence.

Myasthenia gravis is caused by a humoral autoimmune reaction to the α-chain of the acetylcholine receptor (AChR). The aetiology remains obscure, although there are many indications of exogenous initiating factors. Computer search analysis showed a number of virus proteins showing homology to a hydrophilic sequence of the α-chain of the AChR which has been proposed to be a major immunological region. Sera from six out of 40 patients with myasthenia bound, in solid phase ELISA, to a synthetic peptide representing this region of the receptor. Antibodies from these sera, affinity purified to the immobilized receptor peptide, showed binding to the native AChR and important for this discussion was the fact that the antibodies bound equally well to a peptide representing either the receptor or a homologous herpes simplex virus protein (Schwimmbeck, personal communication). Subsequent analysis revealed a six amino acid identical sequence between another hydrophilic region of the AChR α-chain and one of the coat proteins of polio virus in a position known to be exposed to the outside of the virus. Rabbits were immunized with a synthetic peptide representing that sequence, and one out of 11 antisera was shown to react both with the native AChR and the polio virus (Dyrberg & Oldstone, 1987).

With the identification and molecular cloning of autoantigens thought to play a role in the development of autoimmune disease (Table 1), more detailed immunological analysis becomes possible, e.g. search for mimicking microbial epitopes. The insulin receptor, which is the target for autoimmune reaction causing an insulin resistance syndrome, is one such example. The insulin receptor amino acid sequence was reported in 1985 (Ullrich et al, 1985). A number of significant homologies to human virus proteins were demonstrated (Dyrberg & Oldstone, 1986); however, future experiments must show whether these are of aetiopathogenic importance. Other examples of human autoantigens include the thyroid microsomal antigen, identified as the thyroid peroxidase (Ruf et al, 1987; Kimura et al, 1987) associated with autoimmune thyroid disease and the major parietal cell antigen, identified as the H⁺,K⁺ ATPase associated with auto-immune gastritis and pernicious anaemia (Karlsson et al, 1988).

Table 1 Autoantigens and autoimmune disease

Autoantigens	Autoimmune diseases
Acetylcholine receptor	Myasthenia gravis
Insulin receptor	Insulin resistance syndrome type B
Thyroid peroxidase (microsomal antigen)	Thyroid autoimmune disease
H⁺, K⁺-ATPase (parietal cell antigen)	Pernicious anaemia/autoimmune gastritis
HLA-B27??	Ankylosing spondylitis
64,000 Mr islet cell antigen??	Insulin dependent diabetes

In conclusion, the experiments cited above have demonstrated the presence of epitopes shared between known autoantigens and viral proteins, and that synthetic peptides representing such epitopes can induce antibodies cross-reacting with the native proteins. Thus, these data indicate that virus may cause autoimmunity and disease through molecular mimicry.

REFERENCES

Dale J B, Beachey E H 1985 Epitopes of streptococcal M proteins shared with cardiac myosin. Journal of Experimental Medicine 162: 583–591

Dyrberg T, Oldstone M B A 1987 Molecular mimicry between viral proteins and cell antigens—implications for development of autoimmunity. Periodic Biology 89, suppl. 1: 48 (abstract)

Dyrberg T, Oldstone M B A 1986 Peptides as probes to study molecular mimicry and virus induced autoimmunity. Current Topics in Microbiological Immunology 130: 25–37

Fujinami R S, Oldstone M B A 1985 Amino acid homology and immune responses between the encephalotigenic site of myelin basic protein and virus: A mechanism for autoimmunity. Science 230: 1043–1045

Karlsson F A, Burman P, Loof L et al 1988 Major parietal cell antigen in autoimmune gastritis with pernicious anemia is the acid-producing H⁺, K⁺-adenosine triphosphatase of the stomach. Journal of Clinical Investigation 81: 475–479

Kimura S, Kotani T, McBride O W et al 1987 Human thyroid peroxidase: Complete cDNA and protein sequence, chromosome mapping and identification of two alternatively spliced mRNAs. Proceedings of the National Academy of Sciences USA 84: 5555–5559

Notkins A B, Onodera T, Prabhakar B 1984 Virus induced autoimmunity. In: Notkins A B, Oldstone M B A (eds) Concepts in viral pathogenesis. Springer, Heidelberg: 210–216

Oldstone M B A 1987 Molecular mimicry and autoimmune disease. Cell 50: 819–820

Ruf J, Czarnocka B, De Micco C et al 1987 Thyroid peroxidase is the organ-specific 'microsomal' autoantigen involved in thyroid autoimmunity. Acta Endocrinology (Copenhagen) Suppl 281: 49–56

Schwimmbeck P L, Yu D T Y, Oldstone M B A 1987 Autoantibodies to HLA B27 in the sera of HLA B27 patients with ankylosing spondylitis and Reiters syndrome: Molecular mimicry with *Klebsiella pneumoniae* as potential mechanism of autoimmune disease. Journal of Experimental Medicine 166: 173–181

Srinivasappa J, Saegusa J, Prabhakar B S et al 1986 Molecular mimicry: frequency of reactivity of monoclonal antiviral antibodies with normal tissues. Journal of Virology 57: 397–401

Ullrich A, Bell J R, Chen E Y et al 1985 Human insulin receptor and its relationship to the tyrosine kinase family of oncogenes. Nature 313: 756–761

Wood J N, Hudson L, Jessel T M et al 1982 A monoclonal antibody defining antigenic determinants on subpopulations of mammalian neurons and *Trypanosoma cruzi* parasites. Nature 296: 34–38

Discussion: 'Molecular mimicry'
Robert Fujinami and Thomas Dyrberg

Following these two presentations describing the potential induction of autoimmune disease via 'molecular mimicry', several points were raised. It was suggested that the existence of a shared amino acid sequence between microbe and host does not in itself constitute evidence for immunological cross-reactivity, and even evidence of cross-reactive immune responses, although interesting, does not prove any pathogenic link. More rigorous tests, such as the ability to cause disease, and to transfer it, need to be applied. Dr Fujinami agreed, and pointed out that other evolutionary constraints, for example compartmentalization of certain proteins, could lead to maintenance of short amino acid homologies between host and virus proteins. He further stressed the critical role played by host major histocompatibility complex (MHC) molecules in selecting the regions of virus and host proteins to be presented to the immune system. He illustrated this point with the example of how experimental autoimmune encephalomyelitis induced by fragments of myelin basic protein can cause disease in different strains of mouse, and the disease can be transferred by T cells restricted by the murine class II MHC molecules.

The question of induction specificity was brought up: since antibody responses were induced by peptide administered with complete Freund's adjuvant, how certain could one be that the antibody response was to peptide, and not to the mycobacteria in the adjuvant? Dr Dyrberg responded that antibody was specific for purified peptide, and that peptide could block any cross-reactivities exhibited by the antibody. In any case, he said, the fundamental search was for cross-reactivity between microbe (even a mycobacterium!) and host; the identification of such reactivities represented a first step in the quest for a pathological link.

144

8. Picornavirus-initiated chronic inflammation

Paul H. Plotz, Mary E. Cronin, Lori A. Love,
Frederick W. Miller, Patrick McClintock and
David W. Smith

INTRODUCTION

Many human diseases whose cause is still unknown are called autoimmune because they share two features: there is chronic inflammation without known primary cause and, in some patients, autoantibodies are found. The term implies a pathogenetic pathway involving an attack by antibodies and/or lymphocytes specific for the affected tissues. Most investigators now believe that a more proximate cause—genetic, infectious, toxic, or a combination of them—is operating. Although a disorder of the immune system may be present in some of the most flagrant illnesses, in others the well-defined clinical picture and autoantibodies found suggest that a well-defined initiating event must have occurred.

There is direct evidence that drugs and some infections can cause illnesses indistinguishable from those we call autoimmune and, increasingly, there is circumstantial evidence linking particular viruses or bacteria to autoimmune disease. A case in point is the chronic inflammatory disease of muscle known as polymyositis. Picornaviruses have, although rarely, been isolated from or seen in specimens of affected muscles (Tang et al, 1975). Antibody titres against Coxsackie viruses suggest a recent infection in some patients (Christiansen et al, 1986; Travers et al, 1977); in the childhood illness, the onset is frequently in the Fall (Christiansen et al, 1986); in a variety with an abrupt onset and a recently recognized autoantibody to the signal recognition peptide, the onset has been in November in most of the cases we have seen (Leff et al, unpublished observations); several picornaviruses of the enterovirus and cardiovirus groups cause acute myositis or myocarditis in several species including man. Most strikingly, the RNA genomes of some of these same viruses are able to mimic tRNA as a substrate for an aminoacyl-tRNA synthetase (Salomon & Littauer, 1974; Lindley & Stebbing, 1977) and, in patients with myositis, antibodies to histidyl-, threonyl-, or alanyl-tRNA synthetase may occur (Mathews & Bernstein, 1983; Mathews et al, 1984; Bunn & Mathews, 1987).

With this in mind, we undertook to study the human disease and to develop an animal model of myositis (and myocarditis) in mice with the cardioviruses, EMCV and mengo virus, the picornaviruses which are reported to be charged by an aminoacyl-tRNA synthetase. The first major question on which we have focused is whether or not virus must persist in order for chronic inflammation to occur. If the answer turns out to be yes, where and in what form and how? If the answer turns out to be no, what then allows the transition to chronic inflammation: is 'autoimmunity' really involved?

PICORNAVIRUS PERSISTENCE

There is, of course, ample precedent for viral persistence in many viral families. The mechanisms of persistence—the viral strategies—are diverse and fascinating. Measles (Wechsler & Meissner, 1983), herpes simplex (Croen et al, 1987), lymphocytic choriomeningitis virus (Oldstone et al, 1984), reovirus (Verdin et al, 1986) visna (Kennedy et al, 1985), and numerous other viruses are important causes of chronic human or animal illness. Picornaviruses, our myositis candidates, however, are rarely persistent. They mostly enter cells, multiply rapidly, and exit by lysing their host cells.

Foot-and-mouth disease virus (FMDV) can persist for as long as four weeks in cattle (Sutmoller et al, 1968), and can be adapted in tissue culture to produce a chronic, non-lytic infection of BHK-21 cells (De la Torre et al, 1985). In the model *in vitro* infection, which can be cured by ribavirin (De la Torre et al, 1987), the viral genome not only develops point mutations, but it shortens appreciably. By passage 65, virus can no longer be cultured on healthy host cells, but it can be demonstrated by northern blot as a somewhat shortened genome, and at passage 98, genome truncated by about 3 Kb was found, although the sites of deletion are not yet known (De la Torre et al, 1985).

Hepatitis A virus causes only an acute illness in man, but it can be adapted to a chronic tissue culture infection on human fibroblasts (Vallbracht et al, 1984). Interferon, but not antibody cured the culture. A very short (2 Kb) fragment was present by 10 days after infection along with a full-sized virus in a similar culture system with this virus in MRC-5-cells (De Chastonay & Siegl, 1987).

In both of these examples, all the cells in the culture were infected, all remained morphologically normal, and the culture remained susceptible to superinfection by other viruses. A different kind of chronic infection due to the presence of a small number of lytically-infected cells and the presence of a substance in the culture fluid which inhibited viral attachment or penetration has been described with Coxsackievirus B3 (Crowell & Syverton, 1961).

Both poliovirus (Davis et al, 1977) and Echoviruses (Wilfert et al, 1977) can cause a chronic illness in severely immunocompromised human hosts. The Echovirus illness occurs in children with agammaglobulinaemia and may be accompanied by a dermatomyositis-like clinical picture. The virus is generally culturable from cerebrospinal fluid and not usually from muscle. Echovirus 6 has also been adapted to tissue culture to give a chronic infection of a truncated virus, apparently deficient in VP3 (Gibson & Righthand, 1985).

Coxsackievirus B3 causes an acute, followed by a chronic, myocarditis in young mice. The virus ceases to be culturable by two to three weeks. The chronic inflammation appears to be related to the development of antibodies to cardiac myosin in susceptible strains (Neu et al, 1987) or to the development of cellular immunity directed towards normal myocytes (Estrin & Huber, 1987). It is not yet clear how long Coxsackievirus B4 or EMCV-B persists in those mice which develop long-lasting diabetes due to pancreatic destruction (Jordan & Cohen, 1987).

The encephalitis induced in mice by the intercerebral injection of Theiler's virus, a cardiovirus closely related to EMCV (Pevear et al, 1987), may be followed by a chronic demyelinative disease of the spinal cord (Lipton, 1975). In this chronic phase, virus disappears from the brain and can be cultured or located by immunofluorescence or *in situ* hybridization in glial cells in and around the inflammatory lesions for months to years (Lipton et al, 1984; Chamorro et al, 1986). The exact state of the viral genome at these later times is doubtless the subject of intensive study, particularly since the mouse disease clinically and pathologically so closely resembles human multiple sclerosis.

EXPERIMENTAL STUDIES WITH EMCV

We have used, in our studies, a myotropic variant of EMCV, called EMC-221A, and a variant of the mengovirus adapted to G8 myoblasts. EMC 221A causes an acute myositis and myocarditis in susceptible mouse strains (Miller et al, 1987). The myositis has persisted in some experiments and disappeared in others. The myocarditis becomes chronic. A low-grade encephalitis, evidenced by the presence of microglial nodules, is long-lasting. The animals rapidly develop a high-titred, long-lasting antibody response.

In addition to culturing tissues for viruses, we have probed fixed tissues by *in situ* hybridization and sought viral genomes by slot blot and northern blot hybridization of extracted RNA. We used two EMC probes: A8, an approximately 1.4 Kb cDNA clone derived in our laboratory from the 3' end of EMC 221A; and E9-21, from Ann Palmenberg, a 454 base cDNA from near the 5' end. Both were used as templates for the synthesis of ^{35}S- or ^{32}P-labelled single-stranded RNA complementary to the virus + strand. Control probes of mouse β actin and an unrelated phage were included in all experiments to monitor RNA isolation and *in situ* techniques.

For a virus with the life cycle of a typical picornavirus, *in situ* hybridization offers much greater sensitivity for detecting rare but heavily-infected cells present in small quantities of tissue. A single 4 x 4 section of skeletal tissue cut to 5 μm may contain up to 3×10^4 muscle cells in cross-section. One infected cell can easily be found if it contains sufficient virus—in our hands, roughly 10^2-10^3 copies using an ^{35}S-labelled probe representing about 6% of the genome. We have barely been able to detect slot blot signal from RNA extracted from a single section of that size in which roughly 10% of cells contain virus at about 5×10^4 copies per infected cell. With the polymerase chain reaction adapted for RNA we expect to increase sensitivity dramatically, but one does lose interesting histopathological information.

In skeletal muscle of infected animals, the pattern was of an acute myositis. At seven days virus was present in high titre, and there were many degenerating cells and a mononuclear cell infiltration. These disappeared over the next two weeks. Curiously, infected cells were not always adjacent to inflammation, nor was inflammation always associated with positive myocytes, although generally they went hand in hand (Fig. 8.1). Positive cells were present at three or, rarely, four weeks.

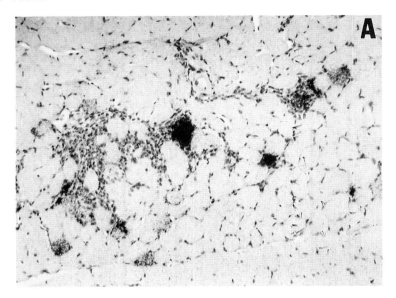

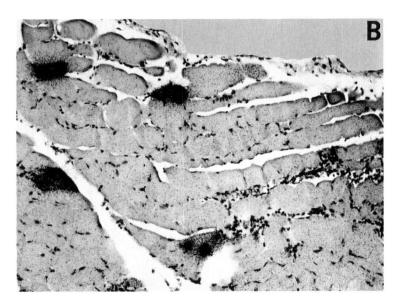

Fig. 8.1 *In situ* hybridization of mouse skeletal muscle in cross-section (A) and longitudinal section (B) one week after infection with EMC-221A, probed with a single-stranded RNA probe

In the heart, a chronic inflammation persisted throughout the 12 week observation period, although a healing process with fibrosis and calcification was also present. As in skeletal muscle, the culturable virus was almost gone at two weeks, but an *in situ* signal remained at least a week longer.

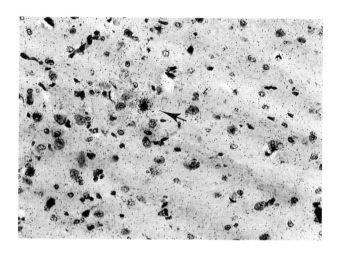

Fig. 8.2 *In situ* hybridization of mouse brain four weeks after infection with EMC-221A. A single cell (arrow) has viral nucleic acid

In the brain a few viruses could be cultured at four weeks, and an *in situ* signal was present in some animals infected with a lower dose of virus (Fig.8.2). These results are summarized in Table 8.1.

Table 8.1 Virus nucleic acid seen by *in situ* hybridization after infection by EMC 221a (number of positives/number tested)

Organ	Week			
	1	2	3	4
Muscle	5/5*	5/6*	5/8+	0/9
Heart	5/5*	5/6*	3/8+	0/9
Brain	5/5*	5/6*	4/6+	2/7+

* Strong signal; many positive areas per section
+ Weak signal; few positive areas per section

In all these tissues, both E9-21 and A8 probes were positive or negative in tandem. By northern blot, besides whole virus there were additional positive bands, presumably representing fragments digested by tissue RNAse. Even in myoblast cultures infected with the virus and extracted in their flasks with all precautions, minor fragments—different for the two probes—were present, along with a major band of intact full-sized viral RNA. We have not yet probed tissues for viral negative strands.

The particle/PFU ratio of picornavirus, even in preparations of whole virus, may be 10^2-10^3 and within an infected cell, much more viral RNA is doubtless present in the form of incompletely synthesized positive strands, negative strands, and breakdown products. It was possible to determine the ratio of viral nucleic acid molecules (E9-21) to PFU from quantitative slot blots at several points. At week one, the ratio ranged from 1 to 10 x 10^5 in skeletal muscle, heart, and brain, and was more than 10^7 in spleen. In brain at four weeks, when few PFU could be cultured, the ratio exceeded 10^8. It is impossible to know now whether the later positive *in situ* signal we have observed represents more than this detritus of the normal viral life cycle.

So far, then, we have found that viral genome can be found in tissues for at least a week beyond the time it can be cultured. What is intriguing is that the inflammatory process has such a different history in the different organs of an animal all exposed to the same humoral and presumably cellular immune response to the virus and the same circulating non-specific mediators of inflammation. With respect to autoimmunity in this animal model, we have subsequently found that EMC-221A and this mengovirus variant, which causes a similar illness, cannot accept an amino acid from any aminoacyl–tRNA synthetase, and antibodies to synthetases, as measured by the immuno-precipitation of tRNA, do not occur following infection by either virus. A search for other autoantibodies is underway.

It will be of great interest to determine by more sensitive means, how long the signal really does persist and whether the remaining viral genetic material is changed. It will also be of interest to know whether viral antigens persist, whether anti-viral therapy is effective in ablating later inflammation, and what does sustain inflammation if virus is well and truly gone.

REFERENCES

Bunn C B, Mathews M B 1987 Autoreactive epitope defined as the anticodon region of alanine transfer RNA. Science 238: 1116–1119
Chamorro M, Aubert C, Brahic M 1986 Demyelinating lesions due to Theiler's virus are associated with ongoing central nervous infection. Journal of Virology 57: 992–997
Christiansen M L, Pachman L M, Schneiderman R, Patel D C, Friedman J M 1986 Prevalence of coxsackie B virus antibodies in patients with juvenile dermatomyositis. Arthritis and Rheumatism 29: 1365–1370
Croen K D, Ostrove J M, Dragovic L J, Smialek J E, Straus S E 1987 Latent herpes simplex virus in human trigeminal ganglia. Detection of an immediate early gene 'anti-sense' transcript by in situ hybridization. New England Journal of Medicine 317: 1427–1432
Crowell R L, Syverton J T 1961 The mammalian cell-virus relationship. VI Sustained infection of HeLa cells by coxsackievirus B3 and effect on superinfection. Journal of Experimental Medicine 113: 419–435
Davis L E, Bodian D, Price D, Butler I J, Vickers J H 1977 Chronic progressive poliomyelitis secondary to vaccination of an immundeficient child. New England Journal of Medicine 297: 241–245
De Chastonay J, Siegl G 1987 Replicative events in hepatitis A virus-infected MRC-5 cells. Virology 157: 268–275
De la Torre J, Davila M, Sobrino F, Ortin J, Domingo E 1985 Establishment of cell lines persistently infected with Foot-and-mouth disease virus. Virology 145: 24–35
De la Torre J C, Alarcon B, Martinez-Salas E, Carrasco L, Domingo E 1987 Ribavirin cures cells of a persistent infection with foot-and-mouth disease virus in vitro. Journal of Virology 61: 233–235

Estrin M, Huber S A 1987 Coxsackievirus B3-induced myocarditis. Autoimmunity is L3T4 and T helper cell and IL-2 independent in BALB/C mice. American Journal of Pathology 127: 335–341

Gibson J P, Righthand V F 1985 Persistence of Echovirus 6 in cloned human cells. Journal of Virology 54: 219–223

Jordan G W, Cohen S H 1987 Encephalomyocarditis virus-induced diabetes mellitus in mice: model or viral pathogenesis. Review of Infectious Diseases 9: 917–924

Kennedy P G E, Narayan O, Ghotbi Z, Hopkins J, Gendelman H E, Clements J E 1985 Persistent expression of Ia antigen and viral genome in visna-maedi virus-induced inflammatory cells. Journal of Experimental Medicine 162: 1970–1982

Lindley I J D, Stebbing N 1977 Aminoacylation of encephalomyocarditis virus RNA. Journal of General Virology 34: 177–182

Lipton H L 1975 Theiler's virus infection in mice: an unusual biphasic disease process leading to demyelination. Infection and Immunity 11: 1147–1155

Lipton H L, Kratochvil J, Sethi P, Dal Cantro M C 1984 Theiler's virus antigen detected in mouse spinal cord 2 1/2 years after infection. Neurology 34: 1117–1119

Mathews M B, Bernstein R M 1983 Myositis autoantibody inhibits histidyl-RNA synthetase: a model for autoimmunity. Nature 304: 177–179

Mathews M, Reichlin M, Bernstein R 1984 Anti-threonyl-tRNA synthetase, a second myositis-related autoantibody. Journal of Experimental Medicine 160: 420–434

Miller F W, Love L A, Biswas T, McClintock P R, Notkins A L, Plotz P H 1987 Viral and host genetic factors influence encephalomyocarditis virus-induced polymyositis in adult mice. Arthritis and Rheumatism 30: 549–556.

Neu N, Beisel K W, Traystman M D, Rose N C, Craig S W 1987 Autoantibodies specific for the cardiac myosin isoform are found in mice susceptible to coxsackievirus B3-induced myocarditis. Journal of Immunology 138: 2488–2492

Oldstone M B A, Southern P, Rodriguez M, Lampert P 1984 Virus persists in B cells of islets of Langerhans and is associated with chemical manifestations of diabetes. Science 224: 1440–1442

Pevear D C, Calenoff M, Rozhon E, Lipton H L 1987 Analysis of the complete nucleotide sequence of the picornavirus Theiler's murine encephalitis virus indicates that it is closely related to cardiovirus. Journal of Virology 61: 1507–1516

Salomon R, Littauer N Z 1974 Enzymatic acylation of histidine to mengovirus RNA. Nature 249: 32–34

Sutmoller P, McVicar J W, Cottral G E 1968 The epizootiological importance of foot-and-mouth disease carriers. I. Experimentally produced foot-and-mouth disease carriers in susceptible and immune cattle. Archiv fur Gesamte Virusforschung 23: 277–235

Tang T T, Sedmak G V, Seigemund K A, McCreadie S R 1975 Chronic myopathy associated with coxsackie virus A9: a combined electron microscopic and viral isolation study. New England Journal of Medicine 292: 608–611

Travers R L, Hughes G R V, Cambridge G, Sewell J R 1977 Coxsackie B neutralization titres in polymyositis-dermatomyositis. Lancet 1: 1268

Vallbracht, A, Hofmann L, Wurster K G, Flehmig B 1984 Persistent infection of human fibroblasts by hepatitis A virus. Journal of General Virology. 65: 609–615

Verdin E M, Maratos-Flier E, Carpentier J L, Kahn C R 1986 Persistent infection with a non-transforming RNA virus leads to impaired growth factor receptors and response. Journal of Cellular Physiology 128: 457–465

Wechsler S L, Meissner H C 1983 Measles and SSPE viruses: similarities and differences. Progress in Medical Virology 28: 65–95

Wilfert C M, Buckley R H, Mohanakumar T, Griffith J F, Katz S L, Whisnant J K, Eggleston P A, Moore M, Treadwell E, Oxman M N, Rosen F S 1977 Persistent and fatal central-nervous-system echovirus infections in patients with agammaglobulinemia. New England Journal of Medicine 296: 1485–1489

Discussion of paper presented by Paul Plotz

Discussant: Stuart Cohen

COMPARISONS BETWEEN ENCEPHALOMYOCARDITIS
VIRUS-INDUCED DIABETES MELLITUS AND
PICORNAVIRUS-INITIATED CHRONIC INFLAMMATION

The pathogenesis of picornavirus infections has been extensively studied using encephalomyocarditis (EMC) virus-induced diabetes mellitus of mice as an experimental model. After briefly describing EMC virus-induced diabetes, I will compare and contrast this model with that of EMC virus-induced myositis as presented by Dr Paul Plotz and colleagues in their paper 'Picornavirus-initiated chronic inflammation'.

The best evidence that a viral infection can cause diabetes mellitus comes from work with EMC virus in mice. In 1968, Craighead and McLane showed that inoculation of genetically susceptible mice with the M-strain of EMC virus would result in hyperglycaemia and insulitis (Craighead & McLane, 1968). This model has been extensively studied but the ability to cause diabetes and the severity of disease caused by the M-strain was inconsistent (Iwo et al, 1983). Therefore, Yoon et al (1980) selected and plaque purified two variants of the M-strain for and against the ability to cause diabetes in SJL/J mice. EMC-D causes diabetes in 100% of susceptible mice, whereas EMC-B is non-diabetogenic. When the variants are co-inoculated in varying proportions, EMC-B interferes with the ability of EMC-D to produce diabetes (Yoon et al, 1980).

The immune response to EMC infection has been systematically studied (Yoon et al, 1980). EMC-B and D are antigenically similar and cannot be distinguished by hyperimmune serum raised against either variant. Antibody titres peak on the seventh day after infection of SJL mice (Yoon et al, 1980). No difference has been noted between the time of appearance or the titre of antibody between EMC-B and D, suggesting that antibody response is not related to the outcome of these infections (Yoon et al, 1980). Cell-mediated immunity will be discussed in detail when comparing EMC virus-induced diabetes with the polymyositis model.

The ability of EMC-B to interfere with the diabetogenicity of EMC-D correlated with the ability of EMC-B to induce high titres of circulating interferon early in the course of infection (Yoon et al, 1980). Maximum circulating interferon titres induced by EMC-B appear within 10 hours post infection and are about three times higher than titres induced by EMC-D which are also delayed in appearance, peaking at 30 hours post infection (Yoon et al, 1980). These data suggested a role for the interferon system in determining the outcome of these infections. Several lines of evidence support this hypothesis. First, interferon or interferon inducers such as polyinosinic-polycytidylic acid (Poly I:C) can prevent EMC-D from causing diabetes in mice (Yoon et al, 1983). Moreover, when anti-interferon globulins are used to pretreat mice infected with EMC-B, 40% of SJL mice die and 40% of the survivors become diabetic (Yoon et al, 1983). Therefore, EMC-B can infect pancreatic beta-cells but viral replication is arrested and tissue destruction is prevented by interferon.

This brief description of the EMC virus-induced diabetes model serves as a background for discussion of the model of chronic inflammation due to EMC. I will examine four issues related to the pathogenesis of these infections: (1) tissue tropism, (2) autoimmunity, (3) the interferon system, (4) persistence.

EMC-221A is a myopathic variant which was a selected variant from the M-strain of EMC virus, the same strain which produced the B and D variants (Miller et al, 1987). EMC-221A causes polymyositis in mice whereas EMC-D causes only minimal myositis (Miller et al, 1987). Different tissue tropism of the two variants is one means of explaining these results. Craighead (1966) first showed that different strains of EMC virus can have different tissue tropisms despite serological similarities. Morishima et al (1982) studied receptor attachment differences between EMC-D and mengovirus-2T. Cardioviruses all belong to a single serotype, therefore these two viruses cannot be distinguished antigenically by hyperimmune serum. The rate of binding to neuroblastoma cells was five to ten times greater for mengovirus-2T when compared with EMC-D. Moreover, binding of homologous virus was blocked whereas heterologous virus was not, suggesting that these viruses bound to different receptors despite their close biological relationship. Therefore, if different receptors are utilized by EMC-221A and EMC-D, tissue tropism is a possible explanation for their differing abilities to cause myositis.

Autoimmunity is an important mechanism of disease in polymyositis and insulin-dependent diabetes mellitus in humans, and therefore requires investigation in this model system. The search for autoantibodies is an interesting one which is actively being pursued. Cellular immunity has been studied extensively in EMC virus-induced diabetes, attempting to define the role of autoimmunity in the destruction of pancreatic beta-cells. Using the M-strain, Huber et al (1985) demonstrated two mechanisms of beta-cell destruction using different strains of mice. In DBA/2 mice, T lymphocyte depletion failed to influence the development of diabetes, suggesting direct beta-cell cytolysis. Whereas, in BALB/cBY mice, four days after infection pancreatic insulin concentrations were depressed, but the mice did not become hyperglycaemic until 11 days post-infection when beta-cell cytolytic T lymphoctye activity was present. It appears that subclinical virus-induced beta-cell damage in a genetically predisposed host can be followed by autoimmune beta-cell cytotoxicity. These results may be explained by the variable mixture of diabetogenic variants present in the M-strain in association with the different strains of mice studied. In contrast, Yoon et al (1985) examined the contribution of autoimmunity to the ability of EMC-D infections to cause diabetes in SJL and DBA/2J mice. They showed no linkage with the H-2 haplotype of the mice, no prevention of diabetes by anti-lymphocyte serum, no difference in the disease in nude or thymectomized mice and that lymphocytes could not passively transfer diabetes. Therefore, immune mechanisms are not important factors in the pathogenesis of these infections. The potential role of cell-mediated autoimmunity in the chronic inflammation model should be pursued in an analogous manner.

Evidence indicating a role for the interferon system as an explanation for the biological differences between EMC-B and D *in vivo* led to studies of the sensitivity to and ability to induce interferon by these variants *in vitro* (Cohen et al, 1983). Marcus et al (1981) first described the interferon-inducing particle (ifp) phenotype by studying two variants of mengovirus. An interferon sensitive mutant of mengovirus (is-1) was isolated after nitrous acid mutagenesis by Simon et al (1976). The interferon sensitivity of this mutant was shown to be due to its ability to induce endogenous interferon which further increased resistance of the cell (Marcus et al, 1981). This property was not seen in the wild type virus. The ifp$^+$ phenotype of the is-1 mutants was associated with interferon sensitivity and is less cytopathic to interferon-pre-treated cells because local interferon production is amplified as a result of the priming effect. The wild type virus demonstrated the ifp$^-$ phenotype which is associated with a relative inability to induce interferon, a relative insensitivity to interferon and cytopathology (Marcus et al, 1981). We determined the ifp phenotypes of EMC-B and D. The B variant carries the ifp$^+$ phenotype whereas EMC-D is ifp$^-$ (Cohen et al, 1983). Furthermore, we have proposed that the ifp phenotype plays an important role in the pathogenesis of EMC virus-induced diabetes (Jordan & Cohen, 1987). Our hypothesis states that EMC-B induces interferon at the site of inoculation which circulates and primes the pancreas for interferon induction very early in the infection. Therefore, when the beta-cells of the pancreas are exposed to the virus of the ifp$^+$ phenotype they produce high titres of local interferon which halts the spread of infection. Because EMC-D induces small amounts of interferon it infects and lyses pancreatic beta cells causing diabetes.

Several other studies raise different questions about the role of interferon in EMC infection related to the timing of the interferon response and the strain of animal being studied. Gould et al (1985) described a greater severity of disease and higher titres of EMC-D on day seven when mice were given interferon on day four. This may relate to a paradoxical immunosuppression which has been seen with interferon based on the timing of the injection (Stewart, 1981). Alternatively, these data may relate in part to the lymphokine properties of interferon and autoimmunity. One further study relates the interferon system to the host in EMC virus-induced diabetes. C57BL/6J mice do not become diabetic after infection with EMC-D. High titres of interferon are present in the serum of these animals despite the relative inability of EMC-D to produce interferon *in vitro* (Gaines et al, 1987). After treatment with anti-interferon globulins 60% of C57BL/6J mice become glucose intolerant (Gaines et al, 1987). These data emphasize the importance of the interferon system in the outcome of EMC infections. It is interesting that the control strain used in studies of the polymyositis model is the 'virulent' strain in the diabetes model. Therefore, it is possible that the interferon system may not be an important factor in the outcome of infection with EMC-221A. Nevertheless, it is important to determine the interferon response of mice infected with EMC-221A as well as the ifp phenotype.

Persistent infection leading to continued inflammation has been demonstrated with picornaviruses *in vivo* and *in vitro* (De la Torre et al, 1985; Gibson & Righthand, 1985; Wilfert et al, 1977). Furthermore, demonstration of viral nucleic acid by *in situ* hybridization in the muscles of animals infected with EMC-221A for at least one week beyond the time the virus can be cultured, argues for further studies directed at the role of persistence in chronic inflammation. More sensitive techniques for detecting viral RNA and viral antigens will help clarify the importance of persistence in EMC virus-induced chronic inflammation.

Our laboratory has been interested in determining the genetic basis for the virulence of EMC-B and D and the ifp phenotype (Jordan et al, 1987). Another variant of EMC virus derived from the same parenteral strain with different biology provides another sensitive probe to relate the genetic structure of picornaviruses to the pathogenesis of infection. Further definition of the biology and genetics of the polymyositis model will therefore be of great interest.

REFERENCES

Cohen S H, Bolton V, Jordan G W 1983 Relationship of interferon-inducing particle phenotype to encephalomyocarditis virus-induced diabetes mellitus. Infection and Immunity 42: 605–611
Craighead J E 1966 Pathogenicity of the M and E variants of the encephalomyocarditis (EMC) virus. I. Myocardiotropic and neurotropic properties. American Journal of Pathology 48: 333–345
Craighead J E, McLane M F 1968 Diabetes mellitus: induction in mice by encephalomyocarditis virus. Science 162: 913–914
De la Torre J, Davila M, Sobrino F, Ortin J, Domingo E 1985 Establishment of cell lines persistently infected with foot-and-mouth disease virus. Virology 145: 24–35
Gaines K L, Kayes S G, Wilson G L 1987 Factors affecting the infection of the D variant of encephalomyocarditis virus in the B cells of C57BL/6J mice. Diabetologia 30: 419–425
Gibson J P, Righthand V F 1985 Persistence of echovirus 6 in cloned human cells. Journal of Virology 54: 219–223
Gould C L, McMannama K G, Bigley N J, Giron D J 1985 Exacerbation of the pathogenesis of the diabetogenic variant of encephalomyocarditis virus in mice by interferon. Journal of Interferon Research 5: 33–37
Huber S A, Babu P G, Craighead J E 1985 Genetic influences on the immunologic pathogenesis of encephalomyocarditis (EMC) virus induced diabetes mellitus. Diabetes 34: 1186–1190
Iwo K, Bellomo S C, Mukai N, Craighead J E 1983 Encephalomyocarditis virus induced diabetes mellitus in mice: long-term changes in the structure and function of islets of Langerhans. Diabetologia 25: 39–44
Jordan G W, Cohen S H 1987 Encephalomyocarditis virus-induced diabetes mellitus: Model of viral pathogenesis. Reviews of Infectious Diseases 9: 917–924
Jordan G W, Cohen S H, Dandekar S, Vanden Brink K M 1987 The genomic RNA of diabetogenic encephalomyocarditis virus: Characterization and molecular cloning. Virology 159: 120–125
Marcus P I, Guidon P T Jr, Sekellick M J 1981 Interferon induction by viruses. VII. Menogovirus: 'interferon-sensitive' mutant phenotype attributed to interferon-inducing particle activity. Journal of Interferon Research 1: 601–611
Miller F W, Love L A, Biswas T, McClintock P R, Notkins A L, Plotz P H 1987 Viral and host genetic factors influence encephalomyocarditis virus-induced polymyositis in adult mice. Arthritis and Rheumatism 30: 549–556

Morishima T, McClintock P R, Aulakh G S, Billups L C, Notkins A L 1982 Genomic and receptor attachment differences between mengovirus and encephalomyocarditis virus. Virology 122: 461–465

Simon E H, Kung S, Koh T T, Brandman P 1976 Interferon sensitive mutants of mengovirus. I. Isolation and biological characterization. Virology 69: 727–736

Stewart W E II 1981 Non-antiviral actions of interferons. In: The interferon system. 2nd ed, New York: Springer-Verlag pp 223–256

Wilfert C M, Buckley R H, Mohanakumar T et al 1977 Persistent and fatal central-nervous-system echovirus infections in patients with agammaglobulinemia. New England Journal of Medicine 296: 1485–1489

Yoon J–W, McClintock P R, Onodera T, Notkins A L 1980 Virus-induced diabetes mellitus XVIII. Inhibition by a nondiabetogenic variant of encephalomyocarditis virus. Journal of Experimental Medicine 152: 878–882

Yoon J-W, Cha C-Y, Jordan G W 1983 The role of interferon in virus-induced diabetes. Journal of Infectious Diseases 147: 155–159

Yoon J-W, McClintock P R, Bachurski C J, Longstreth J D, Notkins A L 1985 Virus-induced diabetes mellitus. No evidence for immune mechanisms in the destruction of B-cells by the D-variant of encephalomyocarditis virus. Diabetes 34: 922–925

Discussion: Picornavirus

Paul Plotz and Stuart Cohen

In response to a comment that the EMC model described did not represent an ideal system for studying diabetes in man, Dr Cohen responded that his major intent was not to develop a model for juvenile onset diabetes, but rather to elucidate mechanisms of picornavirus pathogenesis.

At present there is no molecular evidence (at the sequence level) which ties the interferon-inducing phenotype to viral diabetogenicity; and the molecular structure of the agent makes transfection studies, such as those done with poliovirus, much more difficult.

9. The cytolytic T lymphocyte response to murine cytomegalovirus infection

Ulrich Koszinowski

INTRODUCTION

Recognition of viral antigens by the immune system is followed by the generation of specific humoral and cellular effector mechanisms. In the past years significant advances have been made in the understanding of the structural basis for immune recognition of viral antigens. The crystallographic analysis has provided the three-dimensional structure of some virions and viral proteins and has demonstrated the role of protein conformation for the attack of humoral antibodies. Interest has centred on the analysis of viral structural proteins because the protruding domains of glycoproteins and of virion capsid proteins formed by continuous or discontinuous amino acid sequences are likely to induce and bind neutralizing antibodies.

By comparison, the understanding of viral antigen recognition by protective cellular immune mechanisms has suffered from technical obstacles and from the lack of knowledge of the molecules involved. After characterization of the antigen receptor on T cells (TRC), a heterodimeric structure encoded by genes of the immunoglobulin supergene family (Hood et al, 1985), and after 3D-structure analysis, has provided evidence for the function of major histocompatibility complex (MHC) encoded proteins to present antigen (Bjorkmann et al, 1987), two essential molecules involved in immune recognition of viral antigens by T cells are defined. Cloning procedures for T cells solved the technical difficulty to prepare characterized probes. Recognition of viral antigens by T cells involves the formation of a trimolecular complex consisting of the TCR, the MHC molecule and an antigen. The properties that predispose a viral protein to represent an important antigen for T cells, for instance a cytolytic T lymphocyte (CTL), are unknown. They certainly differ from those important for the generation of neutralizing antibodies.

In this communication interest has been focused on non-structural viral proteins, a class of proteins that has been dismissed so far in concepts of vaccine development. The role of non-structural proteins in immunity is addressed by studying the cellular immune response to murine cytomegalovirus (MCMV), a herpesvirus. Evidence is presented that experimental vaccination using a non-structural protein can induce protective T cell immunity.

158

CMV INFECTION AND THE IMMUNODEFICIENT HOST

Cytomegaloviruses (CMV) constitute a subfamily of herpesviruses, the betaherpesvirinae, which are classified according to biological properties. Despite similar biological properties, CMV of various host species differ with respect to the structural organization of their genomes, the localization of homologous genes and even the function of individual homologous genes. Within the herpesvirus family the CMV contain the largest genomes of double stranded DNA of about 240 kilo base pairs (kbp) in size with the potential to code for at least 80 proteins. To date very few CMV genes and proteins have been analysed in detail. CMV are strictly host specific with the consequence that the biology of the infection with human CMV (HCMV) cannot be studied in animal models.

Typically, the primary HCMV infection occurs in childhood and does not seriously harm the immunocompetent host. As in other herpesviruses, HCMV infection is followed by the establishment of lifelong persistence of the viral genome. Intra-uterine HCMV infection is responsible for several types of organ malformation and for severe neurological disorders, and congential HCMV infection in immunologically immature newborns is associated with alterations in the haematological profile. In the adult, by causing interstitial pneumonia following opportunistic primary or recurrent infection, HCMV is a fatal complication in marrow transplant recipients after iatrogenic immunosuppresion (Meyers et al, 1980). HCMV also represents one of the leading causes of death of acquired immunodeficiency syndrome victims immunocompromised by infection with human immunodeficiency virus (HIV) (Moskovitz et al, 1985).

Humoral immunity is involved in protection against the severity of primary disease and trials to protect marrow recipients by passive antiserum therapy are underway. It is clear, however, that virus reactivation can occur even in the presence of high antibody titres. Cellular immunity is therefore thought to be an important factor in the control of virus spread. It has been suggested that CTL play an essential role in limiting HCMV infection because patients with dysfunction of cellular immunity, as exemplified by the failure to generate cytolytic T lymphocytes (CTL), often succumb to CMV disease (Quinnan et al, 1982).

Of the various animal models murine CMV (MCMV) infection has been most extensively studied. MCMV infection has proved to be a convenient model to investigate aspects of CMV latency, recurrency, pathogenesis and immunity in a natural host. As in the infection of humans with HCMV, immunosuppression correlates with severe MCMV disease, indicating that the establishment of productive infection in the tissues of the host is controlled by the immune system. The availability of characterized murine inbred strains and of specific reagents to identify T lymphocyte subsets provide the means to test the role of specific cellular effector mechanisms in controlling MCMV infection *in vitro* and *in vivo*.

THE ROLE OF T LYMPHOCYTES IN THE CONTROL OF MCMV REPLICATION

In the treatment of patients by irradiation and bone marrow transplantation, serious complications can result from interstitial CMV pneumonia. In mice, irradiation also has a profound effect on the tissue manifestation of CMV infection. When a dose of 10^5 plaque forming units (pfu) of tissue culture grown MCMV is used for infecting immunocompetent mice, infectious virus can be recovered at day 14 p.i. only from the salivary glands. The salivary glands represent a privileged site for MCMV replication. MCMV, formerly named salivary gland virus of the mouse, has originally been isolated from persistently infected salivary glands.

In contrast to immunocompetent mice, high titres of virus are detected not only in salivary glands but also in liver, spleen, adrenal glands and lungs of 6 Gy irradiated recipients (Reddehase et al, 1985). Moderate virus titres are found in the bone marrow. Histological studies demonstrated evidence for a focal interstitial pneumonia, and in situ hybridization and electron microscopic analysis identified interstitial cells, pneumocytes and endothelial cells as targets for MCMV replication. Within the adrenal glands, focal necroses were rare in the medulla but frequent throughout the cortex, with the parenchymal cells in the zona reticularis of the cortex representing the productively infected cells (Reddehase et al, 1988). The bone marrow of irradiated and infected mice was nearly devoid of nucleated cells at day 14 p.i., whereas at the same time the bone marrow of uninfected, irradiated controls was already autoreconstituted (Mutter et al, 1988). Despite the failure of irradiated and MCMV infected mice to reconstitute the bone marrow, only a few of the remaining cells in the bone marrow were productively infected.

The radiation damage could either predispose normally non-permissive cell types to productive infection or could abrogate, due to elimination of lymphocytes, the immune control over the tissue manifestation of the virus. The second alternative was verified by adoptive transfer of lymphoid cells into irradiated and infected recipients. When lymphocytes from immunocompetent MCMV sensitized donors were transferred intravenously into irradiated syngenic recipients that were infected after cell transfer, a significant antiviral effect was observed (Fig. 9.1). Already the transfer of only 10^4 activated lymphocytes reduced the viral titre determined at day 14 in the lung when compared with mice without cell transfer. Non-activated, naive lymphocytes were not active, demonstrating that an antigen specific property acquired in the immunocompetent cell donor was tested. Transfer of 10^7 activated lymphocytes restored the MCMV distribution pattern to the situation seen in immunocompetent mice: only the salivary gland contained infectious virus and the otherwise lethal infection in immunocompromised mice was survived by all adoptive cell transfer recipients (Reddehase et al, 1985).

Graded numbers of activated cells had differential antiviral activity in different tissues. Few lymphocytes were sufficient to limit virus replication in spleen and liver, and a higher number of cells was required to clear the lungs. Clearance of the salivary glands could not be achieved. The antiviral effect in lungs, liver and spleen could be due to either trapping of lymphocytes in lungs and liver or to homing to lymphoid tissues. Direct infiltration of transferred lymphocytes into the infected areas of the adrenal glands and limitation of viral replication in these tissues proved that lymphocytes can specifically migrate to infected areas, and that the effect of transferred cells is not restricted to organs where lymphocytes are trapped or home (Reddehase et al, 1988).

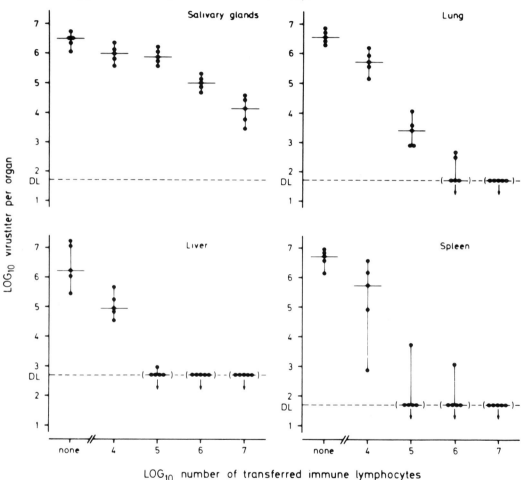

Fig. 9.1 Differential antiviral efficiency of activated donor lymphocytes in the tissues of cell transfer recipients. Irradiated animals received specifically activated donor lymphocytes by intravenous infusion before intraplanatar infection. At day 14 p.i. MCMV titres were measured in the organs of five recipients for each dose of transferred lymphocytes. The median values of the individual titre determinations are shown by horizontal bars. The dashed lines represent the detection levels (DL). (Reproduced with permission from Reddehase et al, 1985 The American Society for Microbiology, The Journal of Virology vol 55 p 264–273)

Mature T lymphocytes comprise two major subsets characterized by the CD4 and CD8 differentiation antigens which are expressed at the cell surface. CD4[+] T lymphocytes recognize antigen presented by major histocompatibility complex (MHC) class II gene encoded molecules and CD8$^+$ T lymphocytes recognize antigen presented by MHC class I molecules. CD4$^+$ lymphocytes are usually associated with helper functions and CD8$^+$ T lymphocytes with the capacity to mediate cytolysis of infected cells (CTL). The antiviral effect of transferred lymphocytes could be assigned to the CD8$^+$ T lymphocyte subset. The CD4$^+$ T lymphocytes had no protective effect on their own and did not improve the antiviral effect of CD8$^+$ T lymphocytes.

From these studies it was concluded that CD8$^+$ T lymphocytes control the tissue distribution of cytomegalovirus during acute infection in the immunocompetent host.

ANTIGENS EXPRESSED DURING THE IMMEDIATE-EARLY PHASE OF MCMV REPLICATION ARE RECOGNIZED BY PROTECTIVE CD8$^+$ T LYMPHOCYTES

Having identified CD8$^+$ T lymphocytes as the T lymphocyte subset involved in immune control of MCMV infection it was of interest to identify the viral antigens recognized. Although CD8$^+$ T lymphocytes, similar to antibodies, can recognize glycoprotein antigens, antigen recognition by T cells is not restricted to intrinsic membrane proteins. Due to the need for presentation of viral protein antigens by MHC molecules the virion structural proteins are not recognized unless taken up by cells or synthesized in cells and processed for antigen presentation. Thus, any protein encoded by the viral genome can perhaps serve as antigen, provided it is efficiently processed and presented. Indeed, it has been shown for other viruses that antigens for CTL can include internal structural proteins and also non-structural regulatory viral proteins (Townsend et al, 1985; Gooding & O'Connell, 1983). Since the 235 kbp genome of MCMV has a very high coding capacity (Ebeling et al, 1983) conditions needed to be employed which allowed the expression of only sets of genes in order to limit the number of potential candidates for further analysis. This was possible because gene expression in CMV is under strict temporal control and coordinately regulated in a cascade fashion (Keil et al, 1984). The first set of genes, the immediate early (IE) or alpha genes, is transcribed by the host cell polymerase II in the absence of any *de novo* viral protein synthesis. IE proteins are non-structural proteins (Keil et al, 1985). Synthesis and the regulatory function (Koszinowski et al, 1986) of at least one IE gene product is required to initiate the transcription of early (E) genes. Early gene products include both structural and non-structural proteins. Most of the structural proteins of the virion are synthesized during the late (L) phase of infection which starts after the synthesis of viral DNA. Using combinations of certain inhibitors the replication cascade in cells can be arrested between phases. For instance, MCMV infection in the presence of the protein synthesis inhibitor cycloheximide (CH) for selective transcription of IE mRNA followed by replacement by the inhibitor of mRNA transcription actinomycin D (Act.D), yields selective translation of IE protein in the absence of *de novo* transcription of early mRNA. Since inhibitor treatment does not interfere with intracellular

162

antigen processing and presentation such cells can then be used as target cells to test antigen recognition by CTL *in vitro*. The presence of at least two populations of MCMV antigen specific CTL was detected (Reddehase et al, 1984). One population was specific for virion structural proteins, as demonstrated by the lysis of cells that presented structural antigens after incubation with inactivated virions. Another population was specific for antigens expressed during the IE phase of MCMV replication.

In order to test the significance of CTL with specificity for IE antigens, their relative frequency within the total population of activated CTL was determined. About 50% of all precursors to cytolytic effector cells generated after MCMV infection were specific for antigens of the IE phase of MCMV and revealed that IE antigens must represent immunodominant antigens of MCMV (Reddehase & Koszinowski, 1984) (Table 9.1).

Table 9.1 High relative frequency of CTL precursors (CTLp) with specificity for MCMV immediate early antigens

Treatment of targets	Frequency f*	f/10⁶ lymphocytes (95% confidence limits)	Comments
—	1/166.0	6 (4–8)	Negative control
Con A	1/2.70	371 (226–516)	Total number of CTLp
IE phase	1/6.90	196 (97–195)	IE antigen specific CTLp
L phase	1/11.30	89 (60–118)	CTLp specific for antigen presented in L phase
UV inactivated virions	1/14.9	69 (48–86)	Structural protein specific CTLp

Effector cells were derived from MCMV activated lymphocytes (CTLp) expanded by interleukins in a limiting dilution assay (Reddehase et al, 1984). Second passage murine embryo fibroblasts were used as targets. The lectin Concanavallin A (Con A) was used at 20 μg ml^{-1} during the cytolytic assay to bypass specific recognition and to assess the progeny of all CTLp with cytolytic activity. CTLp defined that way include MCMV specific CTLp and also activated CTLp with other specificities present in lymphoid tissue. Cells were infected with a multiplicity of 4 pfu per cell. Immediate early (IE) antigen expression was achieved by infection and 3 h incubation in presence of cycloheximide (50 μg ml^{-1}), to be replaced by Actinomycin D (Act.D) (5 μg ml^{-1}). Late (L) phase antigen addition expression was achieved by infection in absence of inhibitors and addition of Act.D 20 hours later. UV irradiation was done at an intensity of 30 m^{-2}8^{-1} for 10 minutes. A dose of UV inactivated virus equivalent to 400 pfu per cell was used. 10³ ³¹Cr-labelled target cells were tested in a standard 3 hours ⁵C release assay. *Precursor frequencies were estimated from the proportion of non-responding microcultures using the minimum chi square and maximum likelihood methods for probability calculation.

The observation that a dominant subset of CD8⁺ T lymphocytes specifically recognized IE antigen suggested, but did not prove, the relevance of this subset in the control of MCMV infection. Evidence was obtained by specific depletion of antigen specific CTL. Depletion of IE antigen specific CTL abolished the capacity of sensitized T cells to limit viral replication *in vivo* after adoptive transfer. Furthermore, IE antigen specific CD8⁺ T lymphocytes, in the absence of T cells specific for viral structural proteins, conferred protective immunity (Reddehase et al, 1987a).

A RECOMBINANT VACCINIA VIRUS EXPRESSING THE NON-STRUCTURAL MAJOR IE PROTEIN OF MCMV PROTECTS AGAINST LETHAL MCMV DISEASE

To ascertain that antigens recognized during the IE phase of infection are indeed virus encoded and not cellular genes induced by the virus, IE genes and gene products were studied in more detail. Transcriptional analysis revealed that abundant transcription during the IE phase is restricted to a region of the MCMV genome of about 12 kbp in size. Three IE transcription units, ie1, ie2 and ie3, are clustered around a long and complex organized enhancer sequence (Keil et al, 1987a; Dorsch-Häsler et al, 1985). Most abundantly transcribed is the transcription unit ie1 from which mRNA species of about 1 to 5 kb in size originate (Fig. 9.2).

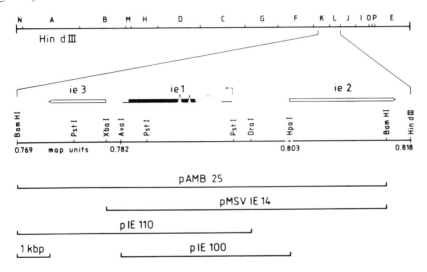

Fig. 9.2 Physical map of the IE region of MCMV. Top: Hind III cleavage sites. Centre: Location of transcription units, direction of transcription, and the structure of the major RNA transcribed from gene ieI in unit ieI. The segmented bar represents the open reading frame, and the hatched box indicates the promotor regulatory region. Units ie2 and ie3 are shown as open arrows to indicate the lack of precise knowledge of structural organization. Bottom: Plasmid-cloned MCMV DNA fragments used for transfection. (Reproduced with permission from Koszinowski et al, 1987[b], The Rockefeller University Press. The Journal of Experimental Medicine, vol 166, p 289–294)

Identification of genes encoding proteins that serve as antigens for CTL can be achieved with CTL clones of defined specificity. Such clones can be used as tools to monitor the expression of the relevant antigen. A CTL clone, termed IE1, was isolated which recognizes a MCMV IE antigen when presented by H-2^d allele of the L glycoprotein (Reddehase et al, 1986a; Reddehase et al, 1987b), one of the three murine MHC class I molecules, K, D and L. The coding region for the viral gene product recognized by clone IE1 cells was identified by co-transfection experiments using the L^d gene and various plasmid cloned DNA fragments of the IE region. Stable transfectants were used as target cells. It was found that expression of the transcription unit ie1 was both necessary and sufficient for recognition by clone IE1 antigen specific CTL (Koszinowski et al, 1987a; Koszinowski et al, 1987b) (Table 9.2).

Table 9.2 Recognition of an ieI product by CTL clone IE1

Construction of target cells			Percent specific lysis at clone IE1/target ratio of				
IE transcription units	Plasmid	Line	10	5	2.5	1.25	0.6
ie3, ie1, ie2	pAMB25	L/IE.B25-L^d/1	30.4	23.8	21.7	14.6	8.5
ie1, ie2	pMSV-IE14	L/IE14-L^d/10	41.4	33.6	32.4	20.9	17.5
ie3, ie1	pIE110	L/IE110-L^d/7	22.0	20.0	18.4	15.9	10.5
ie1	pIE100	L/ie1-L^d/2	49.1	43.2	36.9	25.2	15.4

Data represent mean values of six replicate determinations. Clone IE1 did not lyse the transfectant line L/45/1, which expresses ie1 but lacks L^d (11, 13). Lysis by an L^d specific CTL line ranged between 24 and 69% at an effector/target ratio of 10:1. (Reproduced with permission from U. H. Koszinowski et al, 1987[b], The Rockefeller Press, *Journal of Experimental Medicine*, vol. 166, pp. 289–294.)

The prominent 2.75 kb IE mRNA species is translated into a 89 kD non-structural phosphoprotein with regulatory function, termed pp89 (Keil et al, 1985; Koszinowski et al, 1986). Although transfection of ie1 provided evidence that an ie1 product represents an antigen for CTL, the fact that, due to alternative splicing of mRNA, several related products can be expressed by this unit, it was difficult to identify the protein recognized. Structural analysis of ie1 revealed that the 2.75 kb mRNA originates from four exons. Some mRNA species use the same transcription start site but are spliced onto a fifth or more exons located 3' of the fourth exon and constitute the mRNA's of the transcription unit ie3.

The gene located in transcription unit ie1 encoding the 2.75 kb mRNA was termed ie1. Whereas the first exon serves as a non-translated leader, the second exon contains the translation start site for an open reading frame with the potential to encode a protein of 595 amino acids (Keil et al, 1987b). The introns of ieI were deleted by site directed mutagenesis to provide conditions that only the 2.75 kb mRNA, but no other splice products, could be transcribed from the ieI gene (Fig. 9.3). The continuous open reading frame (orf) of ieI was subjected to the control of the 7.5 promotor of vaccinia virus and this construct was integrated into vaccinia virus. The resulting recombinant vaccinia virus MCMV-ie1-VAC expressed a protein indistinguishable from the authentic pp89 of MCMV with regard to size, post-translational processing and intracellular nuclear localization (Volkmer et al, 1987).

When MCMV-ie1-VAC was used to infect target cells that expressed the L^d molecule, lysis was seen whereas MCMV-ie1-VAC infected cells lacking the L^d glycoprotein were not lysed. Thus, pp89, the product of the ie1 gene provides the epitope recognized by the CTL clone IE1.

The recombinant virus could also sensitize cells *in vivo* for the generation of CTL after secondary re-stimulation *in vitro*. Since MCMV-ie1-VAC was both antigenic and immunogenic, the recombinant vaccinia virus was used as an experimental vaccine (Jonjic et al, 1988). The protective potential of MCMV-ieI-VAC was compared with that of vaccination with a non-lethal dose of MCMV (Fig. 9.4). Three weeks after vaccination mice were challenged with 5 LD$_{50}$ of

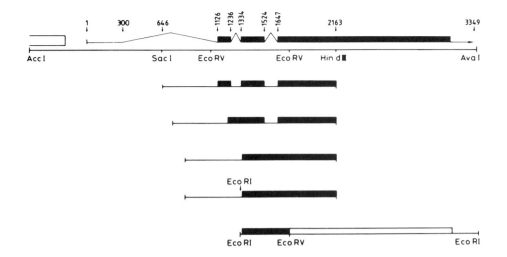

Fig. 9.3 Alteration of gene ieI structure. The structural organization of the ieI gene in the MCMV genome is depicted at the top. The coding sequences of exons are indicated by black bars. The location of the upstream MCMV enhancer is indicated by an open box. The distance (in base pairs) from the transcription start site and the position of exons, introns and some cleavage sites are indicated. Mutagenesis was performed in three sequential steps shown below: First, intron 2 and then intron 3 were removed by using oligonucleotides comprising the flanking exon sequences of the respective intron. The following 20-mers were used for deletion: Intron 2, 5' -CAT CAG ACA AGG TGC CAG CT-3'; intron 3, 5' -CAT GCT GCA GTG AGG AGC GT-3'. The 26-mer 5' -TGA TGA TAA AGA ATT CTA TTT TTT TA-3', with the mismatches underlined, was used to introduce a new Eco RI site 22 bp upstream of the initiation codon by a two basepair exchange. The restructured continuous coding sequence of ieI, consisting of the mutagenized fragment (black bar) joined to the non-mutagenized large fragment of exon 4 (open bar), flanked by Eco RI sites, is shown at the bottom. (Reproduced with permission from Volkmer et al, 1987, The Rockefeller University Press, The Journal of Experimental Medicine 166, p 668–677)

highly virulent salivary gland isolates of MCMV to which non-immunized mice and mice primed with wild-type vaccinia virus succumb within one week. All mice primed with MCMV survived infection. The protection was still effective after *in vivo* depletion of the CD8+ T lymphocyte subset by injection of antibodies to the CD8 antigen at the day of challenge infection. This indicated that protection induced by MCMV was not mediated only by CD8+ T lymphocytes. Vaccination with MCMV-ie1-VAC also protected all animals; however, injection of vaccinated mice with antibodies to the CD8 antigen completely abolished the protective effect. These data confirmed that protection by the experimental vaccine was solely dependent upon the generation of a specific cellular immune response of the CD8+ phenotype. It was also noticed that this vaccine did not protect against primary infection and MCMV disease. By day seven post challenge, however, when non-protected mice died, MCMV-ie1-VAC primed mice started to recover from infection.

Protection by CD8+ T lymphocytes is different from the protective principle of vaccines presently used which induce a long-lasting neutralizing antibody response. It was therefore tested whether MCMV-ieI-VAC could induce a lasting protective immunity. When vaccinated mice were subjected to challenge infection four months after sensitization they were still resistent to lethal infection and proved the longevity of protection induced by MCMV-ieI-VAC.

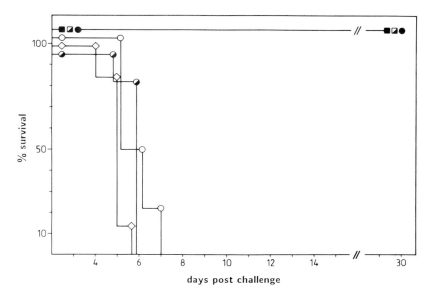

Fig. 9.4 MCMV-ieI-VAC protects against a lethal dose of salivary gland virus. Groups of six to ten mice were immunized 21 days before i.p. challenge with 5 LD_{50} of salivary gland virus. *In vivo* depletion of $CD8^+$ T lymphocytes was performed on the day of challenge. Treatment of mice: (●) MCMV-ieI-VAC sensitization; (◑) MCMV-ieI-sensitization and $CD8^+$ T lymphocyte depletion; (■) MCMCV sensitization; (◪) MCMC sensitization and $CD8^+$ T lymphocyte depletion; (o) VAC sensitization; (◇) naive controls

These results show for the first time that structural viral proteins are not required for the induction of protective immunity against a lethal challenge with a cytolytic virus. It is not surprising that this vaccine cannot protect against infection and disease. Antigen recognition by the $CD8^+$ T effector cells requires presentation of the antigen at the cell membrane, and infection of cells by MCMV and the expression of IE genes is a prerequisite to present a non-structural protein. This delayed start of cellular antiviral activity is advantageous for the infecting virus. Death or survival depends upon the dose of infectious virus, the speed of replication, the viral burst size and, on the other side, on the number of specifically sensitized effector cells and the phase of antigen expression during the viral replication cycle. The speed of CMV replication is rather low. At least in theory, recognition by cellular immune responses of the first viral gene products expressed would be a most effective way of interfering with viral replication.

A HEPTAPEPTIDE OF THE MCMV IE PROTEIN IS RECOGNIZED BY CTL

Recognition of foreign protein antigens by T lymphocytes occurs after formation of a trimolecular complex consisting of T cell receptor, MHC-molecule (the L^d glycoprotein for presenting antigen to the CTL clone IE1) and antigen.

For antigen presentation, the protein is processed which probably involves degradation, fragmentation and transport of short peptides to the cell surface, because this process can be mimicked by adding to target cells synthetic peptides representing the epitope recognized by CTL (Townsend et al, 1986).

Statistical analysis of known epitopes detected by $CD4^+$ and $CD8^+$ T lymphocytes has revealed a common sequence pattern, consisting of a charged amino acid or glycine, followed by two or three hydrophobic amino acids and a charged or polar amino acid (Rothbard & Taylor, 1988). Another property of such epitopes is the capacity to form an alpha helix with amphipathic properties (Margalit et al, 1987). Such small peptides of 8 to 20 amino acids in length could then react with the putative single antigen binding site recently identified by crystallographic structure analysis of a MHC class I molecule (Bjorkmann et al, 1987). The amino acid sequence of pp89 was screened for such sequences and several potential epitopes could be identified in the 595 amino acid sequence of pp89. When six selected synthetic peptides corresponding to different regions of pp89 were tested, all failed to render BALB/C susceptible to lysis by MCMV specific polyclonal CTL.

Because pp89 is recognized after transfection of the gene into eukaryotic cells and after expression of the gene by vaccinia virus, the expression of protein fragments was chosen to identify domains of the protein either essential or irrelevant for CTL induction and recognition by effector cells. One possibility to map such epitopes is to create terminal deletions in the coding sequence. The creation of terminally deleted protein fragments is useful to positively identify epitopes (Whitton et al, 1988) but not to locate protein domains that lack such regions. Therefore, in the case of pp89 a different strategy was followed. The construction of MCMV-ie1-VAC had provided the intron-free open reading frame of gene ieI. First, using this construct, a series of in frame deletions were produced. Second, the deleted genes were introduced into vaccinia virus and the cellular immune response to the expressed products was studied (Del Val et al, 1988) (Table 9.3). It was expected that if multiple epitopes in different domains of the viral protein were detected by CTL, then all deletion mutants of pp89 should present an antigen. This was clearly not the case since deletion mutant F which lacks residues 136 and 249 expressed a protein of the expected size but was not detected by CTL and was also unable to sensitize MCMV specific CTL. The mutant H expressing residues 1 to 249 and the mutant A lacking residues 30 to 135 were both antigenic and immunogenic. Both mutants contain the domain removed from F but lack sequences flanking this region at the N-terminal or at the C-terminal side. This demonstrated that presence or absence of sequences flanking this domain had no effect upon antigen processing and presentation. The mutant J expressing amino acids 1 to 153 failed, as expected, to be recognized and confined the immunogenic and antigenic properties to the domain represented by 95 amino acids between position 154 and 249. Thus, all potential epitopes presented by H-2^d MHC class I molecules and recognized by BALB/C CTL had to be located in a single domain. It should be noted that the synthetic peptides that had failed to identify an epitope for CTL correspond to sequences outside this region.

Table 9.3   Immunogenicity and antigenicity of fragments of pp89 expressed by vaccinia virus recombinants

	Residues expressed	Residues deleted	Calculated m.w.	Apparent m.w.	Recognition by CTL
MCMV-ieI-VAC	1–595	—	67	89	+
MCMV-ieI(A)-VAC	1–29; 136–595	30–135	55	71	+
MCMV-ieI(F)-VAC	1–135; 250–595	136–249	54	74	−
MCMV-ieI(C)-VAC	1–273; 477–595	274–476	44	59	+
MCMV-ieI(H)-VAC	1–249	250–595	30	35	+
MCMV-ieI(J)-VAC	1–153	154–595	17	23	−

In order to positively identify epitopes within this domain the amino acid sequence was again subjected to screening for potential epitopes and some sequences were selected for peptide preparation. A synthetic peptide corresponding to residue 161 to 179, when added to H-2^d cells, rendered them susceptible to lysis by polyclonal MCMV specific CTL (Table 9.4). Further studies revealed that presentation by the L^d molecule is essential for recognition of this peptide and that the epitope is identical with that recognized by CTL clone IE1. An unusual feature of this peptide is the fact it contains two prolines, an amino acid seldomly found in alpha helixes or in epitopes recognized by T lymphocytes, many of which are supposed to adopt an alpha helical conformation.

Table 9.4 Recognition by clone IE1 of MCH L^d targets presenting peptides of pp89

Peptide	Amino acid sequence	Optimal peptide concentration [M]	% specific lysis at IE1/L-L^d ratio of 20
19-mer P(161–179)	GRLMYDMYP*HFMPT*NLGPS	10^{5}–10^{6}	30
16-mer P(161–176)	GRLYMDMYP*HFMPT*NL	10^{6}–10^{7}	38
13-mer P(164–176)	MYDMYP*HFMPT*NL	10^{6}–10^{7}	43
10-mer P(167–176)	MYP*HFMPT*NL	10^{7}–10^{9}	50
9-mer P(168–167)	YP*HFMPT*N	10^{8}–10^{9}	48
9-mer P(167–175)	MYP*HFMPT*N	10^{3}–10^{4}	24
8-mer P(169–176)	P*HFMPT*NL	10^{4}–10^{5}	34
8-mer P(168–175)	YP*HFMPT*N	10^{3}–10^{4}	26
7-mer P(170–176)	*HFMPT*NL	10^{4}–10^{5}	30

Because the amino acid sequence identified represents the epitope detected by CTL clone IE1, this stable clone was used to more precisely analyse the antigenicity of peptides of various length (Reddehase et al, unpublished data). It was clear that the synthetic 19mer (161–179) peptide could not represent the minimal epitope detected by CTL. This peptide contains at residues 170 to 174 the amino acid HFMPT, a sequence pattern of charged and polar amino acids which could represent the core sequence essential for CTL recognition. For preparation of target cells using peptides (161–179), the concentration of 10^{-6} M protein during a 30 minute incubation period of target cells was required.

Shorter peptides corresponding to amino acids 161–179 and 164–176 resulted in optimal antigen presentation already after incubation of target cells with peptides at a 10^{-7} M concentration. The optimal peptide length is represented by the nonapeptide YP-HFMPT-NL (residues 168 to 176) which rendered target cells susceptible for lysis by CTL at a concentration of 10^{-8}–10^{-9} M. The omission of the amino-terminal residue Y did not destroy the capacity of the octamer to be recognized by CTL and also the heptamer sequence HFMPT-NL was detected by the clone. However, to achieve optimal antigen presentation, peptide concentrations (10^{-5} to 10^{-6} M), were required which were three orders in magnitude higher than for presentation of the optimal nonapeptide. The recognition of target cells coated with any of these peptides was still strictly antigen specific and required the presence of the L^d glycoprotein for presentation. Altogether the data show that a heptapeptide can render target cells susceptible for lysis by CTL. Thus, for antigen presentation to be recognized by T lymphocytes, a sequence as short as for recognition by antibody is sufficient.

Evasion of MCMV from IE antigen specific immune surveillance

As discussed above, the capacity to recognize the first viral gene products synthesized after infection of a cell should endow IE specific $CD8^+$ lymphocytes with efficient control functions. Since the complete replication cycle requires about 24 hours, there should be plenty of time for $CD8^+$ T lymphocytes to recognize the virus infected cells and to deliver a lethal hit, long before any infectious progeny or even late phase proteins are synthesized. Similar conditions should apply to the control of human CMV because, as predicted from the studies on MCMV, the homologous IE gene product also represents a dominant antigen for $CD8^+$ T lymphocytes (Borysiewicz et al, 1988). During natural infection of the immunocompetent human host some nucleated blood cells harbour virus that express selectively IE genes (Schrier et al, 1985). This creates the paradox that cells express the antigens against which the most effective T lymphocyte response is generated.

A study was initiated to investigate IE antigen recognition by $CD8^+$ T lymphocytes during the replication cascade of MCMV. The CTL clone IE1 was used as a probe to trace the expression of the antigen during the viral replication cycle (Fig. 9.5). As anticipated by previous studies, presentation of the antigen was most effective when expression of IE genes in infected cells was first selectively enhanced by CH treatment and when consecutive Act.D treatment prevented the expression of early genes. On the other hand, the IE antigen was barely detected by the CTL clone when inhibitors were omitted and IE gene expression was not enhanced. Using natural infection conditions, recognition of pp89 by clone IE1 could not be improved by raising the multiplicity of infection. There was no detection of IE antigen throughout the E phase of viral replication. During the L phase of infection, however, presentation of pp89 antigen for efficient recognition by CTL was detectable (Reddehase et al, 1986b). Similar to the synthesis of most L gene products the L phase expression of the IE antigen could be prevented by infection of cells in the presence of the DNA synthesis inhibitor phosphonoacetic acid (PAA). Further analysis revealed that IE antigen presentation during the late phase was due to reinitiation of ieI gene transcription and *de novo* translation of pp89.

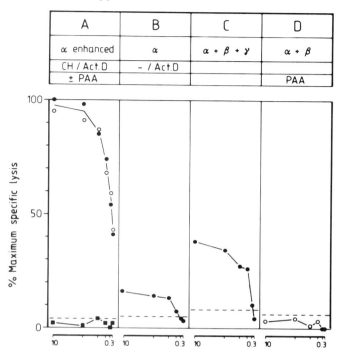

Fig. 9.5 Expression of the epitope of pp89 during the replication cycle of MCMV. CTL clone IE1 was used to detect the epitope presentation. Selective, enhanced synthesis of IE proteins in target cells (column A, ●) was achieved by MCMV infection of mouse embryo fibroblasts in the presence of cycloheximide (CH; 50μg/ml) that was replaced after 3 hours by Act.D (5μg/ml). In the case of non-enhanced expression of genes, Act.D was added 1.5 hours p.i. (column B). PAA (250μg/ml) was added before infection (columns A and D, ○). For mock infection (column A,●), MCMV was inactivated with UV light. Fibroblasts in the late phase of infection were assayed at 24 hours p.i. (column C). For each of the indicated effector/target cell ratios (1000 [51]CR-labelled target cells), specific lysis was determined in six replicates in a standard 3-hour [51]CR-release assay. Mean values are normalized to the maximum specific lysis observed (46% at effector/target cell ratio of 10; column A, ●). The dashed lines represent the upper 5% confidence limit of spontaneous lysis. (Reproduced with permission from Reddehase et al, 1986b, The American Society for Microbiology, The Journal of Virology 60, p 1125–1129)

These data clearly confirmed that pp89 antigen recognition and lysis of productively infected cells is an L phase event. Thus, recognition of pp89 by CTL offers no advantage over recognition of late phase structural proteins with regard to control of virus replication. The hypothesis of a particularly efficient T lymphocyte control due to recognition of productively infected cells already at the IE phase of virus replication was therefore wrong.

Why did IE antigen specific CD8[+] T lymphocytes not detect MCMV infected cells during the IE phase? The observation that selective enhancement of IE gene expression rendered cells susceptible to the recognition by CTL, while natural infection did not, raised the question of whether over–expression of the ie1 gene was required for T cell recognition. As mentioned above, transfected cells that express the ieI gene are susceptible to lysis by CTL clone IE1. Such transfectant cell lines produce a very low amount of pp89 which is comparable with the protein synthesis seen during natural infection. Thus, independent of whether a high or a low amount of pp89 was synthesized in cells, recognition of the antigen did occur when gene expression was restricted to IE genes. This raised suspicions about potential effects of MCMV E genes on IE antigen presentation. Infection of cells under conditions that provided abundant expression of the Ie1 gene, but at the same time allowed expression of MCMV E genes, should provide the pertinent control. Such conditions were achieved by MCMV infection in the presence of CH for enhanced ie1 gene transcription followed by withdrawal of CH to allow IE protein translation and induction of E gene expression. When cells treated that way were tested for IE antigen recognition by CTL clone IE1 no specific lysis was seen. This was despite the presence of pp89 in protein amounts exceeding, by far, the concentration obtained in ieI transfected cells. Therefore, MCMV E genes apparently have a negative effect upon pp89 antigen presentation at the post-translational level. The phase of E gene expression in MCMV takes about 12 hours and no individual MCMV E gene has been characterized so far. To determine the period of E gene expression required to effect the intervention with IE antigen presentation, the protocol was modified to allow first abundant transcription of IE genes in the presence of CH to be followed by only a short phase for IeI mRNA translation and E gene expression. The period of E gene transcription was limited by addition of Act.D at defined times. A 'window' of about 45 minutes of E gene expression was sufficient to effectively intervene with IE antigen presentation and indicated that genes involved in this type of regulation belong to the first E gene expressed during the 12 hour period of the E phase (Del Val, unpublished observations) (Fig. 9.6).

Because antigen presentation requires processing of the antigen and presentation by the MHC molecule, an effect on either the MHC molecule or on the antigen or on both could be responsible for the effect observed.

Reduction of MHC molecule expression is seen after infection with several viruses including herpesvirus, poxvirus, papovavirus, adenovirus, paramyxovirus and retrovirus. For some viruses, this alteration can be explained by the shut off of host cell protein synthesis following infection. During adenovirus infection a direct interaction of viral proteins with certain MHC class I proteins has been observed (Burgert & Kvist, 1985). It should be noted that MCMV does not cause a shut off of cellular protein synthesis. When MHC class I molecule expression in MCMV infected cells was compared with that in non-infected cells, no difference was seen during the early phase. Furthermore, the L^d molecule could be efficiently recognized by H-2^d alloantigen reactive CTL.

Therefore E gene products probably interfere with processing mechanisms independent of L^d expression. This effect could be either a general block of antigen presentation during the E phase or could be restricted to a specific effect on the processing of the epitope sequences of pp89.

If intervention with antigen processing was a general phenomenon then E gene product, expressed during this inhibitory phase, should not be presented as antigens for CTL. To pursue this question, an early gene termed e1 was identified and characterized. This gene is one of the first E genes transcribed after IE gene expression and, after infection, is strictly dependent upon the prior synthesis of IE proteins. The e1 gene produce, a 36 kD protein, is, similar to pp89, a non-structural phosphoprotein and is also accumulated in the nucleus of infected cells. When the plasmid cloned DNA fragment encoding e1 was transfected in cells the isolated gene was stably expressed and expression was independent of the control of IE genes (Bühler unpublished observations). To find out whether this protein serves as antigen for CTL, MCMV specific CTL clones were prepared and screened using the e1 transfected cell line. One CTL clone, termed E1, specifically recognized the cell line transfected with the eI gene. CTL clone E1 also required the L^d molecule for presentation of the eI gene product (Del Val, unpublished observations).

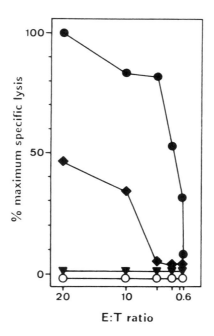

Fig. 9.6 Inhibition of pp89 epitope presentation after MCMV early gene expression. CTL clone IE1 was used to trace presentation of the epitope. Selective, enhanced synthesis of IE proteins in target cells ●) was achieved by infection in the presence of CH that was replaced after 3 hours by Act.D. Target cells with a 'window' of 20 minutes permissive for E gene transcription (■) were prepared by infection in the presence of CH that was washed out after 3 hours, Act.D. was added 20 minutes after removal of CH. Target cells 45 minutes permissive for E gene transcription (▲) were prepared accordingly. Uninfected target cells (○) served as controls. For assay conditions and calculations see legend to Fig. 9.5.

The isolation of MCMV specific CTL clone E1, and the fortuitous finding that antigen presentation for recognition by this clone, also required that the L^d gene product provided the optimal tools to test the alternative of general versus specific intervention of E gene products with IE antigen presentation. Target cells were prepared that expressed only IE or both IE and E proteins. As expected, there was no recognition by clone IE1 at early times of infection due to the co-expression of MCMV E genes. The CTL clone E1, however, was unable to recognize the eI gene product during the E phase and CTL specific for the L^d protein detected the antigen during both phases (Fig. 9.7).

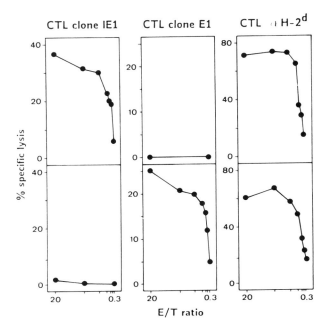

Fig. 9.7 Inhibition of pp89 epitope presentation does not interfere with presentation of the eI gene product by the L^d molecule. CTL clone IE1 was used to trace expression of the pp89 epitope, CTL clone E1 served to detect presentation of the eI gene product and a CTL line with specificity for the L^d molecule was used to control L^d expression. In the upper row targets were prepared for enhanced selective expression of IE antigens. In the lower row targets were prepared by infection in the presence of CH for 3 hours. After removal of CH and before addition of Act.D a window of 2 hours allowed E gene expression

Two conclusions could be drawn from this result. First, as suggested above, MCMV E gene expression neither affected the property of the MHC class I product L^d to be either recognized directly or to present antigen. The MCMV E gene activity is therefore a new phenomenon which differs from the inhibition of antigen presentation due to the viral effects on the expression of MHC gene products. Second, the finding that an E gene product was still correctly processed and presented when the IE gene was not, excluded general inhibition or intracellular antigen processing. Specific inhibition of steps preceding the presentation of the pp89 epitope apparently occurs. The molecular mechanisms of this phenomenon are under study.

CONCLUSIONS

The productive life cycle of murine cytomegalovirus (MCMV) includes several stages such as penetration and uncoding, immediate early, early and late gene expression, DNA replication, virion assembly and release. During all stages the infected cell contains proteins encoded by CMV.

Both viral proteins introduced during penetration and proteins synthesized after gene expression in cells can be processed and presented as antigens for T lymphocytes. T lymphocytes recognize both structural and non-structural antigens of the virus. Antigen recognition by $CD8^+$ T lymphocytes can occur also when only protein fragments as short as a heptamer are presented provided the fragment contains the antigenic epitope. Recognition of a single non-structural viral protein antigen by $CD8^+$ T lymphocytes can control MCMV virus spread. Thus, unless the virus genome can persist in a completely latent stage without any viral protein synthesized, cellular immunity should be able to trace all infected cells harbouring an active viral genome. Remarkably, the virus can escape this immune surveillance by using mechanisms that prevent antigen presentation. This function can be exercised by early viral gene products that intervene with presentation of the dominant, immediate early antigen at the post-translational stage.

Acknowledgements
This study was supported by The Deutsche Forschungsgemeinschaft grant Ko 571/8 and SFB 120. The preparation of the manuscript by I. Bennett is gratefully appreciated.

REFERENCES

Bjorkmann P J, Saper M A, Samraoui B, Bennett W S, Strominger J L, Wiley D C 1987 The foreign binding site and T cell recognition regions of class I histocompatibility antigens. Nature (London) 329: 512–518

Borysiewicz L K, Graham S, Hickling J K, Mason P D, Sissions J G P 1988 Human cytomegalovirus-specific cytotoxic T cells: their percursor frequency and stage specificity, European Journal of Immunology 18: 269–275

Burgert H G, Kvist S 1985 An adenovirus type 2 glycoprotein blocks cell surface expression of human histocompatability class I antigens, Cell 41: 987–997

Del Val M, Volkmer H, Rothbard J B, Jonjic S, Messerle M, Schickedanz J, Reddehase M J, Koszinowski U H 1988 Molecular basis of the recognition by cytolytic T lymphocytes of the murine cytomegalovirus immediate-early protein pp89, Journal of Virology 62

Dorsch-Häsler K, Keil G M, Weber F, Jasin M, Schaffner W, Koszinowski U H 1985 A long and complex enhancer activates trancription of genes coding for the highly abundant immediate early mRNA in murine cytomegalovirus. Proceedings of the National Academy of Sciences USA 82: 8325–8329

Ebeling A, Keil G M, Knust E, Koszinowski U H 1983 Molecular cloning and physical mapping of murine cytomegalovirus DNA. The Journal of Virology 47: 421–433

Gooding L R, O'Connell K A 1983 Recognition by cytotoxic T lymphocytes of cells expressing fragment of the SV40 tumor antigen. Journal of Immunology 131: 2580–2586

Hood L, Kronenberg M, Hunkapiller T 1985 T Cell antigen receptors and the immunoglobulin supergene family. Cell 40: 225–229

Jonjic S, Del Val M, Keil G M, Reddehase M J, Koszinowski U H 1988 A nonstructural viral protein expressed by a recombinant vaccinia virus protects against lethal cytomegalovirus infection. Journal of Virology 62: 1653–1658

Keil G M, Keil-Ebeling A, Koszinowski U H 1984 Temporal regulation of murine cytomegalovirus transcription and mapping of viral RNA synthesized at immediate early times after infection, Journal of Virology 50: 784–795

Keil G M, Fibi M R, Koszinowski U H 1985 Characterization of the major immediate-early polypeptides encoded by murine cytomegalovirus. Journal of Virology 54: 422–428

Keil G M, Ebeling-Keil A, Koszinowski U H 1987a Immediate early genes of murine cytomegalovirus: location, transcripts and translation products. Journal of Virology 61: 526–533

Keil G M, Ebeling-Keil A, Koszinowski U H 1987b Sequence and structural organization of murine cytomegalovirus gene I. Journal of Virology 61: 1901–1908

Koszinowski U H, Keil G M, Volkmer H, Fibi M R, Ebeling-Keil A, Munch K 1986 The 89,000-M_r murine cytomegalovirus immediate early protein activates gene transcription. Journal of Virology 58: 59–66

Koszinowski U H, Reddehase M J, Keil G M, Schickedanz J 1987a Host immune response to cytomegalovirus: products of transfected viral immediate early genes are recognized by cloned cytolytic T lymphocytes. Journal of Virology 61: 2054–2058

Koszinowski U H, Keil G M, Schwarz H, Schickedanz J, Reddehase M J 1987b A nonstructural polypeptide encoded by immediate-early transcription unit 1 or murine cytomegalovirus is recognized by cytolytic T lymphocytes. Journal of Experimental Medicine 166: 289–294

Margalit H, Spouge J L, Cornette J L, Cease K B, Delisi C, Berzofsky J A 1987 Prediction of immunodominant helper T cell antigenic sites from the primary sequence. Journal of Immunology 138: 2213–2229

Meyers J D, Flournoy N, Thomas E D 1980 Cytomegalovirus infection and specific cell-mediated immunity after marrow transplant. Journal of Infectious Diseases 142: 816–824

Moskovitz L, Hensley G T, Chan J C, Adams K 1985 Immediate causes of death in acquired immunodeficiency syndrome. Archives of Pathology and Laboratory Medicine 109: 735–738

Mutter W, Reddehase M J, Busch F W, Bühring H- J, Koszinowski U H 1988 Failure in generating hemopoietic stem cells is the primary cause of death from cytomegalovirus disease in the immunocompromised host. Journal of Experimental Medicine 167 1645–1658

Quinnan G V, Kirmani N, Rook A, Manischewitz J, Jackson L, Moreschi G, Santos G W, Saral R, Burns W H 1982 HLA-restricted T-lymphocyte and non-T-lymphocyte cytotoxic responses correlate with recovery from cytomegalovirus infection in bone-marrow-transplant recipients. New England Journal of Medicine 307: 7–13

Reddehase M J, Keil G M, Koszinowski U H 1984 The cytolytic T lymphocyte response to the murine cytomegalovirus. European Journal of Immunology 14: 56–61

Reddehase M J, Koszinowski U H 1984 Significance of herpesvirus immediate early gene expression in cellular immunity to cytomegalovirus infection. Nature (London) 312: 369–371

Reddehase M J, Weiland F, Munch K, Jonjic S, Lüske A, Koszinowski UH 1985 Interstitial murine cytomegalovirus pneumonia after irradiation: characterization of cells that limit viral replication during established infection of the lungs. Journal of Virology 55: 264–273

Reddehase M J, Bühring H- J, Koszinowski U H 1986a Cloned long term cytolytic T lymphocyte line with specificity for an immediate early membrane antigen of murine cytomegalovirus. Journal of Virology 57: 408–431

Reddehase M J, Fibi M R, Keil G M, Kosinowski U H 1986b Late phase expression of a murine cytomegalovirus immediate early antigen recognized by cytotoxic T lymphocytes. Journal of Virology 60: 1125–1129

Reddehase M J, Mutter W, Munch K, Bühring H- J, Koszinowski U H 1987a CD8-positive T lymphocytes specific for murine cytomegalovirus immediate-early antigens mediate protective immunity. Journal of Virology 61: 526–533

Reddehase M J, Zawatzky R, Weiland F, Bühring H- J, Mutter W, Koszinowski U H 1987b Stable expression of clonal specificity in murine cytomegalovirus-specific large granular lymphoblast lines propagated long-term in recombinant interleukin 2. Immunobiology 174: 420–431

Reddehase M J, Jonjic S, Weiland F, Mutter W, Koszinowski U H 1988 Adoptive immunotherapy of murine cytomegalovirus adrenalitis in the immunocompromised host: CD4-helper-independent antiviral function of CD8-positive memory T lymphocytes derived from latently infected donors. Journal of Virology 62: 1061–1065

Rothbard J B, Taylor W R 1988 A sequence pattern common to T cell epitopes, EMBO Journal 7: 93–100

Schrier R D, Nelson J A, Oldstone M B A 1985 Detection of human cytomegalovirus in peripheral blood lymphocytes in a natural infection, Science 230: 1048–1051

Townsend A R M, Gotch F M, Davey J 1985 Cytotoxic T cells recognize fragments of the influenza nucleoprotein Cell 42: 457–467

Townsend A R M, Rothbard J, Gotch F M, Bahadur G, Wraith D, McMichael A J 1986 The epitopes of influenza nucleoprotein recognized by cytotoxic T lymphocytes can be defined with short synthetic peptides, Cell 44: 959–968

Volkmer H, Bertholet C, Jonjic S, Wittek R, Koszinowski U H 1987 Cytolytic T lymphocyte recognition of the murine cytomegalovirus nonstructural immediate early protein pp89 expressed by recombinant vaccinia virus. Journal of Experimental medicine 166: 668–677

Whitton J L, Gebhard J R, Lewicki H, Thishon A, Oldstone M B A 1988 Molecular definition of major cytotoxic T lymphocytic choriomeningitis virus. Journal of Virology 62: 687–695

Discussion of paper presented by Ulrich Koszinowski

Discussant: J. Lindsay Whitton

VIRAL CHEMOTHERAPY, VACCINES AND INTERACTIONS WITH
THE HOST IMMUNE SYSTEM

Cytotoxic T lymphocytes (CTL) play a critical role in combating virus infections
(reviewed by Zinkernagel & Doherty, 1979). These cells recognize and lyse
virus-infected target cells and exhibit the phenomenon of major
histocompatibility complex (MHC) restriction; CTL from an individual will lyse
a target cell only if the latter presents both specific antigen and matched class
I MHC glycoproteins (Zinkernagel & Doherty, 1974). The biological significance
of CTL is not restricted to the control of virus infection; they are cardinal factors
in the self/non-self discrimination displayed in rejection of tumours and trans-
planted tissues (Smith et al, 1988; Silvers et al, 1987). Thus an understanding of
the mechanisms of induction of, and target cell recognition by, CTL is of
considerable importance. The data from the murine cytomegalovirus (MCMV)
system presented by Dr Koszinowski clearly demonstrate the advances made over
the past three to four years toward this goal; in my role as discussant I will not
reiterate the details of the preceding paper, but rather will attempt to expand
upon the critical points, comment upon relevant work in other virus systems, and
identify some of the many unanswered questions which remain.

Class I MHC proteins select CTL epitopes
One point not raised in the foregoing paper is the profound effect of host class
I MHC genes in determining the response to foreign antigens. Murine CTL
responses to influenza virus infection vary depending on mouse MHC (H2)
haplotype (Vitiello & Sherman, 1983), and we have observed striking mouse
strain differences in studies of lymphocytic choriomeningitis virus (LCMV)
infection. In C57BL/6 mice (H2^{bb}), the CTL responses to LCMV glycoprotein
(GP) and nucleoprotein (NP) moieties are similar in magnitude. In contrast, in
two other mouse strains BALB/C and SWR/J (H2^{dd} and H2^{qq} respectively) there
is no detectable response mounted to the LCMV GP, while the anti-NP response
remains extremely brisk (Whitton et al, 1988a). Use of congenic mouse strains
which differ only at the MHC locus confirm that the pattern of response is
determined by MHC. The observation of MHC-linked low responsiveness to

individual virus proteins is of concern when considering the use of subunit vaccines, and may explain some individual cases of vaccine failure.

CTL often recognize non-membrane proteins

CTL recognition of a target cell requires interaction of membrane-bound proteins; thus until quite recently it was assumed that, to serve as a CTL antigen, a protein would have to be expressed (implicitly intact) on the cell membrane. This reasoning was challenged by the demonstration of CTL activity against influenza virus nucleoprotein (Townsend & Skehel, 1982) which was thought not to be expressed at the cell membrane. Subsequently, many 'internal' proteins, in several virus systems, have been proved to act as CTL target antigens; indeed, in influenza virus infected mice, CTL activity against all internal virus proteins has been demonstrated (Bennink et al, 1987; Yewdell, personal communication). The capacity to present 'internal' proteins to the immune system confers at least two advantages on the infected host. First, it increases the number of potential CTL epitopes, thus diminishing the probability of an MHC-linked low responsiveness to the whole virus; for example, if glycoproteins alone were visible to the cellular immune system then, in the case of LCMV, the $H2^{dd}$ and $H2^{qq}$ mice (which see only NP) might be unable to effectively respond to the infection. Secondly, in some virus infections, integral membrane proteins are expressed only late in the viral life cycle, when cell lysis is imminent; at this stage the lytic activity of CTL would be of minimal apparent value to the host. The ability to recognize virus antigens produced early in infection allows the cells to be destroyed before the production of infectious progeny. In this light the recognition of the MCMV pp89 protein, an immediate-early polypeptide, is interesting, and mirrors the observation that a major proportion of the CTL response to human cytomegalovirus is similarly targeted (Rodgers et al, 1987).

CTL recognize virus antigens as short peptides

Using the influenza virus model, Townsend and his colleagues (1985, 1986a) have shown that truncated NP and GP moities, when expressed within the target cells, can be recognized by CTL. These findings have been confirmed using a variety of LCMV GP deletions expressed in vaccinia virus: recognition appears to be independent of the tertiary structure of the expressed protein, and even the covalent addition of 'foreign' amino acid residues immediately adjacent to the epitope sequence cannot prevent its recognition by CTL (Whitton et al, 1988b). Furthermore, expression from vaccinia virus of a 22 amino acid 'endogenous peptide' containing a CTL epitope allows recognition of infected cells by CTL (Whitton et al, unpublished); this further attests to the flexibility and precision of the system whereby foreign sequences translated within the cell can be detected, and presented by host MHC to the cellular immune system. Together these findings show conclusively that MHC can present short peptides from endogenous proteins to CTL; the recent crystallographic resolution of the structure of a human class I MHC molecule revealed an unidentified density—perhaps a short peptide—in the proposed antigen binding cleft, providing possible physical confirmation of the above conclusions (Bjorkman, 1987a, 1987b). Nevertheless the precise mechanisms of antigen processing, and of presentation by class I MHC, remain enigmatic. As a glycoprotein, MHC is translated on the rough endoplasmic reticulum, and extruded into the extra-cytoplasmic space whence it proceeds by serial vesiculation through the various compartments of the Golgi apparatus and thence to the cell membrane. Where in this process do MHC and potential epitope combine? How, when and where is the foreign protein degraded to peptide? The observation that an MCMV early function can apparently prevent presentation of an IE antigen (despite the continual presence of the IE protein) is extremely interesting and may provide a gateway into the studies of the intracellular processing mechanism. One wonders whether only this IE antigen is affected, or whether all MCMV CTL epitopes are similarly 'suppressed'. Viruses can escape immune surveillance at the target cell level in a variety of ways; for example, by cessation of protein synthesis (possibly the case for latent HSV), by infection of target cells with low or absent MHC class I glycoprotein, or by active intervention in the process of antigen presentation by the infected cell. For instance, adenovirus diminishes the cell surface presentation of CTL epitopes by specifically preventing the transport of class I MHC glycoprotein to the cell membrane (Andersson et al, 1985; Burgert & Kvist, 1985); such a mechanism cannot be invoked for MCMV, however, since Dr Koszinowski's results show that the general ability of the MCMV infected cells to present CTL epitopes is not markedly altered. There is recent tantalizing evidence, of unknown significance, that HCMV encodes a glycoprotein related to HLA (Beck & Barrell, 1988). A role for this molecule in binding of virus to cell has been suggested, possibly by using B2 microglobulin as an intermediary (Grundy et al, 1987); this is presently unproven, and the possibility that this molecule exerts the same effect within the infected target cell remains open.

'Internal' proteins can be effective vaccines
Successful immunization against virus infection often results from induction of neutralizing antibody, which inactivates the organism before infection is es-tablished. In contrast, it is likely that some degree of virus replication may be required to allow CTL to exert their beneficial effects. The MCMV system demonstrates that immunization with a single internal (and non-structural) protein can indeed protect against lethal virus challenge, and that this protection is mediated by the $CD8^+$ lymphocytes i.e. classical CTL surface phenotype. These findings add to the *in vivo* studies showing protection by the internal proteins of influenza virus (Wraith et al, 1987) and lassa virus (Clegg & Lloyd, 1987). We have carried out similar studies using LCMV and found that administration of recombinant vaccinia expressing LCMV NP confers complete protection against lethal challenge.

Thus the potential utility of internal virus proteins as effective immunogens has been amply demonstrated. Since the CTL responses to these proteins are often cross-reactive (that is, CTL are effective across serotypic boundaries), they might appear ideal immunogens. However, natural infection of humans by influenza virus does not confer long-lasting protection against infection by a different serotype, even though the CTL induced against the viral NP are cross-reactive. Furthermore we have found that an animal immunized with LCMV NP may develop immunopathology and subsequently die when challenged with certain LCMV variants which normally establish a non-lethal persistent infection (Klavinskis et al, unpublished).

Can peptides induce CTL responses?

For influenza (Townsend et al, 1986b), LCMV (Whitton et al, 1988b) and now for MCMV (preceding paper), synthetic peptides have been shown to sensitize uninfected target cells to lysis by CTL. Thus, at the level of recognition, exogenous application of peptide can substitute for endogenous synthesis of protein. Can such peptides also induce a CTL response? In general, soluble proteins are poor inducers of CTL; live virus is a much more effective CTL inducer than inactivated virus. One report (Staertz, 1987) suggests that soluble peptides can indeed induce CTL responses. A more detailed study (Carbone et al, 1988) indicates that a peptide containing an influenza virus CTL epitope can induce a response *in vitro*, but the resultant CTL, although peptide specific, have minimal activity against virus-infected cells. Now that CTL epitopes are being precisely identified in other virus systems (LCMV, MCMV) similar experiments on *in vivo* protection using peptides can be undertaken.

Viruses have proved indispensible tools in dissecting the nature of CTL recognition. They will continue to be so in forthcoming studies on antigen processing, presentation by MHC, and induction of effective *in vivo* responses. The insights achieved may pertain not only to virology, but to broader aspects of immunology, cell biology and pathogenesis.

REFERENCES

Andersson M, Paabo S, Nilsson T, Peterson P A 1985 Impaired intracellular transport of class I major histocompatibility complex antigens as a possible means for adenoviruses to evade immune surveillance. Cell 43: 215–222
Beck S, Barrell B G 1988 Human cytomegalovirus encodes a glycoprotein homologous to MHC class I antigens. Nature 331: 269–272
Bennink J R, Yewdell J W, Smith G L, Moss B 1987 Anti-influenza virus cytotoxic T lymphocytes recognize the three viral polymerases and a nonstructural protein. Responsiveness to individual viral antigens is major histocompatibility complex controlled. Journal of Virology 61: 1098–1102
Bjorkman P J, Saper M A, Samraoui B, Bennett W S, Strominger J L, Wiley D C 1987a Structure of the human class I histocompatibility antigen, HLA-A2. Nature 329: 506
Bjorkman P J, Saper M S, Samraoui B, Bennett W S, Strominger J L, Wiley D C 1987b The foreign antigen binding site and T cell recognition regions of class I histocompatibility antigens. Nature 329: 512
Burgert H G, Kvist S 1985 An adenovirus type 2 glycoprotein blocks cell surface expression of human histocompatibility class I antigens. Cell 41: 987–988
Carbone et al (1988) in press.
Clegg J C S, Lloyd G 1987 Vaccinia recombinant expressing lassa-virus internal nucleocapsid protein protects guinea pigs against Lassa fever. Lancet July 25: 186–188
Grundy J E, McKeating J A, Ward P J, Sanderson A R, Griffiths P D 1987 Beta-2 microglobulin enhances the infectivity of cytomegalovirus and when bound to the virus enables class I HLA molecules to be used as a virus receptor. Journal of General Virology 68: 793–804
Rodgers B, Borysiewicz L, Mundin S, Graham S, Sissons P 1987 Immunoaffinity purification of a 72K early antigen of human cytomegalovirus: analysis of humoral and cell-mediated immunity to the purified polypeptide. Journal of General Virology 68: 2371–2378
Silvers W K, Kimura H, Desquenne-Clark L, Miyamoto M 1987 Some new perspectives on transplantation immunity and tolerance. Immunology Today 7: 117

Smith D M, Stuart F P, Wemhoff G A, Quintans J, Fitch F W 1988 Cellular pathways for rejection of class I MHC disparate skin and tumor allografts. Tansplantation 45: 168–175

Staertz U D, Karasuyama H, Garner A M 1987 Cytotoxic T lymphocytes against a soluble protein. Nature 329: 449–451

Townsend A R M, Skehel J J 1982 Influenza A specific cytotoxic T cell clones that do not recognize viral glycoproteins. Nature 300: 655–657

Townsend A R M, Gotch F M, Davey J 1985 Cytotoxic T cells recognize fragments of the influenza nucleoprotein. Cell 42: 457–468

Townsend A R M, Bastin J, Gould K, Brownlee G G 1986a Cytotoxic T lymphocytes recognize influenza hemagglutinin that lacks a signal sequence. Nature 324: 575–577

Townsend A R M, Rothbard J, Gotch F M, Bahadur G, Wraith D, McMichael A J 1986b The epitopes of influenza nucleoprotein recognized by cytotoxic T lymphocytes can be defined with short synthetic peptides. Cell 44: 959–968

Vitiello A, Sherman L A 1983 Recognition of influenza infected cells by cytotoxic T lymphocytes clones determinant selection by class I restriction elements. Journal of Immunology 131: 1635–1640

Whitton J L, Southern P J, Oldstone M B A 1988a Analyses of the cytotoxic T lymphocyte responses to glycoprotein and nucleoprotein components of lymphocytic choriomeningitis virus. Virology 162: 321–327

Whitton J L, Gebhard J R, Lewicki H, Tishon A, Oldstone M B A 1988b Molecular definition of a major cytotoxic T lymphocyte epitope in the glycoprotein of lymphocytic choriomeningitis virus. Journal of Virology 62: 687–695

Wraith D C, Vessey A E, Askonas B A 1987 Purified influenza virus nucleoprotein protects mice from lethal infection. Journal of General Virology 68: 433–440

Zinkernagel R M, Doherty P C 1974 Restriction of in vitro T cell mediated cytotoxicity in lymphocytic choriomeningitis within a syngeneic or semiallogeneic system. Nature 248: 701

Zinkernagel R M, Doherty P C 1979 MHC restricted cytotoxic T cells: studies on the biological role of polymorphic major transplantation antigens determine T cell restriction specificity, and responsiveness. Advances in Immunology 27: 51

Discussion: CMV infections

Ulrich Koszinowski and J. Lindsay Whitton

The preceding papers stressed the recent data which have clearly established a potential role for CD8$^+$ class MHC restricted cells in conferring protection *in vivo*. Furthermore, such cells can recognize synthetic peptide epitopes on H-2 matched target cells. Consequently, the speakers were asked if peptides could be used to induce protective cell-mediated responses. There were known examples of this. However peptides can be used to induce class I MHC restricted responses *in vitro*; such cells rarely have strong anti-viral specificity even when the inducing peptide is a major virus epitope. Peptides are being subjected to a variety of manipulations to try to render them more effective in induction of cellular immunity but such studies are in their infancy, and results are conflicting.

The potential importance of CD4$^+$ (helper phenotype) T lymphocytes was raised; do epitopes recognized by these cells coincide with those seen by CD8$^+$ cells and, if not, might that explain the difficulty in inducing CD8$^+$ responses using short peptides? This was seen as one possibility, although in several systems the *in vivo* depletion of CD4$^+$ (helper) cells had little effect on the ability to induce a CD8$^+$ response. Nevertheless CD4$^+$ cells do play some role in determining the outcome of MCMV infection, in that CD4$^+$-depleted mice tend to harbour MCMV in the salivary gland, while fully immunocompetent mice clear the virus.

Section III
NEW VIRAL VACCINES
Chairman: Erling Norrby

10. The immunobiology of the HIV envelope

Dani P. Bolognesi

INTRODUCTION

The immune response which develops subsequent to infection with HIV consists of both humoral and cellular elements which, when tested *in vitro*, can inhibit virus infection, syncytium formation, and lyse virus infected target cells. If such activities were operative *in vivo*, one would expect that they would be effective in suppressing virus replication and virus induced cytopathic effects. The anti-viral immune response may thus represent one of the primary host defense mechanisms responsible for the protracted asymptomatic phase of the disease which, in most patients, can last several years. An important question to be answered for development vaccine strategies against HIV is whether this response might be an effective barrier to *de novo* HIV infection. Stated otherwise, if the immune response can indeed control the virus even for a limited period of time, then the issue would not be whether or not it is possible to mount a protective immune response against HIV, but that it is necessary to establish it prior to or, possibly, during the very early stages of infection in order for it to be effective.

Information relevant to this issue is becoming available and, although the emerging picture is far from clear, one can begin to visualize certain avenues to pursue that could provide more definitive answers to this question.

NATURAL HISTORY OF HIV INFECTION IN MAN

Both preventive and interventive strategies against HIV will have to take into account what might be termed as the natural history of infection in man, a working model for which is depicted in Fig. 10.1 and the essential concepts could be summarized as follows:

(1)   Exposure to the virus in the absence of any protective barriers would result in its rapid replication in susceptible cells and the development of an early viraemia.

(2)   Within a variable period of time, which depends on several factors

including the infectious dose, the route of infection and the competency of the individual to respond to the virus, an immune defence is established which begins to curtail active viral replication. (It is important to note that the immune response may not be the only factor to impact on virus replication. The accessory genes of HIV which control virus replication may themselves switch off virus expression and latency could be maintained until appropriate activating signals come into play.)

(3)   As the immune response intensifies, viral activity is generally suppressed throughout the asymptomatic phase of the infection. However, several unique properties of HIV, notably its ability to spread by cell to cell transmission, its capacity to exist in latent form, the propensity of the virus to diversify in the face of an immune response, and its potential for suppressing immune function by direct infection or even by indirect means altogether, gradually tip the balance in its favour.

(4)   As virus begins to re-emerge with failing immune responses, clinical symptoms become manifest and gradually progress.

(5)   Profound immune defects follow which render the individual defenceless against other pathogens resulting in the full syndrome of AIDS.

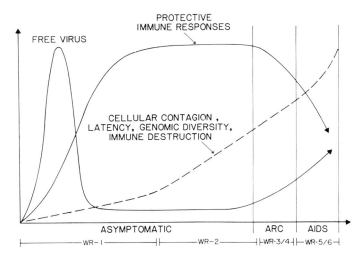

Fig. 10.1 Model of natural history of virus infection in man depicting early viraemia, induction of immunity and suppression of virus during the asymptomatic phase of disease. The dotted line depicts events which permit virus to escape host defences. Eventually, as immune defences fail virus re-emerges and this is accompanied by clinical symptoms progressing to full blown AIDS. Relative levels displayed on the ordinate are only for pictorial purposes and are not associated with specific measurements. The abscissa likewise represents a generalized disease course

There are a few bits of evidence in support of these general concepts which deserve attention. First, the initial phase of virus replication has been noted in a few patients through detection of viral antigens in the circulation prior to the onset of seropositivity (Allain et al, 1986). Also, some individuals experience an influenza-like illness accompanied by swollen lymph nodes during this period which resolves within a matter of days or weeks (Redfield et al, 1986). Precisely when seroconversion occurs after the initial infection is unknown but in some cases this can be a considerable period of time (Ranki et al, 1987). Nonetheless, a vigorous immune response to the virus can be found in many asymptomatic individuals. When this is present, free viral antigen is not detectable (Allain et al, 1986) and gradually emerging is the concept that the virus is more difficult to isolate. One might then consider this period to represent an 'eclipse phase' of the natural infection. However, as clinical symptoms become more severe and immune dysfunction is evident, HIV antigenaemia reappears (Pedersen et al, 1987) and the efficiency of virus isolation increases (deWolf et al, 1987; Redfield, 1987, personal communication). A prognostic marker for the development of these events is a decline in antibodies to one of the core proteins (p24) of HIV (Weber et al, 1987).

If this general premise is correct, it would highlight the importance of determining the course of the infection in an individual following exposure to the virus. For instance, if the immune response which develops is indeed effective in suppressing the virus, the precise characterization of its working parts should be defined. From this information, one could begin to construct some essential components of a vaccine regimen.

Assuming that an effective response to the virus exists but that, in all likelihood, it occurs too late under natural circumstances, it may also be possible through various means to stimulate the process to develop earlier and perhaps more vigorously. This would have important implications for early intervention post-exposure to the virus. Stated otherwise, the amplitude of virus replication might thereby be significantly reduced, the overall degree of infection lowered, and possibly limited to a sub-clinical level. Such manipulations might influence the subsequent rate of progression of the infection, perhaps eliminating it altogether. By reducing the infectious virus pool, one would also curtail the spread of the virus to other individuals. Ample precedents exist for early immunological intervention in retrovirus infections of animals with anti-viral antibodies (Schäfer & Bolognesi, 1987; Thiel et al, 1987) as well as chemical anti-viral agents (Wu et al, 1973, Ruprecht et al, 1986; Sharpe et al, 1987; Tavares et al, 1987) as a means of reducing and even eliminating infection and diseases.

TWO REGIONS OF THE HIV ENVELOPE IMPORTANT FOR VIRUS INFECTION WHICH REPRESENT TARGETS FOR IMMUNE ATTACK

Before embarking on the issue of what constitutes protective immunity against HIV, it is important to define the early phases in virus infection where it might be operative. Three essential steps that stand out in this regard are: (1) binding of the virus to its receptor; (2) fusion of the virus with the cell membrane; and (3) penetration and entry of the virus within the target cell. Of the three processes, the dynamics of HIV binding to its receptor are best understood and involve a very specific interaction between certain regions of the external virus envelope glycoprotein (gp120) and a portion of the CD4 molecule (Dalgleish et al, 1984; Klatzmann et al, 1984; McDougal et al, 1986; Lasky et al, 1987; Kowalski et al, 1987). The process of fusion is also mediated by the HIV envelope. Current evidence suggests that it occurs post-binding and subsequent to rearrangements of both envelope glycoproteins. It may be mediated by insertion of a putative fusogenic domain which is thought to be situated on the gp41 transmembrane component (Gallaher, 1987; Gonzales-Scarano et al, 1987) into the target cell membrane. The process of actual entry is least understood but probably occurs subsequent to fusion.

It is thus not surprising that a great deal of attention has been focused on the HIV envelope as a major target for antibodies that can interfere with infection. A number of studies have been done to define the regions of the envelope glycoproteins that mediate these functions and which might also serve as targets for immune attack. Two of these stand out and will be the focus of this discussion.

When experimental animals are immunized with the full length HTLV-III$_B$ envelope gp160, or with certain recombinant fragments thereof (Rusche et al, 1987) one notes the production of high-titred, isolate restricted, neutralizing and cell fusion blocking antibodies (Table 10.1). Most of the anti-HIV neutralizing activity in these sera is directed against a region of gp120 which can be reproduced with a synthetic peptide of 24 amino acids (Palker et al, 1988; Rusche et al, 1988; Kenealy, 1988, personal communication). Similarly, two neutralizing monoclonal antibodies have also been found to bind the same region of the envelope glycoprotein (Skinner et al, 1988a). Thus, the portion of gp120 lying between residues 307 and 330 is an immunodominant epitope for the development of high-titred, type-specific, neutralizing antibodies against HIV-1.

Table 10.1 Antiviral activities of HIV seropositive human sera and goat sera to HIV envelope subunits

Serum	Inhibition of [1] gp120–CD4 binding	Neutralization[2] III$_B$	RF	Fusion inhibition[3] III$_B$	RF
Infected human A	1,350	56	100	20	10
Infected human B	4,170	235	320	20	20
Infected human C	2,330	320	54	20	20
Goat gp160-III	15	800	0	50	0
Goat gp160-RF[B]	0	0	128	0	80
Goat RP135[4]	0	475	0	40	0
MoAB[5]	0	+	−	+	−

[1] 50% endpoint titre inhibition binding of ^{125}I gp120 to CD4.
[2] 50% endpoint neutralization titre using approximately 100 infectious units of the III$_B$ and RF strains of HIV.
[3] Serum titre that completely blocks fusion between HIV infected MOLT-4 cells and uninfected cells.
[4] RP135 is a 24 amino acid peptide situated within a disulphide bridged hypervariable loop of gp120 (aa 302-337).
[5] Monoclonal antibodies 0.5β (obtained from Dr S. Matsushita) and 9284 (obtained from Dr Robert Ting) which bind to RP135 (Skinner et al., 1988b).

This epitope also constitutes a hypervariable region of the HIV env gene (Starcich et al, 1986). It is thought to exist as a loop formed by two disulphide-linked cysteine residues (Lasky, 1988, personal communication). The two cysteines, residue numbers 302 and 337, are themselves highly conserved within the viral envelope glycoprotein. Thus, although the amino acid sequence within this loop is variable, the loop itself is present in gp120 from different strains of the virus.

While the precise function of this segment of the envelope is unknown, genetic manipulation studies have suggested that the region may be involved in the association of gp120 with the transmembrane component gp41 (Kowalski et al, 1987). This interaction may be important in the process of virus fusion. Interference with fusion may be the mechanism by which these antibodies neutralize the virus. Indeed, our experiments demonstrated that antisera against the hypervariable loop block fusion quite effectively.

Sera taken from HIV-infected humans differ from those raised against envelope components in that human sera generally exhibit broad neutralizing activity and contain a high titre of antibodies which block gp120 binding to CD4 (Table 10.1). Presumably, such antibodies are directed to a conserved region of gp120 which has been identified as a possible binding site (Lasky et al, 1987). One line of circumstantial evidence in support of this is the fact that the aforementioned activities correlate well with the gp120-CD4 blocking titre in such sera.

Whatever the nature of the broader biological activity and gp120-CD4 blocking antibodies recovered from human sera, our experiments indicate that it has been difficult to duplicate this response in animals immunized with viral envelope subunits. This is likely due to the conformational nature of the CD4-binding site of gp120 since naturally occurring antibodies do not react with the molecule following reduction and alkylation, deglycosylation, or denaturation by treatment with ionic detergents (Matthews et al, 1987; Skinner et al, 1988b). However, it is also possible that this region is not easily recognized by the immune system and requires prolonged exposure for appropriate response.

In summary, there are several sharp contrasts between the two epitopes of gp120 discussed here when they are viewed through the effects of antibodies which are biologically active against the virus (Fig. 10.2). One epitope elicits neutralizing antibodies which are isolate restricted and primarily directed to a hypervariable loop structure of gp120 that is not involved in CD4 binding. This site is immunodominant and sensitive epitopes can be reproduced with synthetic peptides. The second class of neutralizing antibodies is apparently directed at a more conserved region which is related to the CD4 binding site of gp120. This domain is conformation-dependent and appears to be less immunogenic.

DEVELOPMENT OF IMMUNE RESPONSES IN A LABORATORY WORKER INFECTED WITH THE HTLV-III$_B$ STRAIN OF HIV

The interplay between HIV and the host response is central to a better understanding of the natural history of HIV infection in man. A unique opportunity to conduct some studies along these lines recently availed itself when infection with the HTLV-III$_B$ strain of HIV could be clearly documented in a laboratory worker (Weiss et al, 1988). Two aspects of this occurrence are particularly noteworthy. The first is that blood samples were collected relatively soon after seroconversion and at various intervals thereafter spanning a period of over 24 months. Several independent virus isolates have been derived from these materials. Secondly, because of the large body of knowledge about this prototype laboratory strain, a number of specific analytical probes are available to study both the emerging viruses and the immune response against them.

Two Disulfide Bridged Loops on gp120 Involved in HIV Infectivity

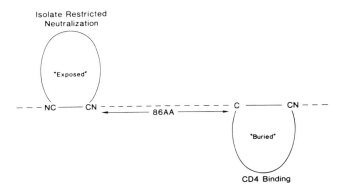

Fig. 10.2 Schematic of two loop structures in HIV gp120 which relate to important biological functions of the virus

We note that early on after seroconversion one finds the presence of neutralizing antibodies, antibodies which inhibit syncytium formation, as well as antibodies which mediate antibody-dependent cell cytotoxicity (ADCC) against virus infected target cells (Table 10.2). The antibodies mediating ADCC are broadly cross-reactive among diverse HIV isolates from the outset. On the other hand, those responsible for virus neutralization or inhibition of cell fusion are highly type specific and remain so for at least 18 months. This latter point was verified by studies which showed that their activity could be completely inhibited by a peptide corresponding to the 24 amino acid hypervariable sequence of HTLV-III_B gp120 described earlier. Within a few months after this peptide was no longer able to mediate its inhibitory action, one began to detect the presence of broadly cross-reactive neutralizing and fusion inhibiting antibodies. These activities coincided roughly with the rising titre of antibodies which blocked the binding of gp120 to CD4.

We interpret the period where the peptide is able to completely inhibit the *in vitro* activities of antibodies against the infecting strain to represent an interval where variants have not yet occurred to a significant degree. By contrast, the subsequent inability of this peptide to inhibit these activities may signal the emergence of a new serotype(s) and the corresponding divergent immune responses. By analogy to various lentivirus models, it is likely that after the initial replication of the infecting virus, type specific neutralizing antibodies are made. This is followed by the emergence of variants which are not susceptible to neutralization and therefore replicate. Only after neutralizing antibodies are formed against the variant epitopes, are these viruses brought under control. Repetitive cycles of this scenario occur which eventually overcome the ability of the host response to deal with the multitude of the variants.

However, this interpretation is obfuscated by the emergence of yet another class of neutralizing antibodies which, rather than being type specific, is broadly cross-reactive with highly diverse HIV strains. These almost certainly are not in response to changes in variable sequences within HTLV-III$_B$ arising during the course of infection. Rather, they are probably directed at a distinct epitope of gp120 which is highly conserved. Because the emergence of this activity occurs when antibodies which block the binding of gp120 to CD4 are increasing in titre (Table 10.2), it is tempting to attribute the *in vitro* broad biological activity to their ability to inhibit this important interaction in virus infection.

Table 10.2 Anti-HIV activities of serum samples from a laboratory worker infected with the III$_B$ strain of HIV

Month: after initial sample	ADCC[1]	Inhibition of fusion (III$_B$)[2]	Blockade of fusion inhibited by RP135[3]	Inhibition of fusion (RF)[4]	Blockade of gp120/CD4 binding[5]
0	13.9	0	NT[6]	0	0
5	21.9	89	85	0	2
6	24.8	83	73	0	0
11	28.0	81	88	NT[6]	4
12	25.5	100	63	0	12
13	24.6	100	6	0	28
17	37.9	100	0	5	41
23	32.1	100	0	88	67

[1] Percent lysis of cells infected with the III$_B$ strain of HIV at a 1/200 serum dilution. Lysis also observed on RF infected cell.
[2] Inhibition of cell fusion between MOLT-4 cells infected with the III$_B$ strain of HIV and uninfected MOLT-4 cells (Matthews et al., 1987).
[3] Blockade of fusion inhibition by the RP135 peptide sequence derived from the BH10 clone of the III$_B$ HIV isolate.
[4] Inhibition of fusion between cells infected with the RF isolate of HIV and uninfected MOLT-4 cells.
[5] Percent inhibition of ^{125}I gp120 (III$_B$) binding to CD4 at a serum dilution of 1:250 (Skinner et al., 1988a).
[6] Not tested.

At this point however, it is difficult to demonstrate that antibodies which block gp120 binding to CD4 are responsible for group specific virus neutralization or inhibition of syncytium formation. To conclude this will require the purification of the respective antibodies using specific fragments of gp120. This may be difficult since a number of studies suggest that the epitope(s) responsible are highly dependent on the conformation of gp120 (Matthews et al, 1987). It is equally important to determine if such antibodies play any role in preventing infection or re-infection *in vivo*.

Clearly, more studies need to be done to unravel these relationships and their roles in the progression of infection and onset of disease. Analysis of the biological and molecular properties of emerging variant viruses in this individual are underway and will be correlated with the humoral immune responses described here as well as cellular immune responses also under study. These and other studies also emphasize the need to initiate similar approaches in cases where early infection can be documented with naturally transmitted HIV.

PASSIVE IMMUNOTHERAPY STUDIES WITH ANTI-HIV IMMUNOGLOBULINS (HIV IG)

In an effort to determine whether the *in vitro* anti-viral activity exhibited by immunoglobulins from HIV seropositive individuals (HIV Ig) is operative *in vivo*, two chimpanzees were inoculated intravenously with HIV Ig and challenged one day later with the HTLV-III$_B$ strain of HIV (Prince et al, 1988). Both animals became viraemic. The amount of HIV Ig administered was in far excess with respect to the challenge dose given and ample quantities of anti-viral antibodies could be verified in the circulation for a number of days. Because of the implications of this result for the development of preventive and interventive measures against HIV, an in-depth analysis of the biological activities in the starting material and circulating antibodies was carried out.

Our findings indicate the presence of broadly cross neutralizing antibodies, antibodies that inhibit cell fusion, antibodies that block binding of gp120 to CD4, and those that mediate antibody dependent cell cytotoxicity (ADCC) in the chimp circulation (Table 10.3). The levels of each are consistent with what one finds in an average HIV seropositive serum. We note, however, that with the exception of ADCC, these activities display a bi-phasic decay curve where the major portion of the activity is lost within three to five days. Thereafter, the levels of biological activity against HIV are generally below those detectable in human sera. One could question whether the three to five days at the higher levels represents a sufficient barrier for the challenge dose given.

Table 10.3 Circulating levels of human anti-HIV immunoglobulins (HIV Ig) in a transfused chimpanzee

Day[4]	Virus[1] neutralization	Cell fusion III$_B$	RH	Blockade[2] binding to CD4	Percent lysis[3] ADCC III$_B$
0	0	0	0	0	0.4
1	190	93	100	2,150	36.3
2	100	87	98	2,100	27.9
7	30	45	63	1,450	26.5
14	0	12	16	520	22.3
Average human HIV seropositive serum 100–300					
	100–300	0–100	0–100	200–500	25–50

[1] 50% neutralization titre using approximately 100 infectious units of the III$_B$ isolate HIV. Roughly similar titres were observed with the RF strains of HIV.
[2] 50% inhibition titre (see Tables 10.1 and 10.2).
[3] Serum dilution was 1:20,000.
[4] Indicates days after HIV Ig administration. Day 0 is immediately prior to addition of HIV Ig. HIV infection occurred on day 1.

A related but distinct issue is whether or not the proper antibodies were present, considering the specific nature of the challenge virus used. We have determined in this study that the HIV Ig contained no reactivitiy with the dominant and specific neutralizing epitope of HTLV-III$_B$. The neutralizing effect demonstrated *in vitro* must then have been due to targets related to the conserved regions of the envelope mentioned earlier, which is consistent with the broad neutralizing spectrum of the serum. One might thus be led to conclude that antibodies which neutralize HIV by such conserved determinants are not effective *in vivo* under the conditions of this experiment. There may be further basis for this from other studies. In a recent report, Fultz et al (1987) were successful in superinfecting chimpanzees with diverse HIV strains long after establishment of the initial infection and the emergence of broad neutralizing activity.

One might then consider the possibility that the hypervariable region, which has proven to be an immunodominant epitope for virus neutralizing antibodies, might prove an effective target for virus neutralization *in vivo*. To test this idea one would have to induce high titres of neutralizing antibodies in chimps using the specific fragment of gp120 harbouring the target epitope and then challenge with the homologous virus. If successful, such a study would focus attention to this region of the envelope as a target for protective antibodies. The remaining formidable problem of how to overcome the hypervariable nature of this region of the HIV envelope would then have to be considered.

Our tentative conclusions from these studies are that there may be a number of reasons why passive immunotherapy failed in this trial. First, it is possible that a sufficient threshold of antibodies was not present long enough to prevent infection by the challenge virus. Secondly, the administered antibodies may have been lacking in terms of activities which effectively block virus infection *in vivo*. Finally, it is possible that the human antibodies which mediate ADCC do not operate efficiently with effector cells in the chimpanzee. The potential role of this mechanism for elimination of infected cells resulting from incompletely neutralized virus would thus be minimized. Additional studies will thus be required to resolve the issue of whether or not protective antibodies against HIV exist and if so what is their exact nature and function.

DISCUSSION

One conclusion that can be drawn from these observations is that much more needs to be learned about the mechanism of virus penetration into the cell. Based on current knowledge, this entails the processes of binding to the CD4 receptor, fusion with the cell membrane, and the entry process itself. Antibodies which effectively block binding or any events requisite for fusion, penetration and perhaps uncoating are likely to be of greatest value in vaccine strategies.

While a great deal is known about binding of HIV and its receptor it has thus far been difficult to artificially induce antibodies to the binding site on gp120 which are biologically active against HIV infection. The high affinity of gp120 for CD4 coupled with the distinct possibility that the binding region is highly conformation dependent, and perhaps exists as a cleft in the molecule which is poorly accessible to antibodies, may explain this problem.

On the other hand, other epitopes exist which may be more effective targets of immune attack. The hypervariable loop appears to be easily accessible and antibodies to it strongly inhibit virus infection as well as virus mediated fusion events. This region of the molecule may somehow be associated with the process of fusion. It has been hypothesized that the gp41 glycoprotein houses the actual fusogenic domain at its N terminus (Gallaher, 1987; Gonzales-Scarano, 1987). The transmembrane glycoprotein also has the function of anchoring the gp120 to the surface of the virus. One could hypothesize that after binding to the receptor, gp120 and gp41 dissociate allowing the gp41 to fuse with the cell membrane. The hypervariable region could represent a portion of the binding region of gp120 to gp41 as suggested from the studies of Kowalski et al (1987). If this is the case, antibodies to the hypervariable region may either prevent the dissociation of the two molecules or sterically hinder the gp41 from associating with the cell surface. Both possibilities could explain the anti-fusogenic activity of such antibodies. The hypervariability of the immunodominant neutralizing epitope of gp120, however, clearly presents a dilemma for vaccine strategies that would employ it as a target. This is, of course, unless the number of variations are not inordinately high so as to preclude approaches with cocktails of peptides that could induce the spectrum of anti-viral immunity necessary to deal with the variation in naturally occurring isolates of HIV.

There are other sites on gp120 and gp41 which are important for virus infection. One of these has recently been reported within the second conserved region of gp120 (Ho et al, 1988). This site, like the hypervariable domain, is not involved in gp120 binding to CD4 but contrasts with it in its ability to induce broadly neutralizing activity. Antibodies to the putative fusogenic domain of gp41 or to other regions of gp41 necessary for binding to gp120 could also exert inhibitory effects and there is evidence to this effect (Chanh et al, 1986; Thomas et al, 1988).

This discussion thus serves to emphasize the need to identify all of the functional domains of the virus envelope and the epitopes that give rise to meaningful immunological responses against HIV. This includes not only those that are effective against the free virus, which most likely will be antibodies, but also those that generate responses that destroy HIV infected cells.

Clearly, much can also be learned from studies which define more precisely the natural history of HIV infection such as described above for the infected laboratory worker. More needs to be done along this line in cases where natural transmission of HIV can be documented early. Likewise, more indepth knowledge of the interplay between HIV and the host is likely to shed light on the immune responses required to control virus infection and replication. Definition of the target epitopes on the virus and the infected cell will facilitate the interpretation of what may constitute a protective response against this devastating pathogen.

Acknowledgements
A number of colleagues are responsible for the work described in this report:

(1) Duke University Medical Center: Drs Thomas J Matthews, Kent J Weinhold, Alphonse Langlois, Barton F Haynes, Thomas Palker, Michael Skinner and Chet Nastala.

(2) Repligen Corporation: Drs James Rusche, Kashi Javaherian, and Scott Putney.

(3) National Cancer Institute: Drs Robert C Gallo, Flossie Wong-Staal and William Blattner

(4) New York Blood Center: Dr Alfred Prince

(5) Southwest Research Foundation: Dr Jorg Eichberg

I am grateful also to Drs Robert C Gallo and Flossie Wong-Staal for their reagents and helpful discussions.

REFERENCES

Allain J P, Laurian Y, Paul D A, Senn D 1986 Serological markers in early stages of human immunodeficiency virus infection in haemophiliacs. Lancet 2: 1233–1236

Chanh T L, Dreesman G R, Kanda P 1986 Induction of anti-HIV neutralising antibodies by synthetic peptides. European Molecular Biology Organization Journal 5: 3065–3071

Dalgleish A G, Beverley P, Clapham P, Crawford D, Greaves M, Weiss R 1984 The CD4 (t4) antigen is an essential component of the receptor for the AIDS retrovirus. Nature 312: 763–767

deWolf F, Goudsmit J, Paul D A et al 1987 Risk of AID related complex and AIDS in homosexual men with persistent HIV antigenaemia. British Medical Journal 295(6598): 569–572

Fultz P N, Srinivasan A, Greene C, Butler D, Swenson R B, McClure H M 1987 Superinfection of a chimpanzee with a second strain of human immunodeficiency virus. Journal of Virology 61(12): 4026–4029

Gallaher W R 1987 Detection of a fusion peptide sequence in the transmembrane protein of human immunodeficiency virus. Cell 50: 327–328

Gonzales-Scarano F, Waxham M N, Ross A M, Hoxie J A 1987 Sequence similarities between human immunodeficiency virus gp41 and paramyxovirus fusion proteins. AIDS Research and Human Retroviruses 3(3): 245–252

Ho D D, Kaplan J C, Rackauskas I E, Gurney M E 1988 Second conserved domain of gp120 is important for HIV infectivity and antibody neutralization. Science 239: 1021–1023

Klatzmann D, Champagne E, Chamaret S et al 1984 T-lymphocyte T4 molecule behaves as the receptor for human retrovirus LAV. Nature 312: 767–768

Kowalski M, Potz J, Basiripour L et al 1987 Functional regions of the envelope glycoprotein of human immunodeficiency virus type 1. Science 237: 1351–1355

Lasky L A, Nakamura G, Smith D H et al 1987 Delineation of a region of the human immunodeficiency virus type 1 gp120 glycoprotein critical for interaction with the CD4 receptor. Cell 50: 975–985

Matthews T J, Weinhold K J, Lyerly H K, Langlois A J, Wigzell H, Bolognesi D P 1987 Interaction between the human T-cell lymphotropic virus type III$_B$ envelope glycoprotein gp120 and the surface antigen CD4: Role of carbohydrate in binding and cell fusion. Proceedings of the National Academy of Sciences 84: 5424–5428

McDougal J S, Kennedy M S, Sligh J N, Cort S P, Mawle A, Nicholson J K A 1986 Binding of HTLV-III/LAV to T4+ cells by a complex of the 110K viral protein and the T4 molecule. Science 231: 382–385

Palker T J, Clark M E, Langlois A J et al 1988 Type-specific neutralization of the human immunodeficiency virus with antibodies to env-coded synthetic peptides. Proceedings of the National Academy of Sciences 85: 1932–1936

Pedersen C, Nielsen C M, Vestergaard B F, Gerstoft J, Krogsgaard K, Nielsen J O 1987 Temporal relation of antigenaemia and loss of antibodies to core antigens to development of clinical disease in HIV infection. British Medical Journal 295(6598): 567–569

Prince A M, Horowitz B, Baker L et al 1988 Failure of an HIV immune globulin to protect chimpanzees against experimental challenge with HIV. Proceedings of National Academy of Sciences, in press

Ranki A, Krohn M, Allain J P, Franchini G, Valle S L, Antonen J, Leuther M, Krohn K 1987 Long latency precedes overt seroconversion in sexually transmitted human immunodeficiency virus infection. Lancet (September 12): 589–593

Redfield R R, Wright D C, Tramont E C 1986 The Walter Reed staging classification for HTLV-III/LAV infection. New England Journal of Medicine 314: 131–132

Ruprecht L G, O'Brien G, Rossoni L D, Nusinoff-Lehrman S 1986 Suppression of mouse veremia and retroviral disease by 3'-azido-3'deoxythymidine. Nature 323: 467–469

Rusche J R, Lynn D L, Robert-Guroff M et al 1987 Humoral immune response to the entire human immunodeficiency virus envelope glycoprotein made in insect cells. Proceedings of National Academy of Sciences 84: 1–5

Rusche J R, Javaherian K, McDanal C 1988 Antibodies that inhibit fusion of HIV infected cells bind a 24 amino acid sequence of the viral envelope. Proceedings of the National Academy of Sciences 85: 3198–3202

Schafer W, Bolognesi D P 1987 Mammalian C-type oncornaviruses: Relationships between viral structural and cell-surface antigens and their possible significance in immunological defense mechanisms. Contemporary Topics in Immunobiology 7: 127–167

Sharpe A H, Jaenisch R O, Ruprecht A 1987 A rapid model for neurovirulence and transplacental antiviral therapy. Science 236: 1671–1674

Skinner M A, Langlois A J, McDanal C B, Bolognesi D P, Matthews T J 1988a Serum from HIV infected humans prevents gp120 binding to CD4 and this activity is not elicited in animals immunized with envelope protein components. Journal of Virology, in press

Skinner M A, Ting R, Matthews T J 1988b Characteristics of a neutralizing monoclonal antibody HTV-III$_B$ envelope glycoprotein. AIDS Research and Human Retroviruses 4(3): 187–198

Starcich B R, Hahn B H, Shaw G M et al 1986 Identification and characterization of conserved and variable regions in the envelope gene of HTLV-III/LAV, the retrovirus of AIDS. Cell 45: 637–648

Tavares L, Roneker C, Johnston K, Nusinoff-Lehrman S, de Noronha F 1987 3'-azido-3'-deoxythymidine in feline leukemia virus-infected cats: A model for therapy and prophylaxis of AIDS. Cancer Research 47: 3190–3195

Thiel H J, Schwarz H, Fischinger P, Bolognesi D, Schafer W et al 1987 Role of antibodies to murine leukemia virus p15E transmembrane protein in immunotherapy against AKR leukemia: A model for studies in human acquired immunodeficiency syndrome. Proceedings of the National Academy of Science 84: 5893–5897

Thomas E K, Weber J N, McClure J et al 1988 Neutralizing monoclonal antibodies to the AIDS virus. AIDS 2: 25–29

Weber J N, Clapham P R, Weiss R A et al 1987 Human immunodeficiency virus infection in two cohorts of homosexual men: neutralizing sera and association of anti-gag antibody with prognosis. Lancet 1: 119–122

Weiss S H, Goedert J J, Gartner S 1988 Risk of human immunodeficiency virus (HIV-1) infection among laboratory workers. Science 239: 68–71

Wu A M, Ting R C, Gallo R C 1973 RNA-directed DNA polymerase and virus-induced leukemia in mice. Proceedings of the National Academy of Sciences 70: 1298–1302

Discussion of paper presented by Dani Bolognesi

Discussant: Robin A. Weiss

TOWARDS AIDS VACCINES

Dr Bolognesi has illustrated some of the problems of developing vaccines protective against the AIDS virus, HIV, by reviewing the immunobiology of the HIV envelope, and the lack of adequate animal models for testing not only safety but efficacy. In this brief commentary, I shall extend the discussion by posing the following three questions: What types of vaccine may be developed? What target antigens of HIV are appropriate? Does the receptor binding site on the outer envelope glycoprotein, gp120, provide a common target?

Types of vaccine
The possible approaches to AIDS vaccines may be listed as follows:

(1) Live, attenuated virus
(2) Killed virus
(3) Purified antigen subunits and complexes
(4) Recombinant antigens
(5) Synthetic peptides
(6) Live, recombinant vectors
(7) Anti-idiotypic antibodies

All of these methods, except for the first, are pursued as plausible reagents. A live, attenuated vaccine, as used for polio, is a most doubtful option because we do not understand the basis for attenuation of retroviruses. Besides, for any virus with such a long incubation period and with chronic infection that, once acquired, cannot be eliminated, it would be difficult to determine attenuation; moreover, retroviruses readily undergo genetic recombination with related strains, and new virulent forms may arise. Killed, whole virus is an option but it should be realized that the HIV envelope incorporates host cell antigens during the budding process, including MHC antigens, so that the purity of the vaccine preparation is unlikely ever to be sufficient. That leaves purified subunit reagents, or better, complexes of subunits; immunostimulatory complexes (iscoms) are currently attracting more interest because of their previous use in feline retrovirus vaccines.

For the generation of sufficiently large amounts of pure subunit vaccines, recombinant DNA methods will almost certainly be required for immunogen production, whether produced by bacteria, yeast, or animal cells. Many preparations of recombinant envelope antigens are already being tested, but, as Bolognesi has already mentioned, none has yet protected chimpanzees from subsequent HIV challenge. Where small, linear antigenic epitopes are identified, for example in stimulating cell mediated immunity, it is possible that chemically synthesized peptides, coupled with appropriate carriers or adjuvants may afford some protection. But this takes us into a new technology that has not yet proved practicable for such well known viruses as foot and mouth disease or polio.

Live, recombinant vaccines are in fashion, particularly those based on vaccinia vectors. While vaccinia recombinants bearing HIV envelope antigens have not yet protected chimpanzees, the first human trial is in progress (Zagury et al, 1988). Anti-idiotypic immunogens have been much talked about and appear to be protective for hepatitis B virus.

For HIV, anti-idiotypic approaches have been confined thus far to mirror-image anti-idiotypes to antibodies recognizing the site on the cell surface receptor, CD4, to which HIV binds (Dalgleish et al, 1987). Some of these anti-idiotypic antibodies afford weak, though broadly cross-specific, neutralization of HIV *in vitro*, as illustrated later.

HIV antigens

Bolognesi has discussed the HIV envelope and its antigenic variability. We have studied common and variable neutralizing properties of human and animal antisera to HIV (Weiss et al, 1986; Berman et al, 1988). Clearly there are shared neutralization antigens, even a one-sided cross-neutralization of HIV-1 by antisera to HIV-2 (Weiss et al, 1988), yet we do not know on what antigen or precisely where these epitopes reside. On the other hand, a dominant, strain-specific neutralization epitope has now been defined on gp120 (Thomas et al, 1988; Palker et al, 1988).

While envelope components will almost certainly be incorporated into HIV vaccines, it is worth mentioning that core components should not be ignored. With hepatitis B virus, both core and surface antigen are important, and with influenza virus, too, cell mediated cytotoxicity of infected cells directed against the nucleocapsid epitopes represents a significant part of the host's immune response to infection. In longitudinal studies of HIV-infected subjects a low or falling humoral response to the p24 core protein presages early development of AIDS (Weber et al, 1987).

It is not clear yet whether the high anti-p24 levels are simply a marker of sustained health or whether they play a role in it, but such observations emphasize the desirability of seeking to enhance anti-core immunity, either before or following HIV infection. Neither should such investigations be restricted to p24; other gag antigens, such as p17, may be even more important. In addition, reverse transcriptase and non-structural, regulatory proteins might also be considered as targets in a multi-component vaccine.

The receptor binding site

By and large, viruses keep their receptor-binding sites on the surface of the virus well protected. Thus with polio and influenza viruses, the dominant epitopes eliciting neutralizing antibodies cluster around a receptor-binding pocket, but are not part of it. HIV is no exception, as both Bolognesi's and my collaborators have shown in analysing neutralizing epitopes (Palker et al, 1988; Thomas et al, 1988).

Since we identified the CD4 lymphocyte antigen as the receptor for HIV (Dalgleish et al, 1984), the interaction between HIV gp120 and CD4 has been intensively studied and the recognition sites on either molecule are becoming increasingly well defined (Sattentau & Weiss, 1988). Because the receptor recognition site on CD4 is shared by all strains of HIV-1, HIV-2 and simian immunodeficiency viruses (SIV) studied (Sattentau et al, 1988), the blocking of gp120/CD4 interaction might be exploited in therapy, and antibodies to those sites useful for vaccine development.

Table 1 summarizes our own studies on the potency and specificity for neutralization of diverse HIV and SIV strains by anti-gp120, anti-CD4 anti-idiotype and recombinant soluble CD4 molecules. The results show that a highly potent monoclonal antibody to gp120 (Thomas et al, 1988) is strain specific, whereas the activity of the receptor site anti-idiotype is universal but weak. Somewhat stronger as a cross-reactive reagent is soluble CD4 itself. Interestingly, the HIV-2 isolates are considerably less susceptible than HIV-1 or SIV.

Table 1 HIV neutralization: specificity and potency

Virus		Origin	Anti-gp120	Anti-CD4 anti-id	Soluble CD4
HIV-1	LAV-1	France	500,000[a]	10	300
	SF33	USA	—	50	1,000
	RF	Haiti	—	50	300
	CBL4	Tanzania	—	10	300
HIV-2	LAV-2	Guinea-Bissau	—	10	15
	CBL20	Gambia	—	10	150
SIV	SIV$_{mac}$	Macaque	—	10	150
	SIV$_{smm}$	Mangabey	—	25	200

[a] The titres represent the reciprocal of the highest dilution of Ig or soluble CD4 (100 μg/ml) causing >80% inactivation of infectivity when incubated with 1,000 infectious units of HIV 1 hour prior to plating on C8166 T-cells.

These 'neutralizing' reagents block infection *in vitro* not only of CD4-positive lymphocytes, but also of monocytes and macrophages. It remains to be seen whether HIV infects brain and gut cells by the same mechanism and whether receptor-blocking reagents can be applied clinically in preventing infection or progression to disease.

REFERENCES

Berman P W, Groopman J E, Gregory T et al 1988 Human immunodeficiency virus type 1 challenge of chimpanzees immunised with recombinant envelope glycoprotein gp 120. Proceedings of the National Academy of Sciences USA 85: 5200–5204
Dalgleish A G, Beverley P C L, Clapham P R et al 1984 The CD4 (T4) antigen is an essential component of the receptor for the AIDS retrovirus. Nature 312: 763–767

Dalgleish A G, Thompson B T, Chan L T, Malkovsky M, Kennedy R C 1987 Anti-idiotypic antibodies which mimic the T4/CD4 epitope neutralise a broad range of HIV isolates—a potential AIDS vaccine. Lancet 2: 1047–1050

Palker T J, Clark M E, Langlois A J et al 1988 Type-specific neutralization of the human immunodeficiency virus with antiboides to *env*-coded synthetic peptides. Proceedings of the National Academy of Sciences USA 85: 1932–1936

Sattentau Q J, Weiss R A 1988 The CD4 antigen: Physiological ligand and HIV receptor. Cell 52: 631–633

Sattentau Q J et al 1988 The human and simian immunology viruses HIV-1, HIV-2 and SIV interact with similar epitopes on their cellular receptor, the CD4 molecule. AIDS 2: 101–105

Thomas E K, Weber J N, McClure J et al 1988 Neutralizing monoclonal antibodies to the AIDS virus. AIDS 2: 25–29

Weber J N, Clapham P L, Weiss R A et al, 1987 Human immunodeficiency virus infection in two cohorts of homosexual men: neutralizing sera and association of anti-gag antibodies with prognosis. Lancet 1: 119–122

Weiss R A, Clapham P R, Weber J N, Dalgleish A G, Lasky L A, Berman P W 1986 Variable and conserved neutralization antigens of HIV. Nature 324: 572–575

Weiss R A, Clapham P R, Weber, J N et al 1988 HIV-2 antisera cross-neutralize HIV-1. AIDS 2: 95–100

Zagury D, Bernard J, Cheynier R et al 1988 A group specific anamnestic immune reaction against HIV-1 induced by a candidate vaccine against AIDS. Nature 332: 728–731

Discussion: HIV

Dani P. Bolognesi and Robin Weiss

Three main topics were discussed. One topic concerned the failure of the experiment to use intravenous HIV human hyperimmune globulin for prevention of infection in chimpanzees. It was suggested that as an alternative approach the immunoglobulin and virus might be allowed to interact *in vitro* whereupon the presumed neutralized virus would be injected into animals. If neither passive nor active immunization can be demonstrated to have any effect on virus replication in chimpanzees the possibility would remain to try a combination of the two.

A second topic for discussion was the kinetics of the antibody response to the p24 protein. It is now well documented that at the terminal stage of infection the antibody titres to envelope antigens remain whereas antibodies against the gag proteins disappear and are followed by antigenaemia. It was pointed out that the latter situation represents a true antigenaemia and not a reflection of circulating immune complexes. If p24 antigen excess is the cause of the disappearance of antibodies against this antigen AZT treatment, suppressing virus replication might possibly lead to a resumed antibody protection. However, this need not necessarily be the outcome. It might be that the p24 antibody response is relatively more T-cell dependent than the antibody response to the envelope antigens (the occurrence of shared carbohydrate and protein epitopes in the latter antigens may play a role in this context). If this is so, a resumed antibody production to p24 would require a restoration of T-cell functions consequential to the AZT treatment.

The final topic discussed concerned post-exposure vaccination. It was noted that in this situation one would have to stimulate not only a vigorous antibody response but also a strong cellular immune response to deal with infected cells. The question then is whether such a cellular immune response could be detrimental. Could it for example cause irreversible damage to brain endothelial cells? It was argued that the consequences of immune-mediated cell damage would depend on the possibilities for continuous replacement of cells by division. Still to be demonstrated is the pathogenic role of a possible infection of neuronal cells and genuine glial cells (expressing the GFAP protein) in AIDS dementia, and hence what the consequences of immune destruction of these cells might be. It was mentioned that interferon treatment of HIV antibody positive but not negative hepatitis B virus carriers has led to the appearance of markedly abnormal psychomotor and other cognitive functions. If a subclinical HIV brain infection can become disease-causing in this situation caution needs to be taken not to activate the brain infection by other means.

11. Redesigning poliovirus for vaccine purposes

Jeffrey W. Almond, Karen L. Burke,
Michael A. Skinner, Morag Ferguson,
Eric D. A. D'Souza, Glynis Dunn,
Vincent R. Racaniello and Philip D. Minor

INTRODUCTION

The live attenuated vaccines against poliomyelitis in current use were developed by Albert Sabin in the 1950s by continuous passage of wild type strains (Sabin & Boulger, 1983). These vaccine viruses replicate in the recipient and induce a mucosal as well as a systemic immune response and thereby provide protection against infection and disease. Widespread use of the vaccines has had a major impact on the incidence of poliomyelitis and in many countries of the world epidemic poliomyelitis has been eliminated (for a review see Melnick, 1980). However, a few sporadic cases are still observed in well vaccinated communities and over recent years evidence has accumulated that these are caused by the vaccines themselves (Assaad & Cockburn, 1982). The viruses isolated from these cases can often be designated 'vaccine-like' on the basis of serology and RNA analysis (Nottay et al, 1981; Minor, 1980). Almost all such isolates are serotypes 2 and 3 whereas the type 1 vaccine by contrast has rarely, if ever, been implicated as a cause of disease and must be regarded as one of the safest vaccines used in humans (Assaad & Cockburn, 1982). This paper describes the modification of poliovirus vaccines to address the following questions:

(1)   Can the existing type 3 vaccine be further attenuated to the point where it is comparable in safety to the presently used type 1 strain?

(2)   Can the existing type 1 vaccine strain be modified antigenically using protein engineering techniques so that it resembles the type 2 and 3 viruses and therefore potentially be used as a vaccine against these two serotypes?

(3)   Can the very safe type 1 poliovirus vaccine be used as a vehicle for antigenic determinants from other pathogenic micro-organisms, particularly in cases where a good mucosal immunity is required for protection from disease?

The poliovirus particle is composed of a single-stranded positive sense RNA genome of approximately 7450 nucleotides enclosed in an icosahedral particle of 27 nm diameter (for review see Rueckert, 1985). The three dimensional crystallographic structure of the capsid of poliovirus type 1 has been determined at 2.9A resolution, providing a detailed knowledge of the folding and arrangement of the individual virus proteins VP1-VP4 (Hogle et al, 1985). From this structural information and from the characterization of monoclonal antibody resistant mutants and immune responses to synthetic peptides (Minor et al, 1983, 1985, 1986a, 1986b; Emini et al, 1983; Nomoto & Wimmer, 1986), the amino acids constituting antigenic sites have been identified and located on the surface of the virus particle (Table 11.1). The complete nucleotide sequence of all three serotypes of poliovirus, including the three Sabin vaccine strains have been determined (for review see Almond, 1987). Site-directed mutagenesis of poliovirus RNA is made possible by the fact that a full length DNA copy of the genome cloned in *Escherichia coli* is infectious for mammalian cells in culture (Racaniello & Baltimore, 1981).

Table 11.1 Location (amino acid number) of antigenic sites in poliovirus type 3

Site	Location
1	VP1; 89–100
2a	VP1; 220–222
2b	VP2; 164–172
3a	VP1; 286–290
3b	VP3; 58–60, 70, 71, 77, 79

MODIFICATION OF THE POLIOVIRUS TYPE 3 SABIN VACCINE STRAIN P3/LEON 12_a1_b

As discussed above, the Sabin types 2 and 3 vaccines can cause rare cases of paralysis in vaccines, with most cases attributable to the type 3 strain (Assaad & Cockburn, 1982). Results of early trials with this virus suggested that it was the least stable of the three vaccine strains and this is supported by results in tissue culture (see Almond, 1987). The type 3 strain has been investigated extensively in an attempt to determine the molecular basis of its attenuation. Comparative nucleotide sequence analysis has revealed that this vaccine strain differs from its neurovirulent progenitor P/Leon/37 by just 10 point mutations in their 7432 nucleotides (Stanway et al, 1984). Evidence from several lines of investigation suggest that two of these mutations are primarily responsible for the attenuation phenotype. These are the C-U change at position 2034 in the virus genome which causes a serine to phenylalanine amino acid substitution in virus protein VP3 (Westrop et al, 1987, unpublished). Our evidence (unpublished) suggests that this mutation also confers a temperature sensitive phenotype on this virus. The second mutation which contributes to the attenuated phenotype is a C-U change at position 472 in the non-coding region of the virus genome (Evans et al, 1985). The mechanism by which this mutation gives rise to the attenuation phenotype is unknown although it has been suggested that it may act via an effect on the secondary structure of the virus RNA. Studies on viruses excreted by vaccinees have indicated that this mutation rapidly reverts to the wild type C upon passage of the virus in the human gut, and that this reversion is associated with an increase in neurovirulence (Evans et al, 1985; Minor et al, 1986a). It has also been shown, using a series of recombinants based on the mouse adapted poliovirus P2/Lansing and incorporating the 5' non coding region of either the type 3 vaccine strain, its neurovirulent progenitor, or a vaccine revertant, that the presence of C at 472 is obligatory for growth in the CNS of mice (La Monica et al, 1987). Growth in tissue culture, however, is unaffected by the mutation at this position. It is interesting to note that the type 1 and type 2 vaccine strains also contain mutations in this region of their RNA when compared with their neurovirulent progenitor or revertant strains respectively (Nomoto et al, 1982; Pollard et al, unpublished). In the case of the type 1 virus there is direct evidence that this is an attenuating mutation (Nomoto et al, 1987). It has also been shown that the type 1 vaccine strain has further multiple attenuating mutations as compared with its neurovirulent progenitor, thus providing an explanation for the relative stability of this strain (Omata et al, 1986).

It seems then that the non-coding region of the genome around position 470–490 has a crucially important function in replication of poliovirus in cells of the CNS and probably also the gut. We have therefore attempted to introduce further mutations into this region to try to (a) define its function, and (b) produce a derivative of the vaccine which may be less likely to revert to neurovirulence upon replication in humans. Fig. 11.1 indicates the mutations that we have introduced into this region of the type 3 genome, linked to the coding region of P2/Lansing as described previously (La Monica et al, 1987). Of the 10 infectious DNAs manipulated four gave rise to viable virus and these mutants have been tested for neurovirulence in mice. Mutations 7 and 13 clearly attenuate the virus in terms of LD50 (Table 11.2) as compared with the wild type, whereas mutation 14 has little or no effect. Having identified new mutations which attenuate the virus we were interested to construct a double mutant containing two independently attenuating mutations. Mutant 8 contains the mutation found in the vaccine strain of type 3, i.e. U at 472, plus the A at 482 present in mutant 7. This double mutant has been tested in mice and preliminary results suggest that it is more attenuated than either of the single mutant strains (Table 11.2). We are presently investigating this double mutant further to determine whether it is genetically more stable than the vaccine strain. The ability to introduce further attenuating mutations into this region, possibly including deletion mutations, raises the prospect of constructing very stable, completely safe, strains which may be more stable than the existing type 3 vaccine strain. The functional analysis of the effects of these mutations on virus functions such as RNA translation, replication and encapsidation are currently under investigation.

PROTEIN ENGINEERING OF THE SABIN TYPE 1 STRAIN

As stated above, in contrast to the types 2 and 3 vaccine the Sabin type 1 vaccine strain is rarely, if ever, associated with paralysis in vaccinees and is probably the safest vaccine ever used in humans (Assaad & Cockburn, 1982). The knowledge of the three dimensional crystal structure of type 1, plus the availability of infectious Sabin 1 cDNA, has raised the possibility of the redesign of the poliovirus particle for vaccine purposes (Almond et al, 1984; Burke et al, 1988; Murray et al, 1987). In particular we have been interested in the prospect of

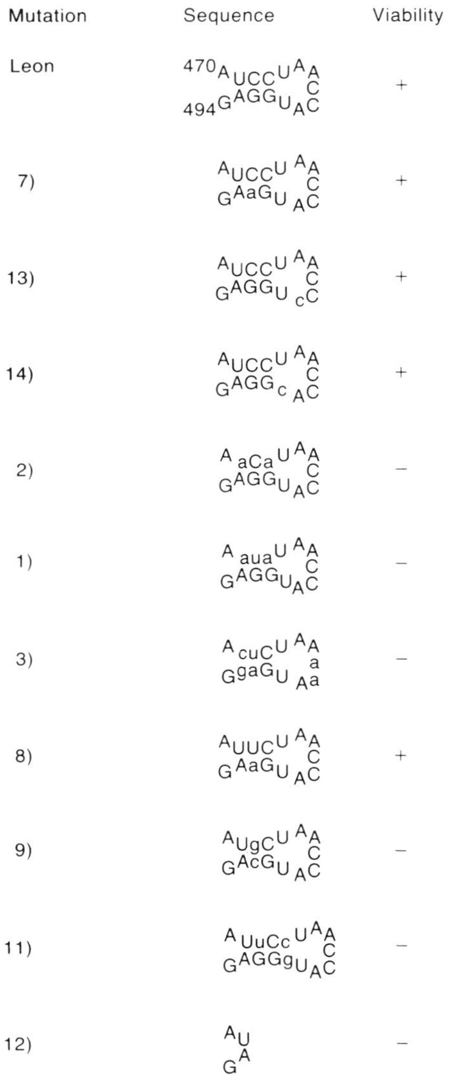

Mutation	Sequence	Viability
Leon	$^{470}A_{UCC}U^A_A{}_C$ $_{494}G^{AGG}U_{A}C$	+
7)	$A_{UCC}U^A_A{}_C$ $G^{AaG}U_{A}C$	+
13)	$A_{UCC}U^A_A{}_C$ $G^{AGG}U_{c}C$	+
14)	$A_{UCC}U^A_A{}_C$ $G^{AGG}c_{A}C$	+
2)	$A_{aCa}U^A_A{}_C$ $G^{AGG}U_{A}C$	−
1)	$A_{aua}U^A_A{}_C$ $G^{AGG}U_{A}C$	−
3)	$A_{cuC}U^A_A{}_a$ $G^{gaG}U_{A}a$	−
8)	$A_{UUC}U^A_A{}_C$ $G^{AaG}U_{A}C$	+
9)	$A_{Ugc}U^A_A{}_C$ $G^{AcG}U_{A}C$	−
11)	$A_{UuCc}U^A_A{}_C$ $G^{AGGg}U_{A}C$	−
12)	A_{U} G^A	−

Fig. 11.1 Nucleotide sequence of bases 470–484 and RNA folding as described in Evans et al (1985) of P3/Leon/37 and ten site-directed mutants. Mutations are indicated by lower case letters. Number 12 is a deletion mutant missing bases 472–482 inclusive

modifying the antigenic sites of Sabin 1 so that they resemble those of the more problematical type 2 and type 3 viruses (Almond et al, 1984). The antigenic sites involved in neutralization of poliovirus type 3 have been identified (Minor et al, 1986b) (Table 11.1). We have extensively modified the counterparts of these sites in Sabin 1 in an attempt to change the antigenic structure of the virus (Burke et al, 1988, unpublished). In early experiments site-directed mutagenesis was

Table 11.2 LD$_{50}$ values in mice (La Monica et al., 1987) for parenteral mouse adapted strain P2/Lansing, the type 3 vaccine and progenitor recombinants (PRV7.3 nd PRV6.1) and various site-directed mutants of PRV6.1 (SFPs)

Virus	LD$_{50}$	
P2/Lansing		1.6×10^3–1×10^5 pfu
PRV 6.1 (Leon)	472 C	$< 6 \times 10^2$
7.3 (Sabin)	472 U	$> 2 \times 10^7$
SFP 7	482 A	7.5×10^6
8	472 U, 482 A	1.6×10^8
13	479 C	9.1×10^6
14	480 C	$< 7 \times 10^4$

carried out on a 1174 base pair restriction endonuclease fragment of cDNA. This resulted in the coding region for eight amino acids from site 1 of the type 1 vaccine strain (SASTKNKD) being replaced by the corresponding amino acids from a poliovirus type 3 strain 3.370 (EQPTTRVQ) (Burke et al, 1988). Chimaeric virus was recovered from a full length cDNA incorporating this modified restriction fragment by transfection of Hep2C cells in culture. This virus, designated S1/3.10, was shown to contain an altered RNA as determined by direct nucleotide sequence analysis through the region 2762–2785. Moreover, the virus had antigenic and immunogenic properties of type 3 poliovirus as well as type 1. In a standard typing assay an unknown poliovirus is incubated with pairs of immune specific antiserum (i.e. type 1 plus type 2, type 2 plus type 3, and type 1 plus type 3) to neutralize all but one serotype of virus in each test. The chimaera S1/3.10 was neutralized by all three combinations of antisera by the type 1 and type 3 antisera alone but not by the type 2 antiserum (Table 11.3). This demonstrates that the virus chimaera has antigenic characteristics of both type 1 and type 3 but is not a mixture of these viruses. The antigenicity of S1/3.10 was also examined using panels of Sabin 1 and Sabin 3 specific monoclonal antibodies in both antigen blocking and neutralization tests (Ferguson et al, 1984; Minor et al, 1986b). These results confirmed that the particle has composite antigenicity. All type 3 antibodies against site 1, which reacted with the 3.370 strain, also reacted with the chimaeric virus, whereas type 3 antibodies against other sites failed to react with the chimaeric virus. As expected, antibodies against site 1 of type 1 failed to react with the chimaera (since this site had been replaced), whereas monoclonal antibodies against sites 2 and 3 of type 1 reacted as well with the chimaeric virus as they did with Sabin type 1 (Burke et al, 1988).

Table 11.3 Neutralization of chimaeric virus by monospecific polyclonal antisera

Antiserum	Sabin 1	Sabin 2	Sabin 3	S1/3.10
Type 1	> 5.75	0.0	0.0	> 6.5
Type 2	0.0	> 5.25	0.0	0.0
Type 3	0.0	0.0	> 5.25	4.0

Reductions in titre (log$_{10}$) of infectious virus were determined by challenging 10-fold dilutions of virus with a fixed dilution of antiserum in a standard microtitre assay (Burke et al., 1988).

The immunogenicity of the chimaera was tested in mice, rabbits, and monkeys following a single inoculation of the virus. As can be seen from Table 11.4, animals inoculated with this virus showed a good immune response against type 3 p.iiovirus (strain 3.370) as well as against type 1. In contrast mice immunized with Sabin type 1 produced antibody against the chimaera and the homologous virus but failed to produce antibody against 3.370. Because of the sensitivity of antigenic site 1 to trypsin digestion (Icenogle et al, 1986; Minor et al, 1987), it was possible to analyse further the type 3 antibody induced by the chimaera S1/3.10. All S1/3.10 antisera showing neutralization of intact type 3 virus failed to react with trypsin cleaved type 3 virus, indicating that the type 3 response was against the intact site 1 in the configuration found in normal infectious virus. It was of interest to note that the monkey used in these experiments developed anti-type 3 antibody response following infection via feeding. It has been shown previously that antigenic site 1 of excreted viruses is in a cleaved form, presumably as a result of action of intestinal proteases (Minor et al, 1986b). This implies that virus in the gut differs antigenically from that grown in tissue culture in respect of the presence of site 1. The fact that anti-site 1 antibodies were observed in the serum of the monkey suggests that at least some of the virus presented to its immune system was in the uncleaved form and therefore likely to have undergone replication in body sites other than the gut.

Table 11.4 Antibody titres against intact and trypsin cleaved virus in antigen-blocking tests

Animal	Immunized with	S1/3.10	S1/3.10 TRP	Antibody titre to virus Sabin type 1	Sabin type 1	3.370	3.370 TRP
Mouse							
1	Sabin type 1	160	160	320	160	< 10	< 10
2		160	160	160	160	< 10	< 10
3		640	640	640	640	< 10	< 10
4		640	640	640	320	< 10	< 10
5		160	160	160	160	< 10	< 10
6	S1/3.10	160	160	160	160	10	< 10
7		2,560	2,560	2,560	2,560	1,280	< 10
8		80	80	80	80	< 10	< 10
9		80	80	80	80	20	< 10
10		160	160	160	160	20	< 10
Rabbit							
1	S1/3.10	80	80	80	80	10	< 10
2		320	320	80	80	80	< 10
3		160	160	40	40	160	< 10
Monkey							
1	S1/3.10	160	160	160	160	20	< 10

Animals were immunized with 0.1 ml of sucrose purified poliovirus of titre approximately 10^8 $TCID_{50}$ per ml. Mice were inoculated twice by the intraperitoneal route, and rabbits twice by the intramuscular route. A cynomolgus monkey was fed 1 ml of virus tissue culture fluid and blood samples and faecal specimens taken twice a week for four weeks. Antibody titres were measured in the antigen blocking test (17) and are expressed as the end point dilution which inhibits the diffusion of virus. Viruses were treated with trypsin as described (5). TRP = trypsin treated virus (from Burke et al., 1988).

In summary, these results indicate that after exchange of one of its antigenic sites the very safe poliovirus type 1 vaccine can induce neutralizing antibodies against poliovirus type 3. This modification involves a region of the genome of the type

1 strain which is unlikely to contain attenuating mutations (Nomoto et al, 1982; Omata et al, 1986). It is therefore reasonable to expect that the chimaera should retain the stable attenuation phenotype of the parenteral vaccine strain. Work is in progress to assess the antigenic and immunogenic properties of several other polio type 1/3 and type 1/2 chimaeras. To date we have constructed thirteen viable viruses with sequences derived from more than one poliovirus serotype. Chimaeras of this sort could well prove to be serious alternatives to the existing type 3 and type 2 vaccine strains. They should also provide valuable tools to study further both cellular and humoral immunity to poliomyelitis.

USE OF THE SABIN TYPE 1 VACCINE STRAIN AS A VEHICLE FOR ANTIGENIC DETERMINANTS FROM OTHER PATHOGENIC MICRO-ORGANISMS

The success in constructing antigenic chimaeras of poliovirus discussed above prompted us to explore the possibility of using the poliovirus to stimulate immunity against other pathogenic micro-organisms. This idea is particularly attractive where the pathogen in question infects via a mucosal surface and where secretory antibodies are believed to play an important role in protection (Ogra et al, 1980). The known safety record and efficacy of the Sabin poliovirus type 1 strain, plus 25 years' experience of its use, manufacture and control, make this a particularly attractive vector of foreign immunogens. We have therefore attempted to engineer antigenic determinants from a whole range of pathogenic micro-organisms into the Sabin 1 strain with a view to (a) determining the structural and antigenic flexibility of the virus particle, and (b) assessing the configuration of foreign determinants in relation to whether the manipulation viruses could constitute candidate vaccines. To facilitate experiments of this sort, a modified poliovirus cDNA was constructed which obviates the need for oligonucleotide directed mutagenesis. Thus a cassette for changing antigenic site 1 of the type 1 vaccine strain was constructed as follows: A 3594 base pair partial Kpn 1 restriction endonuclease fragment of the Sabin 1 cDNA containing the coding regions for antigenic site 1 was sub-cloned into the single stranded phage vector M13 mp18.

The nucleotide sequence flanking the antigenic site was altered by site-directed mutagenesis which resulted in the introduction of unique Sal 1 and Dra 1 sites at nucleotides 2753 and 2783 respectively. This mutated fragment was introduced into a full length copy of the Sabin 1 genome carried in a derivative of vector pBR332 lacking Sal 1 or Dra 1 sites and containing a T7 promoter in front of the cDNA. Using this mutagenesis cassette the alteration of antigenic site 1 is a simple procedure requiring the synthesis of two complementary oligonucleotides incorporating the new sequence plus a Sal 1 sticky end and a flush-end, and ligation of this DNA into the double digested cassette. It can be arranged that the incorporated fragment destroys the Sal 1 or Dra 1 sites of the vector to facilitate screening of recombinant plasmids. Live virus is recovered from a T7 transcript of the cDNA which is infectious for cells in tissue culture. Our preliminary results so far suggest that antigen chimaeras of poliovirus, which contain putative B cell epitopes from foot and mouth disease virus (Bittle et al, 1982), rhinovirus (McCray & Werner, 1987), hepatitis A virus (Baroudy et al, 1985), human immunodeficiency virus (Gnann et al, 1987; Modrow et al, 1987) and chla·ıydia trachomatis (Baehr et al, 1988) are viable. The antigenic characterization of these viruses is presently in progress.

CONCLUSION

Site-directed mutagenesis of poliovirus cDNA based on existing knowledge of the molecular determinants of neurovirulence and the three dimensional structure of the virus particle, offers several possibilities for the construction of very, completely safe, poliovirus vaccines against serotypes 2 and 3. Antigenic modification of the Sabin poliovirus type 1, which is a very safe and effective vaccine and known to induce a good secretory immune response, raises the possibility of using this strain as a vehicle to induce immune responses against immunogenic proteins of other pathogens. Preliminary results look encouraging and suggest that antigenic site 1 of the virus can be modified in a variety of ways. The flexibility of this and other regions of the poliovirus capsid proteins in terms of the size and structure of peptides which can be accommodated and their antigenicity and immunogenicity are presently under investigation.

REFERENCES

Almond J W 1987 The attenuation of poliovirus neurovirulence. Annual Review of Microbiology 987; 41:153–180
Almond J W, Stanway G, Cann A J et al 1984 New poliovirus vaccines: a molecular approach. Vaccine 2: 177–184
Assaad F, Cockburn W C 1982 The relation between acute persisting spinal paralysis and poliomyelitis vaccine—results of a ten-year enquiry. Bulletin of World Health Organization 60: 231–242
Baehr W, Zhang Y-X, Joseph T et al 1988 Mapping protective antigenic domains expressed by C. trachomatis major outer membrane protein (MOMP) genes. Proceedings of the National Academy of Sciences, USA 85: 4000–4004
Baroudy B M, Ticehnurst J R, Miele T A, Maizel J V Jnr, Purcell R H, Feinstone S M 1985 Sequence analysis of hepatitis A virus cDNA coding for capsid proteins and RNA polymerase. Proceedings of the National Academy of Sciences USA, 82: 2143–2147
Bittle J L, Houghton R A, Alexander H et al 1982 Protection against foot and mouth disease by immunization with a chemically synthesised peptide predicted from the viral nucleotide sequence. Nature 298: 30–33
Burke K L, Dawn G, Ferguson M, Minor P D, Almond J W 1988 Antigenic chimaera of polio virus as a potential new vaccine. Nature 382: 81–82
Emini E A, Jameson B A, Wimmer E 1983 Priming for and induction of anti-poliovirus neutralizing antibodies by synthetic peptides. Nature 304: 699–703
Evans D M A, Dunn G, Minor P D et al 1985 Increased neurovirulence associated with a single nucleotide change in a non-coding region of the Sabin type 3 poliovaccine genome. Nature 314: 548–550
Ferguson M, Minor P D, Magrath D I, Yi-Hua Q, Spitz M, Schild G C 1984 Neutralization epitopes on poliovirus type 3 particles: an analysis using monoclonal antibodies. Journal of General Virology 65: 197–201
Gnann J W, Nelson J A, Oldstone M B A 1987 Fine mapping of an immunodominant domain in the transmembrane glycoprotein of human immunodeficiency virus. Journal of Virology 61: 2639–2641

Hogle J M, Chow M, Filman D J 1985 The three-dimensional structure of poliovirus at 2.9A resolution. Science 229: 1358–1365

Icenogle J P, Minor P D, Ferguson M, Hogle J M 1986 Modulation of humoral response to a 12-amino-acid site on the poliovirus virion. Journal of Virology 60: 297–301

La Monica N, Almond J W, Racaniello V R 1987 A mouse model for poliovirus neurovirulence identifies mutations that attenuate the virus for man. Journal of Virology 61: 2917–2920

McCray J, Werner G 1987 Different rhinovirus serotypes neutralized by antipeptide antibodies. Nature 329: 736–738.

Melnick J L 1980 Poliomyelitis vaccines: an appraisal after 25 years. Comprehensive Therapeutics 5: 6–14

Minor P D 1980 Comparative biochemical studies of type 3 poliovirus. Journal of Virology 34: 73–84

Minor P D, Schild G C, Bootman J et al 1983 Location and primary structure of a major antigenic site for poliovirus neutralization. Nature 301: 674–679

Minor P D, Evans D M A, Ferguson M, Schild G C, Westrop G, Almond J W 1985 Principal and subsidiary antigenic sites involved in the neutralization of poliovirus type 3. Journal of General Virology 66: 1159–1165

Minor P D, Ferguson M, Evans D M A, Almond J W, Icenogle J P 1986a Antigenic structure of polioviruses of serotypes 1, 2 and 3. Journal of General Virology 67: 1283–1291

Minor P D, John A, Ferguson M, Icenogle J P 1986b Antigenic and molecular evolution of the vaccine strain of type 3 poliovirus during the period of excretion by a primary vaccinee. Journal of General Virology 67: 693–706

Minor P D, Ferguson M, Phillips A, Magrath D I, Huovilainen A, Hovi T 1987 Conservation in vivo of protease cleavage sites in antigenic sites of poliovirus. Journal of General Virology 68: 1857–1865

Modrow S, Hahn B H, Shaw G M, Gallo R C, Wong-Staal F, Wolf H 1987 Computer assisted analysis of envelope protein sequences of seven human immunodeficiency virus isolates: prediction of antigenic epitopes in conserved and variable regions. Journal of Virology 61: 570–578

Murray M G, Kuhn R J, Wimmer E 1987 Poliovirus type 1/type 3 antigenic hybrid virus: characterization and properties. Abstract of the VII International Congress of Virology, Edmonton, Canada R16.40

Nomoto A, Omata T, Toyloda H, Kuge S et al 1982 Complete nucleotide sequence of the attenuated polio virus, Sakin-1 strain genome. Proceedings of the New York Academy of Sciences 79: 5793–5795

Nomoto A, Kohara M, Kuge S et al 1987 Study on virulence of poliovirus type 1 using in vitro modified viruses. In: Brinton MB, Rueckert RR (eds). Positive strand RNA viruses (UCLA Symposia on Molecular and Cellular Biology, (in press)

Nomoto A, Wimmer E 1986 Genetic studies of the antigenicity and the attenuation phenotype of poliovirus. In: Russell WC, Almond J W (eds). Molecular basis of virus disease (SGM Symposium) 40: 107–134

Nottay B K, Kew O, Hatch M, Heyward J, Obijeski T 1981 Molecular variation of type 1 vaccine related and wild polioviruses during replication in humans. Virology 108: 405

Ogra P L, Fishaut M, Gallagher M R 1980 Viral vaccination via the mucosal routes. Reviews of Infectious Diseases 2: 352–369

Omata T, Kohara M, Kuge S et al 1986 Genetic analysis of the attenuation phenotype of poliovirus type 1. Journal of Virology 58: 348–358

Racaniello V R, Baltimore D 1981 Cloned poliovirus complementary DNA is infectious in mammalian cells. Science 214: 916–919

Rueckert R R 1985 Picornaviruses and their replication. In: Fields B N et al (eds). Virology Raven Press, New York: 705–738

Sabin AB, Boulger LR 1983 History of Sabin attenuated poliovirus oral live vaccine strains. Journal of Biological Standards 1: 115–118

Stanway G, Hughes P J, Mountford R C, Reeve P, Minor P D 1984 Comparison of the complete nucleotide sequences of the genomes of the neurovirulent poliovirus P3/Leon/37 and its attenuated Sabin vaccine derivative P3/Leon12a$_1$b. Proceedings of National Academy of Sciences USA 81: 1539–1543

Westrop G D, Evans D M A, Minor P D, Magrath D, Schild G C, Almond J W 1987 Investigation of the molecularbasis of attenuation of the Sabin type 3 vaccine using novel recombinant polioviruses constructed from infections cDNA. In: Rowlands DJ, Mahy BWJ, Mayo M (eds). The molecular biology of positive strand viruses. Academic Press, London 53–60

Discussion of paper presented by Jeffrey Almond

Discussant: Vincent R. Racaniello

Poliomyelitis has been successfully controlled in many countries through the use of live, attenuated vaccines developed by Albert Sabin. Although poliovirus vaccines of all three serotypes are among the safest known, they are not perfect. Cases of poliomyelitis arise at a very low rate which appears to be due mainly to the type 2 and 3 components of the vaccine. The occurrence of vaccine-associated poliomyelitis has led to efforts to develop a new, more stable vaccine strain. In addition, given the success and safety of the type 1 poliovaccine, experiments have been conducted to determine whether neutralizing antigenic epitopes of polioviruses types 2 and 3 as well as epitopes from other medically important micro-organisms can be expressed in the type 1 poliovirion. The results of these experiments are described in the presentation by J. W. Almond.

One approach to improving the existing poliovirus vaccines is to identify new, more stable attenuating mutations. Previous studies conducted in a number of laboratories have shown that sequences around nucleotides 470–480 of the 5'-non-coding regions of the vaccine strains contain important determinants of attenuation. For example, in the type 3 vaccine, attenuation is conferred by a U at position 472 while a C at this position is associated with a neurovirulent phenotype. Viruses isolated from cases of vaccine-associated poliomyelitis have reverted from U to C at this position, explaining the increased neurovirulence of these strains.

To construct new poliomyelitis vaccines that do not revert to neurovirulence, Almond and his co-workers took advantage of the observation that mutations known to attenuate poliovirus in humans also attenuate the mouse-adapted P2/Lansing strain in mice. A variety of base changes were introduced into the region around nucleotides 470–480, using cloned infectious cDNA, and the neurovirulence of the resulting viruses was determined in mice. Of 10 mutations introduced to this region, four resulted in viable viruses, three of which were markedly attenuated when compared to the wild-type virus. Attenuation was conferred by specific mutations at base 482 (G to A) or 479 (A to C); in addition, a virus containing a U at 472 and an A at 482 was more attenuated than viruses carrying the individual mutations. These studies show that it is possible to identify new attenuating mutations in the 5'-non-coding region, and to produce viruses that are less neurovirulent than the existing vaccine strain. The next important step will be to determine the stability of these new strains.

Another approach to improving the poliovirus vaccines employs the observation that the type 1 component appears to be the most stable. Would it be possible to introduce neutralization sites of the less stable type 2 and 3 components into a type 1 vaccine virus? Previous studies had indicated that a sequence of VP1 amino acids 89–100 is a major neutralization antigenic site in the type 3 strain. Therefore, Almond and his colleagues constructed a chimaeric virus in which an eight amino acid sequence from the P1/Sabin virus, respresenting antigenic site 1, was replaced by the corresponding sequence from the P3/Sabin strain. The resulting chimaeric virus was recognized by antibodies against type 1 and type 3, and in addition elicited neutralizing antibodies against type 1 and type 3 viruses when inoculated into mice, rabbits and monkeys. These results clearly demonstrate the feasibility of constructing poliovirus antigen chimaeras. Since variants resistant to neutralization with monoclonal antibodies can be isolated at relatively high frequency, an important question is whether antibodies generated against such chimaeras would be protective. Clearly it will be important to determine whether monkeys vaccinated with the type 1/3 chimaera can withstand oral challenge with wild type virus.

Since it is possible to construct chimaeras in which poliovirus antigenic sites are exchanged among different serotypes, an interesting question is whether poliovirus sequences can be substituted with antigenic determinants derived from other pathogens. This approach could be valuable for production of vaccines against micro-organisms which are effectively controlled by mucosal antibodies. Such chimaeras would be particularly attractive in cases where it has not been possible to produce vaccines, since many years of experience working with poliovaccine would be combined with the appropriate antigenic specificity. Almond and his colleagues have found that viable viruses can be isolated in which antigenic site 1 of poliovirus P1/Sabin can be replaced with amino acid sequences from foot-and-mouth disease virus, rhinovirus, hepatitis A virus, HIV and *Chlamydia trachomatis*. These are exciting findings, although it remains to be determined whether such foreign sequences are expressed in the poliovirus background, and whether the chimaeras induce protective immunity.

It should be noted that the utility of antigenic chimaeras goes beyond their potential use as new vaccines. It is known that the ability of the mouse-adapted P2/Lansing to infect mice maps to the capsid proteins, and recently it was shown that the mouse-adapted phenotype can be conferred to another strain by substitution of antigenic site 1 from P2/Lansing. The ability to manipulate the poliovirus genome by using cloned infectious cDNA, coupled with knowledge of the three-dimensional structure of the capsid, makes possible not only the design and construction of new and improved vaccines but detailed investigation of structure–function relationships.

Discussion: Poliomyelitis
Jeffrey W. Almond and Vincent R. Racaniello

The recent advance in poliovaccine research opens new possibilities not only to make the use of live poliomyelitis vaccine safer but possibly also to simplify its application. The reason for the dominating replicative capacity and superior immunizing effect of poliovirus type 2 was discussed. At present no explanation for this observation is available. Currently oral polio virus consists of a mixture of all three viral serotypes and in some cases interference of replication occurs. By use of antigenic mosaics it might be possible to use only virals displaying antigenic determinants of all three serotypes. Potentially one could also use live poliovaccine as a vehicle for heterologous viral or other microbial antigens targeted for inducing a local immunity in the gut. One may also consider other enteroviruses as a vehicle for antigens, e.g. ECHO virus type 1 which in clinical trials has been documented to be non-pathogenic.

It was discussed to what extent modification of genomic RNA around nucleotide position of 472 might have general effects of attenuation. Mutations in this area that lead to a reduction of poliovirus neurovirulence have been identified, and an interesting question is whether these might affect completely distinct enteroviruses.

At a recent meeting on poliomyelitis by the U.S. National Academy of Sciences the possibilities for testing new candidate strains for oral poliovaccines was discussed. In view of the low frequency of vaccine-associated cases with the current vaccine (one case of paralysis per 1.2 million distributed doses) there would be a requirement for immunization of a very large cohort. However, in view of the markedly improved possibilities for *in vitro* and *in vivo* (in mice and monkeys) evaluation of poliovirus neuropathogenicity (new genetic markers) it would seem that the requirement for large clinical trials may not have to be met. The availability of methods for generation of a variety of chimeric viruses means the opening of a new chapter in the history of poliovaccine research.

Eventually it was pointed out that even with the next generation of live poliovaccines some problems concerning their use in developing countries may remain. The problems involve the efficacy of dispatching the vaccine by ensuring the availability of a cold chain and the interference by co-infecting other enteric viruses.

12. Prospects for development of a rotavirus vaccine against rotavirus diarrhoea by a Jennerian and a modified Jennerian strategy

Albert Z. Kapikian, Jorge Flores, Kim Y. Green, Yasutaka Hoshino, Mario Gorziglia, Kazuo Nishikawa, Robert M. Chanock and Irene Perez-Schael

INTRODUCTION

It is somewhat paradoxical in a publication which embraces 'Frontiers of Infectious Diseases' as its major theme that a new 'frontier' vaccine aimed at preventing diarrhoeal morbidity and mortality caused by rotaviruses should espouse a strategy pioneered by Edward Jenner almost 200 years ago. In this approach, a related rotavirus strain which causes diarrhoea in an animal host is used as an attenuated vaccine for humans in an attempt to induce protective immunity. Although the Jennerian strategy was well known for almost two centuries it could be applied only recently to rotaviruses because they were discovered less than 20 years ago. Knowledge of rotavirus genetics obtained in the last 10 years has allowed the development of a modified Jennerian approach. In this discussion, I describe: (1) the importance of rotaviruses as aetiological agents of diarrhoeal illnesses; (2) some properties of the virus which are important for development of vaccine strategies; (3) efficacy trials employing the Jennerian approach; and (4) the development of a modified Jennerian approach aimed at achieving broad protection against rotavirus diarrhoea.

THE IMPORTANCE OF ROTAVIRUSES AS AETIOLOGICAL AGENTS OF DIARRHOEAL ILLNESSES IN INFANTS AND YOUNG CHILDREN

Diarrhoeal disease is an important cause of morbidity in developed countries, and of both morbidity and mortality in developing countries (Kapikian & Chanock, 1985a; Kapikian et al, 1986a). For example, in the Cleveland, USA, family study of over 25,000 illnesses over a span of almost 10 years, infectious gastroenteritis (considered at that time to be non-bacterial) was the second most common disease experience after common respiratory disease (Table 12.1)

(Dingle et al, 1964). However, the impact from diarrhoeal diseases in developing countries is overwhelming, with estimates of mortality in a single year ranging from 4.6 to 10 million with the greatest toll in infants and young children (Table 12.2) (Synder & Merson, 1982; Walsh & Warren, 1979).

Table 12.1 Incidence of major classes of illness

Class of illness	Number of illnesses	Illnesses per person-year	% of all illnesses
Total illnesses	25,155	9.4	100
Common respiratory diseases	14,990	5.6	60
Specific respiratory diseases	793	0.3	3
Infectious gastroenteritis	4,057	1.5	16
Other infections	1,931	0.7	8
Other illnesses	3,384	1.3	13

From: Dingle, Badger and Jordan (1964).

Table 12.2 Estimate of morbidity and mortality from acute diarrhoeal illnesses in children < 5 years of age in Africa, Asia (excluding China) and Latin America

Estimate	Number
Population < 5 years of age	338,000,000
Median diarrhoeal episodes/child/year	2.2
Diarrhoeal illnesses/year	744,000,000
Median diarrhoeal mortality rate/1,000 children	13.6
Diarrhoeal deaths/year	4,600,000*
Diarrhoeal deaths/day	12,600
Diarrhoeal deaths/hour	525
Case fatality ratio (deaths/100 episodes)	0.6

* 80% in ≦2 year olds
Adapted from Snyder and Merson (1982).

Despite the importance of diarrhoeal diseases, the aetiology of most episodes remained obscure (Yow et al, 1970) until the early 1970s when discovery of the 27 nm Norwalk virus and its association with epidemic viral gastroenteritis in older children and adults (Kapikian et al, 1972), followed by the discovery of the 70 nm human rotavirus and the elucidation of its important role in severe diarrhoea of infants and young children (Bishop et al, 1973), marked the first major advances in understanding the aetiology of what were presumed for decades to be diarrhoeas of viral aetiology (Fig. 12.1). Although the Norwalk virus is considered to be the cause of some 40% of community-type outbreaks of non-bacterial gastroenteritis (and the Norwalk group with about 10% of all gastroenteritis outbreaks) in older children and adults, it and related agents are not implicated as a cause of severe diarrhoea of infants and young children (Kapikian et al, 1974; Greenberg et al, 1979; Kaplan et al, 1982a; Kaplan et al, 1982b; Kapikian & Chanock, 1985b).

Rotavirus are consistently found to be the single most important aetiological agents of severe diarrhoea in infants and young children in both developed and developing countries (Kapikian & Chanock, 1985a; Kapikian et al, 1986a). Its role in a developed country was shown convincingly in an eight-year cross-sectional study in Washington, DC, of children hospitalized with a diarrhoeal illness (Fig. 12.2) (Brandt et al, 1983). Over this period, approximately 35% of over 1,500 children shed rotavirus in faeces. The peak prevalence of rotavirus infections occurred during the cooler months of each year. In a similar study in Japan, 45% of over 1,900 children hospitalized with diarrhoea shed rotavirus; a comparable temporal pattern was observed (Konno et al, 1983). This striking seasonality is not observed in countries in which major temperature fluctuations do not occur (Kapikian & Chanock, 1985a).

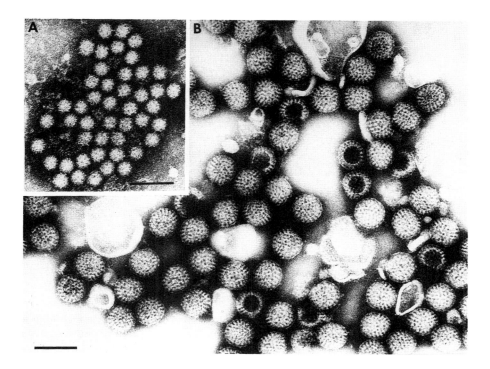

Fig. 12.1 (A) A group of Norwalk virus particles observed after incubation of 0.8 ml. of Norwalk stool filtrate (prepared from a stool of a volunteer administered the Norwalk agent) with 0.2 ml. of 1:5 dilution of a volunteer's prechallenge serum and further preparation for EM. The quantity of antibody on these particles was rated as 1+. The bar = 100 nm. From Kapikian et al (1988) (bar added). (B) Human rotavirus particles observed in a stool filtrate (prepared from a stool of an infant with gastroenteritis) after incubation with PBS and further preparation for EM. The particles have a double-shelled capsid. Occasional 'empty' particles are seen. The bar = 100 nm. From Kapikian et al (1988)

Overall, in the USA, prevalence studies indicate that by three years of age, 90% of the population has been infected with rotavirus (Kapikian & Chanock, 1985a). In addition, it is estimated that in the USA approximately 3 million infants and young children develop rotavirus diarrhoea annually, with 82,000 hospitalizations and 150 deaths (Prospects for Immunization Against Rotaviruses, 1985b).

In developing countries, rotaviruses have emerged consistently as the major aetiological agents of severe diarrhoeal illnesses of infants and young children (Kapikian et al, 1986a). In a hallmark study in Bangladesh, rotaviruses were the

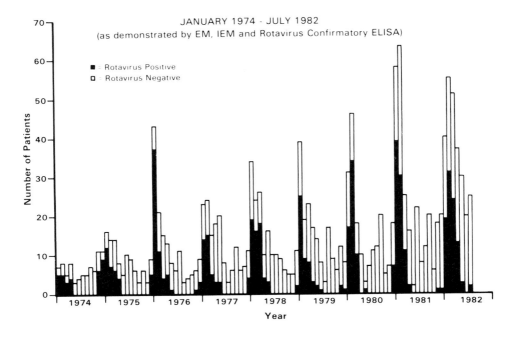

Fig. 12.2 Rotavirus infections in in-patients with gastroenteritis. From: Brandt et al (1983)

most frequent cause of diarrhoea which resulted in visits to a treatment centre for in-patients under two years of age with 46% of this age group experiencing rotavirus diarrhoea (Black et al, 1980). The next most frequently detected pathogens associated with diarrhoea were the enterotoxigenic *Escherichia coli*, occurring in 28% of this age group. In a more recent study in Egypt of children admitted to a hospital with fatal or potentially fatal diarrhoea, rotaviruses were the single most frequently detected pathogen with the enterotoxigenic *E. coli* ranking second (Table 12.3) (Shukry et al, 1986).

Overall, in developing countries prevalence studies reveal that by three years of age about 90% of children acquire serum antibodies to rotavirus, a figure similar to that observed in developed countries (Kapikian & Chanock, 1985a). In addition, it is estimated that in a single year the burden from rotavirus infection in the developing countries is comprised of over 125 million cases of diarrhoea (including some 18 million moderately-severe to severe episodes) and over 870,000 deaths (Prospects for Immunizing Against Rotavirus, 1985a).

Thus, with rotavirus established as the major pathogen responsible for severe diarrhoea in infants and young children worldwide, it is clear that an effective vaccine is needed to prevent this severe toll during the first two years of life. Since animal studies revealed that resistance to rotavirus disease was mediated primarily by local intestinal immunity (Snodgrass et al, 1976), major emphasis has been placed on the development of a live, attenuated oral vaccine rather than one administered parenterally. The efficacy of oral rehydration salt solutions in alleviating the morbidity of diarrhoeal disease does not reduce the need for a rotavirus vaccine since the widespread implementation of this treatment remains a major problem.

Table 12.3 Enteropathogens isolated from infants with severe diarrhoea according to the presence or absence of complications in Cairo from 1982 to 1983

Agent sought	Patients with complicated diarrhoea		Patients with uncomplicated diarrhoea		All patients	
	No. tested	No. (%) positive	No. tested	No. (%) positive	No. tested	No. (%) positive
Rotavirus	137	47 (34)	131	41 (31)	268	88 (33)
Shigella	142	8 (1)	133	1 (1)	275	2 (1)
Salmonella	142	11 (8)	133	4 (3)	275	15 (5)
Campylobacter	145	1 (1)	135	4 (3)	280	5 (2)
EPEC*	137	13[b] (9)	129	8 (6)	266	21 (8)
LT ETEC	137	12[b] (9)	129	18 (14)	266	30 (11)
ST ETEC	49	9 (18)	77	16 (21)	126	25 (20)
E. histolytica	118	0	118	0	236	0
None[c]	40	9 (23)	66	17 (26)	106	26 (25)

* Determined by serotype.
[b] One patient had both EPEC and LT ETEC in the stool.
[c] Results given for specimens examined for all agents.
From: Shukry et al. (1986).

PROPERTIES OF ROTAVIRUSES RELEVANT TO VACCINE DEVELOPMENT

Rotaviruses are classified as a new genus in the family Reoviridae. These viruses cause diarrhoea not only in humans but also in almost all animal species studied. They are 70 nm in diameter, non-enveloped and possess a distinctive double capsid (Fig. 12.1B). Located within the inner capsid is the core which contains the genome consisting of 11 segments of double-stranded ribonucleic acid (RNA) (Kapikian & Chanock, 1985a). The name rotavirus (rota=wheel) was suggested because the smooth outermost margin gives the appearance of the rim of a wheel placed on short strokes radiating from a wide hub when the virus is observed by electron microscopy (Flewett et al, 1974).

Rotavirus have three important antigenic specificities group, subgroup and serotype, which are mediated by three viral proteins: group and subgroup antigens are located on VP6, the major inner capsid protein (encoded by RNA segment 6); and serotype antigens are located on both VP7, the major neutralization protein located on the outer capsid (encoded by RNA segment 8 or 9) and VP3 also on the outer capsid (encoded by RNA segment 4) (Fig. 12.3) (Kapikian & Chanock, 1985a). Most human and animal rotaviruses share a common group antigen and are thus classified as group A rotaviruses (Bachmann et al, 1984). Four epidemiologically important human rotavirus serotypes are recognized by neutralization (Wyatt et al, 1984; Hoshino et al, 1984); however, two new serotypes were recently described but their importance is yet to be determined (Matsuno et al, 1985; Albert et al, 1987; Clark et al, 1987). Only recently have the human group A rotaviruses been grown efficiently in tissue culture directly from faecal specimens (Sato et al, 1981; Urasawa et al, 1981).

The non-group A rotaviruses (also known as pararotaviruses) do not share the common group antigen and have been recovered from humans and various animal species (Bridger, 1987); one member of this group has been implicated in large gastroenteritis outbreaks in China (Hung et al, 1984).

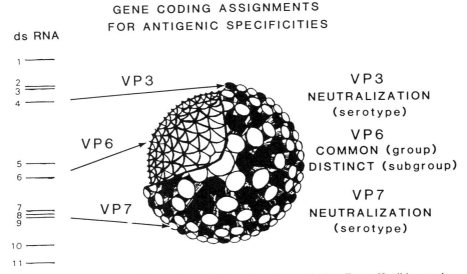

Fig. 12.3 Rotavirus—gene coding assignments for antigenic specificities. From: Kapikian et al (1986a)

EFFICACY TRIALS OF ROTAVIRUS VACCINES BY THE JENNERIAN APPROACH

Techniques used for the development of rotavirus vaccines range from conventional cell culture cultivation of human or animal strains to the use of molecular biology. The most promising and most extensively evaluated vaccination strategy for rotaviruses is based on the concept pioneered by Edward Jenner in 1798 for human smallpox vaccination in which a related live attenuated agent from a non-human host is used as the immunizing agent. Early rotavirus studies were instrumental in exploring this approach since it was found that human and animal rotaviruses share a common group antigen which makes them indistinguishable in various serological assays (such as CF) (Flewett et al, 1974; Kapikian et al, 1975, 1976; Woode et al, 1976).In addition, children undergoing human rotavirus infection developed a serological response (by CF) to both human and various animal rotavirus strains (Kapikian et al, 1976). Later studies established the rationale for this approach when calves inoculated *in utero* with a bovine rotavirus were protected against challenge with a human rotavirus at birth (Wyatt et al, 1979). In contrast, most control animals developed diarrhoea following the human rotavirus challenge.

Efficacy trials of bovine rotavirus vaccine (RIT 4237), developed by Smith Kline—RIT, in children one year of age or less, in a developed country demonstrated a protection rate of over 80% against clinically significant rotavirus diarrhoea (Vesikari et al, 1984, 1985). However, recent efficacy trials with this vaccine in several developing countries were disappointing and thus further field trials were not planned (De Mol et al, 1986; Hanlon et al, 1987). Another bovine rotavirus strain (WC 3) developed at the Wistar Institute has undergone phase I and early phase II studies with encouraging results (Clark et al, 1986).

We have evaluated a different animal rotavirus—the rhesus rotavirus strain MMU 18006—as a vaccine candidate (Kapikian et al, 1985, 1986b, 1988). This strain was isolated from the stool of a rhesus monkey with diarrhoea (Stuker et al, 1980) and is similar to human rotavirus type 3 by neutralization (Wyatt et al, 1984; Hoshino et al, 1984). It has been passaged nine times in primary or secondary monkey kidney cell culture and seven times in DBS FRhL 2 cells, a semi-continuous diploid cell strain from rhesus monkey lung (Fig. 12.4) (Kapikian et al, 1985). The latter cells were developed by the Office of Biologics, FDA,

Passage No in indicated type of cell culture	Cell Culture
(1)	CMK (original isolation)
(2)	CMK (passage sent to NIH)
(1)	AGMK
(2)	AGMK (1st plaque purification)
(3)	AGMK (2nd plaque purification)
(4)	AGMK (3rd plaque purification)
(5)	AGMK (amplification in roller tube cultures)
(6)	AGMK (amplification in flask culture)
(7)	AGMK (Flow laboratories)
(1)	DBS-FRhL-2 (rhesus monkey diploid cell strain)
(2)	DBS-FRhL-2
(3)	DBS-FRhL-2
(4)	DBS-FRhL-2 (harvest ether treated)
(5)	DBS-FRhL-2
(6)	DBS-FRhL-2 (prevaccine seed [passage 22 of FRhL-2 cells])
(7)	DBS-FRhL-2 (vaccine lot designated RRV-1 [passage 24 of FRhL-2 cells] RRV-1 titer 10^7 PFU/ml after clarification)

Summary: Passage history of RRV-1 vaccine candidate CMK2 AGMK7 DBS-FRhL-2 7.

Fig. 12.4 Passage history rhesus rotavirus (RRV) candidate vaccine Lot RRRV-1 (Strain MMU 18006).
From: Kapikian et al (1989)

as a potential cell substrate for vaccine production (Wallace et al, 1973). Following extensive phase I studies, beginning in adults and progressing in stepwise fashion to neonates, in which variable reactogenicity was observed with different dosages at various locations, a 10^4 PFU oral dose was found to be antigenic and acceptably reactogenic; overall this dose induced a transient febrile response in about one third of the vaccinees (Kapikian et al, 1985, 1986b, 1988; Perez-Schael et al, 1987; Vesikari et al, 1986; Losonsky et al, 1986; Anderson et al, 1986; Wright et al, 1987; Christy et al, 1986; Rennels et al, 1987a; Flores et al, 1988a). In a recent controlled phase I trial in 40 neonates in Venezuela this dose of rhesus rotavirus vaccine was non-reactogenic (Flores et al, 1988a). Whether this is a result of high levels of passively acquired maternal antibodies or to intrinsic neonatal host factors is not known.

Table 12.4 Protective efficacy of rhesus rotavirus (RRV) vaccine against RV diarrhoea in infants 1–10 months of age* at time of vaccination in Venezuela

Inoculum	No. in each group	No. with RV diarrhoea**
RRV vaccine	151	8
Placebo	151	22

Protection rate = 64%; P < 0.01
* Mean age 4.9 mo.
** ≥ 3 loose or watery stools in 24 hours.
Adapted from: Perez-Schael et al. (1989b).

Over 1,000 infants have been studied in 11 placebo-controlled field trials of the rhesus rotavirus vaccine (Kapikian et al, 1988). The five completed trials have yielded inconsistent findings. The most encouraging results were observed in the Caracas, Venezuela trial in which 302 children 1–10 months of age were administered either rhesus rotavirus vaccine or a placebo. In this study vaccine efficacy was 64% (Table 12.4) (Kapikian et al, 1988; Flores et al, 1987; Perez-Schael et al, 1989a). Moreover, among vaccinees 1–4 months of age, the vaccine efficacy was 82% (Table 12.5). In addition, when diarrhoeal episodes were classified according to severity, vaccine efficacy reached 90% for severe diarrhoeal illnesses (a rating of ≥8) in the entire study group (Kapikian et al, 1988; Flores et al, 1987; Perez-Schael et al, 1989a). The vaccine also appeared promising in trials in Maryland, Sweden and Finland in infants predominantly over six months of age (Kapikian et al, 1988; Rennels et al, 1987b; Gothefors et al 1989). However, in two studies of infants aged two to five months in Rochester and Arizona vaccine efficacy was nil; in the latter study the RIT bovine rotavirus vaccine was also evaluated and it, too, failed to protect against rotavirus diarrhoea (Kapikian et al, 1988).

The reason for such inconsistent rhesus rotavirus vaccine efficacy appears to be related to the serotype of the circulating infecting strains. In the Venezuelan study, in which protection was observed, the predominant infecting strains belonged to serotype 3 (13 of 23 typeable strains), the same serotype as the vaccine (Kapikian et al, 1988; Flores et al, 1987; Perez-Schael et al, 1989a). However, in the Rochester study, the prevalent infecting strains (29 of 30) belonged to serotype 1, whereas in the Arizona study only 1 of 15 typeable strains belonged to serotype 3 (Kapikian et al, 1988; Christy et al 1989). Thus, serotype specific immunity appears to be necessary to protect against rotavirus diarrhoea in children who have not experienced a previous rotavirus infection. Such individuals do not appear to develop a broadened antibody response following immunization.

Table 12.5 Protective efficacy of rhesus rotavirus (RRV) vaccine against RV diarrhoea in infants 1–4 months of age at time of vaccination in Venezuela

Inoculum	No. in each group	No. with RV diarrhoea*
RRV vaccine	76	3
Placebo	75	17

Protection rate = 82%; P < 0.001
* ≥ 3 loose or watery stools in 24 hours.
Adapted from: Perez-Schael et al. (1989b).

PURSUIT OF A MODIFIED JENNERIAN APPROACH TO ROTAVIRUS VACCINATION

Since the rhesus rotavirus vaccine failed to induce protection against rotavirus diarrhoea caused by heterotypic rotavirus strains in vaccinees under six months of age, we have modified our course by developing a multivalent rotavirus vaccine containing components representing each of the four epidemiologically important serotypes. This was accomplished by taking advantage of the ability of rotaviruses to undergo genetic reassortment during co-infection. By co-infecting cell cultures with both rhesus rotavirus and a human rotavirus belonging to a different serotype (i.e. 1, 2 or 4) in the presence of neutralizing antibody to the former, single gene substitution human-rhesus rotavirus reassortants have been isolated (Midthun et al, 1985, 1986). These reassortments derive 10 genes from the rhesus rotavirus parent (which attenuates the virus for humans) and a single gene from the human rotavirus parent, namely the gene which encodes VP7, the major outer capsid protein (Fig. 12.5). Thus, the single gene substitution reassortants have the neutralization specificity of human serotype 1, 2 or 4. The ideal vaccine should contain reassortants with serotype 1, 2 or 4 specificity (the modified Jennerian approach) and the rhesus rotavirus as the representative of serotype 3 (the Jennerian approach).

Clinical studies of each of the reassortants in adults and in progressively younger infants has revealed reactogenicity and antigenicity comparable with those of the rhesus rotavirus parent. For example, in a recently completed phase I study in Venezuela, a serotype 1 (D x RRV) or serotype 2 (DS1 x RRV) reassortant, or rhesus rotavirus vaccine were studied individually along with a bivalent serotype 1 reassortant-rhesus rotavirus vaccine for reactogenicity and antigenicity in infants aged from one to five months (Flores et al, 1988b). Table 12.6 shows that these vaccines tended to induce a low grade fever (38.1–38.5°C) in less than 20% of the infants overall, and loose stools in about 10%. Antigenicity studies were encouraging as over 80% of each group developed a sero-response (Table 12.7). The antigenicity of the VP3 component of rhesus rotavirus vaccine

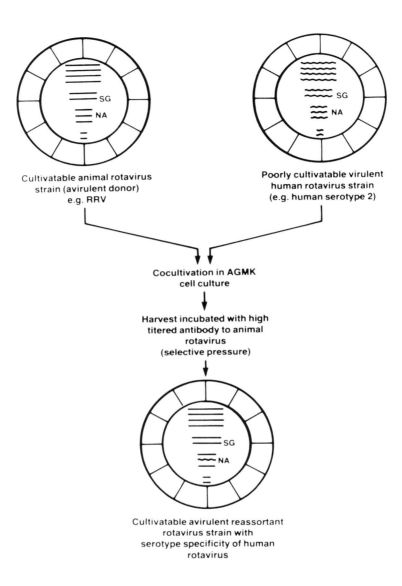

Fig. 12.5 Production of reassortant rotavirus vaccine. Adapted from: Kapikian et al (1986b)

was evident since the number of antibody responses to rhesus rotavirus exceeded those to the human P strain which has a related VP7 and an unrelated VP3 protein. Other studies have shown that the VP3 protein can induce protection independent of the VP7 protein (Offit et al, 1986; Hoshino et al, 1988). This may be of importance in future vaccine formulations if the current emphasis on VP7 does not lead to satisfactory protection.

Since the individual reassortant vaccines as well as bivalent formulations were acceptably reactogenic and antigenic, a quadrivalent vaccine consisting of a mixture of equal titres of rhesus rotavirus vaccine (serotype 3) and each of three

Table 12.6 Reactions to RRV vaccine or human-RRV vaccine reassortants in Venezuelan infants during the week following vaccination

Clinical manifestations	Inoculum administered				
	Placebo N = 23†	D × RRV N = 24†	DS1 × RRV N = 25	RRV N = 21	D × RRV + RRV N = 23‡
Fever 38.1–38.5°C	0	4 (1 × 38.3)* (3 × 38.5)	2 (38.4)	4 (2 × 38.3) (2 × 38.5)	4 (3 × 38.2) (1 × 38.4)
>38.5°C	1 (39.3)	2 (1 × 39.0)** (1 × 40.5)	0	1 (38.7)	0
Diarrhoea***	0	2	3	3	2
Coughing****	1	7	7	6	2

† 1 child not followed.
‡ 2 children not followed.
* Figures in parenthesis represent highest temperature observed.
** Both infants had upper respiratory infections, one of them with pharyngitis. Illness in one of them started on the day of vaccination, the other one on day 6 after vaccination.
*** Defined as 3 or more liquid or semi-liquid stools passed within a 24 hour period. Diarrhoea in 4 of the 10 infants started the day of vaccination. Six of the 10 episodes lasted only 1 day.
**** 12 cases of coughing started on day 1, 4 started on day 2.
From: Flores et al. (1988b).

Table 12.7 Seroresponses to rotavirus after administration of RRV vaccine or human-RRV reassortant vaccines in Venezuelan infants

Inoculum	By plaque reduction neutralization against indicated antigen				By IGA ELISA	By Any test
	WA	DS1	P	RRV		
Placebo	nt*	nt*	1/19 (5)**	nt*	2/21 (10)	2/22 (9)
D × RRV	9/23 (39)	4/16 (25)	5/20 (25)	11/23 (48)	13/23 (57)	20/23 (87)
DS1 × RRV	nt*	12/23 (52)	nt*	15/23 (65)	21/24 (88)	24/24 (100)
RRV	4/12 (33)	1/12 (8)	6/19 (32)	12/20 (60)	11/19 (58)	18/21 (86)
D × RRV + RRV	12/21 (57)	7/20 (35)	9/19 (47)	12/19 (63)	16/22 (73)	20/22 (91)

* Not tested.
** Number of infants exhibiting a four-fold antibody response/number of infants tested. Percentage of seroresponders in each group shown in parenthesis.
From: Flores et al. (1988b).

human rotavirus-rhesus rotavirus reassortants representing serotypes 1, 2 and 4 was recently evaluated in phase I studies in Venezuela employing two different dose schedules: 0.25 x 10⁴ PFU of each component and in a later study 0.5 x 10⁴ of each component (Perez-Schael et al, 1989b). Significant vaccine reactions were not observed except for a mild transient fever lasting 1–2 days in 10–28% of the infants (Table 12.8). Serological results are being evaluated but it appears that the antibody response to the higher dose was greater than that to the lower dose but that neither was sufficient to warrant a field trial. Therefore, a 'full' dose of each component (1 x 10⁴ PFU/ml) as used in the individual reassortant or rhesus rotavirus studies must be evaluated.

Various phase II studies with individual reassortant vaccines are in progress and several with the quadrivalent vaccine are awaiting an acceptable formulation of its components. The outcome of these trials should determine the future course of this combined Jennerian, modified Jennerian approach. However, epidemiological as well as molecular biological evidence support the view that this strategy may prove successful. The epidemiological evidence comes mainly from two sources: (1) the Venezuelan field trial which demonstrated that homotypic immunity was achieved with the rhesus rotavirus vaccine, whereas vaccine failure in two other locations was attributable to prevalence of infecting heterotypic strains; and (2) the elegant longitudinal study of Chiba et al (1986) demonstrating that, even under natural conditions, homotypic immunity could be achieved only when serum antibody levels of 1:128 or greater were present and that heterotypic infection rarely induced this level of antibody.

Table 12.8 Clinical reactions to a low or high dose of quadrivalent* rotavirus vaccine representing the four human rotavirus serotypes in 10–20 week-old Venezuelan infants during the week post-vaccination

	Low dose study		High dose study	
	Control	Vaccinees $(0.25 \times 10^4$ PFU)†	Control	Vaccinees $(0.5 \times 10^4$ PFU)†
No. of infants studied	23	27	20	20
No. of infants with fever $\geqslant 38.1°C$	0	8**	3	4
Day of fever onset and (duration) if over 1 day	—	2, 2, 2(2) 3, 3, 3(2) 3(2), 4	1, 2(2), 5	1, 1, 3, 5(2)
No. of infants with liquid stools	4	3	1***	2
No. of infants with coughing	12	10	5	5
No. of infants with rhinorrhoea	4	1	2	1

* Quadrivalent vaccine contained D × RRV (serotype 1), DS1 × RRV (serotype 2), RRV (serotype 3), and ST3 × RRV (serotype 4).
** The highest temperatures observed were 39.7°C in one infant and 39.1°C in another.
*** Infant had campylobacter diarrhoea with fever maximum of 40°C.
† Amount of virus in each component.
Adapted from: Perez-Schael et al. (1989a).

The molecular biological observations pertinent to our vaccine studies indicate that there was marked conservation of amino acid sequence in the two major neutralization domains of the VP7 of the rhesus rotavirus and human rotavirus serotype 3 strains isolated in the Venezuela study (Fig. 12.6) (Kapikian et al, 1988). In contrast, heterotypic strains isolated in the Rochester study failed to show such conservation of amino acid sequences. As expected, reassortant rotavirus vaccines for serotypes 1, 2 and 4 demonstrate a high degree of conservation of these domains with the corresponding strains of serotypes 1, 2 or 4 (latter strain not shown). Such data is consistent with recent studies demonstrating marked amino acid conservation (greater than 85%) in the VP7 of different strains of the same serotype (Green et al, 1987).

CONCLUSION

Although the Jennerian approach to vaccination has been modified by more recently developed genetic techniques in an attempt to achieve protection against rotavirus diarrhoea caused by all four epidemiologically important serotypes, it is hoped that the broad concept pioneered by Edward Jenner some 200 years ago, along with its modern genetic modification, may prove successful. Studies aimed to answer this question are in progress and perhaps within the next year or two we will be able to determine the feasibility of this time-proven strategy to prevent a major cause of morbidity in infants and young children in developed countries, and morbidity and mortality in developing countries.

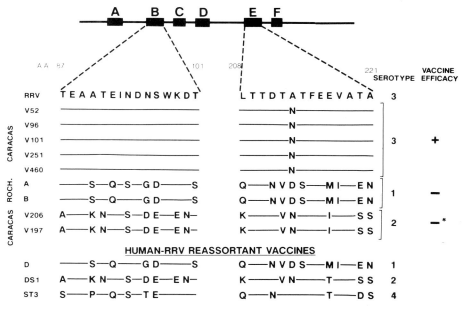

Fig. 12.6 Neutralization domains in RV VP7. From: Kapikian et al

Acknowledgements

We thank H.D. James Jr, A.L. Pittman, M. Finbloom, J. Sears, J. Valdesuso, M. Sereno, R. Jones, J. Jackson, C. Banks, E. Williams and S. Chang for assistance.

REFERENCES

Albert M J, Unicomb L E, Bishop J F 1987 Cultivation and characterization of human rotoviruses with 'supershort' RNA patterns. Journal of Clinical Microbiology 25: 1635–1640
Anderson E L, Belshe R B, Bartram J, Crookshanks-Newman F, Chanock R M Kapikian A Z 1986 Evaluation of rhesus rotavirus vaccine (MMU 18006) in infants and young children. Journal of Infectious Diseases 153: 823–831
Bachmann N P, Bishop R F, Flewett T H, Kapikian A Z, Mathan M M, Zissis G 1984 Nomenclature of human rotaviruses: designation of subgroups and serotypes. Bulletin of the World Health Organization 62: 501–503

Bishop R F, Davidson G P, Holmes I H, Ruck B J 1973 Virus particles in epithelial cells of duodenal mucosa from children with viral gastroenteritis. Lancet 2: 1281–1283

Black R E, Merson M H, Mizanur Rahman A S M et al 1980 A two-year study of bacterial, viral and parasitic agents associated with diarrhea in rural Bangladesh. Journal of Infectious Diseases 142: 660–664

Brandt C D, Kim H W, Rodriguez W J et al 1983 Pediatric viral gastroenteritis during eight years of study. Journal of Clinical Microbiology 18: 71–78

Bridger J C, (1987) Novel rotaviruses in animals and man. In: Ciba Foundation Symposium 128 'Novel Diarrhoea Viruses'. J. Wiley and Sons, New York 5–15

Chiba S, Yokoyama T, Nakata S et al 1986 Protective effect of naturally acquired homotypic and hetertypic rotavirus antibodies. Lancet 2: 417–421

Christy C, Madore H P, Treanor J J et al 1986 Safety and immunogenicity of live attenuated monkey rotavirus vaccine. Journal of Infectious Diseases 154: 1045–1047

Clark A F, Offit P A, Dolan K T et al 1986 Responses of adult human volunteers to oral administration of bovine and bovine/human reassortant rotaviruses. Vaccines 4: 25–31

Clark H F, Hoshino Y, Bell L et al 1987 Rotavirus isolate WI 61 representing a presumptive new human serotype. Journal of Clinical Microbiology 25: 1757–1762

De Mol P, Zissis G, Butzler J P 1986 Failure of live attenuated oral rotavirus vaccine. Lancet 2: 108

Dingle J H, Badger G F, Jordan W S 1964 Illness in the home: A study of 25,000 illnesses in a group of Cleveland families. Cleveland, Ohio: Western Reserve University Press 19–32

Flewett T H, Bryden A S, Davies H, Woode G N, Bridger J C, Derrick J M 1974 Relationship between virus from acute gastroenteritis of children and newborn calves. Lancet 2: 61–63

Flores J, Perez-Schael I, Gonzalez M et al 1987 Protection against severe rotavirus diarrhea by rhesus rotavirus vaccine in Venezuelan infants. Lancet 1: 882–884

Flores J, Daoud G, Daoud N et al 1988a Reactogenicity and antigenicity of rhesus rotavirus vaccine (MMU 18006) in newborn infants in Venezuela. Pediatric Infectious Disease Journal, in press

Flores J, Perez-Schael I, Blanco M et al 1988b Reactogenicity and antigenicity of two human-rhesus rotavirus reassortant vaccine candidates serotypes 1 and 2 in Venezuelan infants, submitted

Gothefors L, Wadell G, Judo P et al 1988 Prolonged efficacy of rhesus rotavirus vaccine in Swedish children, submitted

Green K, Midthun K, Gorziglia M et al 1987 Comparison of the amino acid sequences of the major neutralizing protein of four human rotavirus serotypes. Virology 160: 153–159

Greenberg H B, Valdesuso J, Wolken R H et al 1979 Role of Norwalk virus in outbreaks of non-bacterial gastroenteritis. Journal of Infectious Diseases 139: 564–568

Hanlon P, Hanlon L, Marsch V et al 1987 Trial of an attenuated bovine rotavirus vaccine (RIT 4237) in Gambian infants. Lancet 1: 1342–1345

Hoshino Y, Wyatt R G, Greenberg H B, Flores J, Kapikian A Z 1984 Serotypic similarity and diversity of rotaviruses of mammalian and avian origins as studied by plaque reduction neutralization. Journal of Infectious Diseases 694–702

Hoshino Y, Saif L J, Sereno M, Chanock R M, Kapikian A Z 1988 Infection immunity of piglets to either VP3 or VP7 outer capsid protein confers resistance to challenge with a virulent rotavirus bearing the corresponding antigen. Journal of Virology 62: 744–748

Hung T, Chen G, Wang C et al 1984 Waterbourne outbreak of rotavirus diarrhea in adults in China caused by a novel rotavirus. Lancet 1: 1139–1142

Kapikian A Z, Chanock R M 1985a Rotavirus. In: Fields B N et al (eds.) Raven Press, New York 863–906

Kapikian A Z, Chanock R M 1985b Norwalk group of viruses. In: Fields B N et al (eds.) Raven Press, New York 1495–1517

Kapikian A Z, Kim H W, Wyatt R G et al 1974 Reovirus-like agent in stools: association with infantile diarrhea and development of serologic tests. Science 185: 1049–1053

Kapikian A Z, Cline W L, Mebus C A et al 1975 New complement-fixation test for the human reovirus-like agent of infantile gastroenteritis. Nebraska calf diarrhea virus used as antigen. Lancet 1: 1056–1061

Kapikian A Z, Wyatt R G, Dolin R, Thornhill T S, Kalica A R, Chanock R M 1972 Visualization by immune electron microscopy of a 27nm particle associated with acute infectious non-bacterial gastroenteritis. Journal of Virology 1075–1081

230

Kapikian A Z, Cline W L, Kim H W et al 1976 Antigenic relationships among five reovirus-like (RVL) agents by complement fixation (CF) and development of a new substitute CF antigen for the human RVL agent of infantile gastroenteritis. Proceedings of the Society for Experimental Biology and Medicine 152: 535–539

Kapikian A Z, Flores J, Hoshino Y et al 1988b Rationale for the development of a rotavirus vaccine for infants and young children. In: Talwar G (ed) Progress in Vaccinology. Springler-Verlag Publishers, in press

Kapikian A Z, Midthun K, Hoshino Y et al 1985 Rhesus rotavirus: a candidate vaccine for prevention of human reovirus disease. In: Lerner R A, Chanock R M, Brown F (eds.) Vaccines 85. Molecular and chemical basis for resistance to parasatic, bacterial, and viral diseases. New York: Cold Spring Harbor Laboratory, 357–367

Kapikian A Z, Flores J, Hoshino Y et al 1986a Rotavirus: the major etiologic agent of severe infantile diarrhea may be controllable by a 'Jennerian' approach to vaccination. Journal of Infectious Diseases 153: 815–822

Kapikian A Z, Hoshino Y, Flores J et al 1986b Alternative approaches to the development of a rotavirus vaccine. In Holmgren J, Lindbury A, Molldy R (eds) Recent advances in vaccine and drugs against diarrhea 11th Nobel Conference, 1988 Student Literature, Lund, Sweden: pp192–214

Kapikian A Z, Flores J, Midthun K, et al 1988 Development of a rotavirus vaccine by a 'Jennerian' and a modified 'Jennerian' approach. In: Vaccines 88, Ginsberg H, Brown F, Lerner R A, Chanock R M (eds.) Vaccines 88. Cold Spring Harbor Laboratory, 151–159

Kaplan J E, Gary G W, Baron R C et al 1982a Epidemiology of Norwalk gastroenteritis and the role of Norwalk virus in outbreaks of acute nonbacterial gastroenteritis. Annals of Internal Medicine 96: 756–761

Kaplan J E, Feldman R, Campbell D S, Lookabaugh C, Gary G W 1982b The frequency of a Norwalk-like pattern illness in outbreaks of acute gastroenteritis. American Journal of Public Health 12: 1329–1332

Konno T, Suzuki H, Kutsushima N et al 1983 Influence of temperature and relative humidity on human rotavirus infection in Japan. Journal of Infectious Diseases 147: 125–128

Losonsky G A, Rennels M B, Kapikian A Z et al 1986 Safety, infectivity, transmissibility, and immunogenicity of rhesus rotavirus vaccine (MMU 18006) in infants. Pediatric Infectious Diseases 5: 25–29

Matsuno S, Hasegawa A, Mukoyama A, Inoye A 1985 A new candidate for a new serotype of human rotavirus. Journal of Virology 54: 623–624

Midthun K, Greenberg H B, Hoshino Y, Kapikian A Z, Wyatt R G, Chanock R M 1985 Reassortant rotaviruses as potential live rotavirus vaccine candidates. Journal of Virology 53: 949–954

Midthun K, Hoshino Y, Kapikian A Z, Chanock R M 1986 Single gene substitution rotavirus reassortants containing the major neutralization protein (VP7) of human rotavirus serotype. Journal of Clinical Microbiology 24: 822–826

Offitt P A, Clark F H, Blavat G, Greenberg H B 1986 Reassortant rotaviruses containing structural proteins VP3 and VP7 from different parents induce antibodies protective against parental serotype. Journal of Virology 60: 491–496

Perez-Schael I, Gonzalez M, Daoud N et al 1987 Reactogenicity and antigenicity of the rhesus rotavirus vaccine MMU 18006 in Venezuelan children. Journal of Infectious Diseases 155: 334–337

Perez-Schael I, Blanco M, Vilar M et al 1989a Clinical studies of a quadrivalent rotavirus vaccine in Venezuelan infants, in preparation

Perez-Schael I, Daoud N, Perez M et al 1989b A longitudinal study of acute diarrhea in Venezuelan infants and young children receiving rhesus rotavirus vaccine MMY 18006, in preparation

Prospects for immunizing against rotavirus 1985a In: New Vaccine Development. Establishing Properties. Vol. II. Diseases of Importance in developing countries. National Academy Press, Washington, DC, 308–318

Prospects for immunizing against rotavirus 1985b In: New Vaccine Development. Establishing Properties. Diseases of Importance in the United States. National Academy Press. Vol. 1. Washington, DC 410–423

Rennels M B, Losonsky G A, Shindledecken F N P et al 1987a Immunogenicity and reactogenicity of lowered doses of rhesus rotavirus vaccine strain MMU 18006 in young children. Pediatric Infectious Diseases Journal 6: 260–264

Rennels M B, Losonsky G A, Levine M M et al 1987b Preliminary evaluation of the efficacy of rhesus rotavirus vaccine strain MMU 18006 in young children. Pediatric Infectious Diseases 5: 587–588

Sato K, Inaba Y, Shinozaki T, Fujii R, Matumoto M 1981 Isolation of human rotavirus in cell culture. Archives of Virology 69: 155–160

Shukry S, Zaki A M, Shoukry I, Tagi M E, Hamed Z 1986 Detection of enteropathogens in fatal and potentially fatal diarrheas in Cairo, Egypt. Journal of Clinical Microbiology 24: 959–962

Snodgrass D R, Smith W, Gray E W, Herring J A 1976 A rotavirus in lambs with diarrhea. Research Veterinary Science 20: 113–114

Snyder J D, Merson M H 1982 The magnitude of the global problem of acute diarrhoeal disease: a review of active surveillance data. Bulletin of the World Health Organizaton 60: 605–613

Stuker G, Oshiro L, Schmidt N L 1980 Antigenic comparisons of two new rotaviruses from rhesus monkeys. Journal of Clinical Microbiology 11: 202–203

Urasawa T, Urasawa S, Taniguchi K 1981 Sequential passages of human rotavirus in MA-104 cells. Microbiology and Immunology 25: 1025–1035

Vesikari T, Isolauri E, D'Hondt E, Delem A, Andre F E, Zissis G 1984 Protection of infants against rotavirus diarrhea by RIT 4237 attenuated bovine rotavirus strain vaccine. Lancet 1: 977–981

Vesikari T, Isolauri E, Delem A et al 1985 Clinical efficacy of the RIT 4237 live attenuated bovine rotavirus vaccine in infants vaccinated before a rotavirus epidemic. Journal of Pediatrics 107: 189–194

Vesikari T, Kapikian A Z, Delem A, Zissis G 1986 A comparative trial of rhesus monkey (RRV-1) and bovine (RIT 4237) oral rotavirus vaccines in young children. Journal of Infectious Diseases 153: 832–839

Wallace R E, Vasington P J, Petricciani J C, Hopps H E, Lorenz D E, Kadanka Z 1973 Development of a diploid cell line from fetal rhesus monkey lung for virus vaccine production. In vitro 8: 323–332

Walsh J A, Warren K S 1979 Selective primary health care: an interim strategy for disease control in developing countries. New England Journal of Medicine 301: 967–974

Woode G N, Bridger J C, Jones J M et al 1976 Morphological and antigenic relationships between viruses (rotaviruses) from acute gastroenteritis of children, calves, piglets, mice and foals. Infection and Immunity 14: 804–810

Wright P F, Tajima T, Thompson J, Kokubun K, Kapikian A Z, Karzon D T 1987 Candidate rotavirus vaccine (rhesus rotavirus strain) in children: an evaluation. Pediatrics 80: 473–480

Wyatt R G, Mebus C A, Yolken R H et al 1979 Rotaviral immunity in gnotobiotic calves: heterologous resistance to human virus induced by bovine virus. Science 203: 548–550

Wyatt R G, Greenberg H B, James W D et al 1984 Definition of human rotavirus serotypes by plaque reduction assay. Infection and Immunology 37: 110–115

Yow M D, Melnick J L, Blattner R J, Stephenson W B, Robinson N M, Burkhardt M A 1970 The association of viruses and bacteria with infantile diarrhea. American Journal of Epidemiology 92: 33–39

Discussion of paper presented by Al Kapikian

Discussant: Göran Wadell

This discussion centres around the question of whether the same approach to rotavirus vaccination can be adopted in North America and Europe as in South America, Africa, and Asia.

The oral rhesus rotavirus vaccine was evaluated in Umea, Sweden, in two studies, A and B, which started in 1985 and 1986, respectively, involving 104 and 23 children. Somewhat surprisingly it was noted that 42 children in group A had significant diarrhoea as a reaction to the rhesus rotavirus vaccine. In addition, a number had significant fever of a degree which would not be accepted by most mothers. These responses were analysed by age and some of the infants of 5 to 12 months old had unacceptable fever. In the younger age group (group B, below four months), 29% had fever, whereas at four to five months it had risen to 75%. So there is a clear indication that the younger the child, the less severe the adverse reactions. It is clearly very important to recognize the possibility of inducing diarrhoea when using this vaccine as it is sometimes difficult to explain to the mother why this is so when it is being given supposedly as a protection against this possibility.

Does buffer make a difference? We used a sodium carbonate buffer with citrate to improve the taste. In this small study, giving $10^{4.8}$ PFU, without buffer there was 56% seroconversion and, with buffer, 83%. In group A given $10^{5.8}$ PFU we obtained 92% seroconversion in the vaccinated children and 2% when using placebo. This is an improvement compared with the bovine NCDV derived RIT 4237 vaccine that yielded 75% seroconversion (Vesikari et al, 1987). However, the question is whether seroconversion is needed—the Finnish studies showed protection without complete seroconversion.

We then evaluated efficacy by recording episodes of rotavirus associated diarrhoea in Umea during an 18-month period. The aim was to analyse whether protection would last for at least two seasons in a developed country until the child is two years old. There was a very slight difference in the total episodes of diarrhoea (75 versus 79) but there was, overall, an efficacy of protection against rotavirus infection of 49% in the study (Table 1). The rhesus rotavirus vaccine is a rotavirus 3 serotype. All the viruses recovered were typed, rotavirus type 1 represented 21 of 23 typed rotavirus strains. This would be indicative of heterotypic protection in an 18-month study (Gothefors et al, 1988).

Table 1 Episodes of rotavirus diarrhoea in children in Umea during the follow-up period, February 1985–June 1986

	Children receiving vaccine (N = 53)	Placebo (N = 51)
Total episodes of diarrhoea	75	79
Rotavirus diarrhoea*	9	17
Indicators of severity		
Days with diarrhoea		
1–2	4	3
3–4	4	5
≧ 5	1	9
Mean	2.9	3.7
Maximum number of motions in 24 hours		
0–3	5	5
4–7	4	9
≧ 8	0	3
Mean	3.7	4.7
Vomiting	6 (67%)	6 (94%)
Physician's visits	0	2
Severity scores		
WHO criteria	2	10
NIH ≦ 3	2	0
4–6	5	10
≧ 7	2	7
Mean	5.0	6.2

Efficacy = 49%, p = 0.07 by chi-square.
For other indicators of severity determined by Mann-Whitney test of T test were not significant (Gothefors et al., 1988).

How should vaccine efficacy be monitored? It could be by seroresponse, measured by complement fixation, ELISA, neutralization, or by means of RIPA (Fig. 1). The gel displays both pre-immune and post-vaccination results, the first six children having been immunized with a rhesus rotavirus vaccine, the next six were immunized with bovine RIT 4237 vaccine and numbers 13 to 16 are naturally infected children. Child 13 and 14 were not infected prior to exposure. Although most of these children were negative by ELISA and by complement fixation all children but one had antibodies reacting with rotavirus when analysed by RIPA.

On the first rotavirus exposure (13 and 14) there is a limited but significant response against VP3 and VP7. However, in the two children (15 and 16) who had had a previous exposure to natural infection, there was an enormous boost following a natural infection. With either the rhesus rotavirus or RIT 4237 vaccine, there is some reactivitiy, primarily to the core proteins with a significant reactivity to VP6. There was no qualitative difference between the two vaccines; but the RRV vaccine was more immunogenic (Fig. 2) (Svensson et al, 1987). This correlates with the difference in efficacy between the two vaccines. RIT 4237 is no longer used but the rhesus rotavirus carried with it all our hopes. A crucial question concerns protection at the gut level and, from these studies, it could be guessed that such protection is indeed important. It is likely that a cell-mediated immune response in the gut could recognize core proteins, i.e. VP6 of rotavirus in analogy with hepatitis B and influenza A.

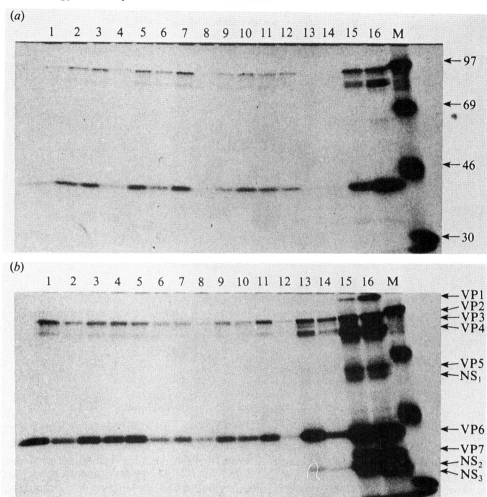

Fig. 1 Immunoprecipitation of ^{35}S methionine-labelled human rotavirus S-1 polypeptides with (a) pre-immune and (b) convalescent sera from rotavirus-vaccinated (lines 1 to 12) or naturally infected children (lines 13 to 16). All sera were tested at 1:10 dilution. Children 1 to 6 were vaccinated with RRV-1 and 7 to 12 were vaccinated with RIT 4237. Mol wt. markers (M); phosphorylase b (97 000), bovine serum albumin (69 000), ovalbumin (46 000), carbonic anhydrase (30 000), lactoglobulin (18 000). Reproduced from Svensson et al (1987)

To evaluate the degree of heterotypic protective efficacy it is necessary to wait for evidence of protection to every circulating serotype after vaccination but this requires an enormous effort in both resources and time.

It is essential to discuss the efficacy of this vaccine in the very different settings found in developing and in developed countries. Mortality is very high in developing countries and while it exists elsewhere—e.g. there were 150 cases in one year in the United States—this cannot be compared with the situation which exists in developing countries. Morbidity, of course, is pronounced in both areas, particularly expressed as a lack of weight gain. It is said that 40% of the children have an abnormal weight gain in developing countries.

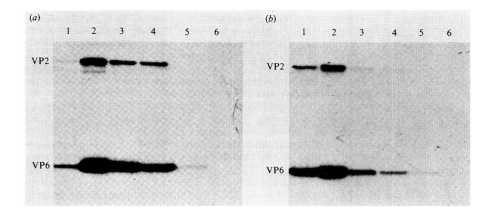

Fig. 2 Comparison of immune responses (by RIPA) to various DS-1 polypeptides in pre- and post-vaccination sera and titrations of post-vaccination sera. (*a*) Child 1; recipient of RRV-1 vaccine; pre 1:50 lane 1. post 1:100 (lane 2), 1:500 (lane 3), 1:1000 (lane 4), 1:5000 (lane 5), 1:10 000 (lane 6), (*b*) Child 7; recipient of RIT 4237 vaccine; pre 1:50 (lane 1), post 1:100 (lane 2), 1:500 (lane 3), 1:1000 (lane 4), 1:5000 (lane 5), 1:10 000 (lane 6). Reproduced from Svensson et al (1987)

The degree of exposure to rotaviruses is restricted in developed countries while it is water-borne and massive in the developing countries, which is of great importance when considering protection. Maternal immunity may be reduced, which was the situation in Finland, and may explain the high seroconversion ratio after vaccination even in comparison with the United States in phase 1 studies. The age at vaccination may be allowed to differ in developed countries with seasonal outbreaks of rotavirus infections while, in the developing countries, the ideal would be to have vaccination at birth because that is probably the only time when most children are seen by the medical staff.

It would be advantageous to combine the oral poliovirus vaccine (OPV) with the oral rotavirus vaccine. From the evidence of one study the rotavirus vaccine does not interfere with the take of poliovirus vaccine, but the poliovirus vaccine does interfere with the take of the rotavirus, and this holds true for both settings. On the other hand, enteroviruses would not interfere with rotavirus vaccines in developed countries but they might, to a significant extent, do so in developing countries where many of the 72 enterovirus serotypes circulate.

Protection is primarily homotypic. The Scandinavian experience of vaccination with rhesus rotavirus was a vigorous response including adverse reactions, that resulted in heterotypic protection, which is unusual. Chiba et al (1986) have followed 18 outbreaks of diarrhoea in an orphanage in Sapporo during a ten-year period. Three consecutive outbreaks due to rotavirus type 3 were recorded. Out of 38 children with homotypic antibody titres up to 64, 35 were infected and 32 fell ill. Protection against illness required homotypic neutralizing antibody titres of 256. The majority of the children had concomitant antibody responses against rotavirus serotypes 1 and 4 but fewer reacted with serotype 2.

The next question to be resolved is whether a rotavirus infection will sensitize for entero adherent, entero pathogenic or other *Escherichia coli*. This has not been definitely established as there are few double infections by *E. coli* and rotavirus—9 of 416 children in a prospective one-year study (1986)—in Sweden (Uhnoo et al, 1986). Double infections are common in developing countries and if sensitization occurs after natural rotavirus infection it is essential to establish whether this happens also after infection by the vaccine virus.

When considering vaccination against rotavirus it is necessary to know whether there is a detectable effect on the overall frequency of diarrhoea. There is obviously some effect but, if the overall incidence of diarrhoea is reduced by only 10% to 20%, it may be difficult to persuade mothers and authorities to use the vaccine. Rotavirus diarrhoea is not smallpox, i.e. clinically it is not possible to identify the child with or without the rotavirus diarrhoea, and he/she may have something else, whereas smallpox usually was well recognized. This is a great problem in practical global medicine.

In conclusion the following aspects of rotavirus vaccines have to be evaluated: (*a*) the take rate in the child; (*b*) the length of protection; (*c*) acceptance by the mother concerning adverse reactions; (*d*) the effectiveness in relevant populations; and (*e*) endorsement by society.

REFERENCES

Chiba S, Yokoyama T, Nakata S. et al 1986 Protective effect of naturally acquired homotypic and heterotypic rotavirus antibodies. Lancet 2: 417–421
Gothefors et al 1988 Prolonged efficacy of rhesus rotavirus vaccine in Swedish children. Journal of Infectious Diseases, submitted
Svensson L, Sheshberadaran H, Vesikari T, Norrby E, Wadell G 1987 Immune responses to rotavirus polypeptides after vaccination with heterologous rotavirus vaccines RIT 4237, RRV 1. Journal of General Virology 68: 1993–1999
Uhnoo I, Wadell G, Svensson L, Olding-Stenkvist E, Ekwall E, Mollby R 1986 Aetiology and epidemiology of acute gastroenteritis in Swedish children. Journal of Infection 13: 73–89
Vesikari T, Isolauri E, Ruuska T, Routanen T 1987 Clinical trials of rotavirus vaccines. In: Bishop (ed) Ciba foundation Symposium 128. Novel diarrhoea viruses. p. 218–231

Discussion: Rotavirus infection

Albert Kapikian and Göran Wadell

Dr Plotkin opened the discussion by presenting some data from his and his colleagues' studies of a live rotavirus vaccine. They also use the Jennerian approach but the cross-reacting animal virus they employ is a type 6 bovine strain called WC3. The objective is to have facilities for producing large amounts of virus retaining its original immunogenicity. For this purpose the virus was passaged 12 times in different established cell lines. The resulting virus material has been given to children in phase 1 and 2 trials. There was no increase, compared with a control group, in reactions and therefore this bovine strain like the RIT vaccine candidate strain (recently withdrawn) is highly attenuated. It produces an antibody response primarily against bovine strains, with less antibodies against human rotavirus type 3 and limited amounts of antibody to type 1. Nevertheless in a type 1 outbreak near Philadelphia, pre-immunized children, i.e. given either WC3 virus or placebo, were observed to be protected at a rate of approximately 76% (3 cases of rotavirus diarrhoea in the vaccine group compared with 14 in the placebo group). When only severe or moderate to severe disease was considered there was 100% protection. This appears as a clear demonstration of heterotypic response active at the gut level but poorly reflected in the presence of circulating antibodies. Whether the local immunity is humoral or cell mediated is currently being evaluated. Bovine strains should be useful against human type 1 and 3 strains but not against 2 and 4 strains, which are antigenically distinct. Studies using monoclonal antibodies and sequencing of the VP3 gene have shown that there is a good deal of cross-reaction between certain serotypes and induction of cross-reactivity therefore may be useful in vaccine strains. It was remarked that a requirement for monotypic immunity may be particularly important under the age of four months. After this the ubiquitous occurrence of rotaviruses, combined with their capacity for causing re-infection cause a complex picture as concerns heterotypic immunity. In a study in Umea, Sweden, there was a protection against human serotype 1 with the rhesus rotaviruses vaccine probably because the children had pre-existing antibodies.

A concern was expressed whether reassortment *in vivo* might lead to emergence of new strains. This was concluded not to represent a risk since the vaccine virus genome is totally rhesus rotavirus except for the VP7 gene. Further it remains to demonstrate the extent of spread of vaccine attenuated virus.

Since the future vaccine product will contain reassortants representing all four human types of rotaviruses it was inquired whether there was a risk for interference between these viruses. So far preliminary studies with a quarter of the normal dose of each virus type have been carried out. Under these conditions all virus types were detected in the stools, but the problem needs to be studied further under full dose conditions. Since breast milk has a certain protective effect against rotavirus infection it was discussed whether immunization of mothers might be a useful avenue. This appears not to be a simple approach since mothers normally have pre-existing antibody at high levels. In order to boost these antibodies a potent inactivated antigen would be required.

13. Vaccination against varicella

Stanley A. Plotkin, Stuart E. Starr,
Anne A. Gershon, Barbara A. Zajac and
Barbara J. Kuter

INTRODUCTION

In vaccinating against varicella with a live attenuated virus we face two problems never before faced in vaccine development. First, contrary to all other vaccines, a group at high risk of vaccine reaction is being expressly singled out for vaccination and indeed, is being used to validate the safety of the product for use in normal children. Second, the vaccine strain virus, like the wild type virus, will occasionally induce an expected reaction, zoster, that may occur 50 years later.

Nevertheless, these problems are being faced, and the licensure of the Oka strain in Europe and Japan may be followed soon by licensure in the United States. If so, it is probable that an attempt will be made to make it a routine vaccine for children. In this paper we will examine the current knowledge on which such a decision might be based.

Table 13.1

Complications of varicella	
Appendicitis	Optic neuritis
Arthritis	Orchitis
Glomerulonephritis	Pneumonitis
Hepatitis	Purpura
Myocarditis	Secondary bacterial infections
Cerebellar ataxia	Uveitis
Diffuse encephalomyelitis	Reye syndrome
Guillain-Barré syndrome	Transverse myelitis

Complications of herpes zoster	
Motor deficit neuralgia	Ocular complications:
Herpes gangrenosa	Uveitis
Pneumonia	Keratitis
Meningoencephalitis	2° Glaucoma
Unilateral deafness	Iridocyclitis
	Panophthalmitis

Varicella-zoster has had the reputation of being a trivial disease, but this is far from true. Although the rates of complications are relatively low, when the fact that virtually 100% of the population gets the disease is taken into account, one's perspective of the disease changes. Table 13.1 lists some of the complications of varicella and zoster that have been reported in the medical literature (Fleisher et al, 1982; Guess et al, 1984; Plotkin, 1985). Recently, American investigators have sought to define the epidemiology of complications, using either national reporting or a comprehensive study of all the residents of Olmstead County, Minnesota (Preblud, 1986; Guess et al, 1986). Some interesting data emerged. In an average year there are 364,000 physician visits for varicella and 3,800 hospitalizations.

Table 13.2 Age specific incidence of varicella and hospitalization due to varicella

Age	Incidence*	% of total cases	Hospitalizations per 10,000 cases	% of total hospitalized
<1	3,377	3.3	10	9
1–4	8,214	32.3	9	29
5–9	9,027	49.9	8	29
10–14	1,753	11.1	12	10
15–19	291	1.9	42	6
>20	33	1.5	127	17

* Cases per 100,000 persons per year.

Overall the rate of hospitalization, as shown in Table 13.2, is 1/1000 varicella cases, and the principal contributors to that rate are bacterial skin infections, CNS disease and pneumonia (Guess et al, 1986).

Table 13.3 Varicella cases and costs without and with a childhood varicella vaccination programme

Parameter	Without a programme	With a programme	Reduction (%)
No. of cases	3,292,750	729,253	77.9
Cost ($)			
Disease			
Medical	16,881,227	4,523,165	73.2
Home care	384,565,683	88,737,092	76.8
Subtotal	399,446,960	93,260,257	76.6
Vaccine			
Medical		81,125	
Home care		45,286	
Vaccine		44,009,900	
Subtotal		44,136,311	
Total	399,446,960	137,396,568	65.6

These days it is considered desirable to calculate economic as well as human costs of disease. Preblud (1986) has made extensive analyses of the cost of varicella, summarized in Table 13.3, from which it can be seen that an effective vaccine would save millions of dollars in the United States alone.

VACCINE DEVELOPMENT

Several attenuated vaccine strains of VZV have been developed (Neff et al, 1981; Hediard et al, 1983) but only the Oka strain is now being widely tested. This strain was isolated by Takahashi in 1970 (Takahashi et al, 1974; Takahashi, 1986), and was attenuated by passage in human and guinea pig embryo fibroblasts as shown in Table 13.4. The vaccine pools currently being used were prepared in MRC-5 cells.

Table 13.4 History of Oka VZV strain

Vesicle fluid of 3-year-old boy with varicella
Inoculated into human embryo lung (HEL)
Passages 1–11 in HEL
Passages 12–13 in guinea pig embryo fibroblasts
Passages 24 in WI–38
Passages 25–30 in MRC-5

Oka can be distinguished from wild strains by its better growth in guinea pig cells, better immunogenicity in guinea pigs, and lesser ability to grow at 39°C (Hayakawa et al, 1984; Takahashi et al, 1985). Its restriction-endonuclease pattern differs from American wild isolates (Fig. 13.1), which enables its identification and differentiation from wild-type varicella in clinical studies. In part, this difference is due to geographical differences between American and Japanese strains (Hayakawa et al, 1984; Martin et al, 1985). The Oka vaccine strain is fully sensitive to acyclovir, which is an important safety factor (Preblud et al, 1984).

VACCINATION OF NORMAL CHILDREN

In this paper we will concentrate on the results of American clinical trials. Data from Japan and Europe will be mentioned only in passing.

Several thousand normal children have already received the Oka strain vaccine in the United States, with excellent tolerance. About 5.5% have had local reactions at the injection site; a similar percentage showed a mild rash

Table 13.5 FAMA antibody responses and their persistence after Oka vaccine in healthy seronegative children

	FAMA antibody			LPR*		
	N	>1:2	GMT	N	S.I. >2.0	Mean S.I.
6 w	91	100%	34.0	67	97%	13.6
9–12 m	61	100%	14.5	57	46%	10.3
3–4 y	54	100%	9.6	28	89%	24.7

* Varicella-specific lymphocyte proliferation measured as stimulation index.

consisting of one to five papules which lasted one to three days, were negative when cultured and disappeared without trace. About 10% of children had fever, but few were higher than 39°C (Arbeter et al, 1986).

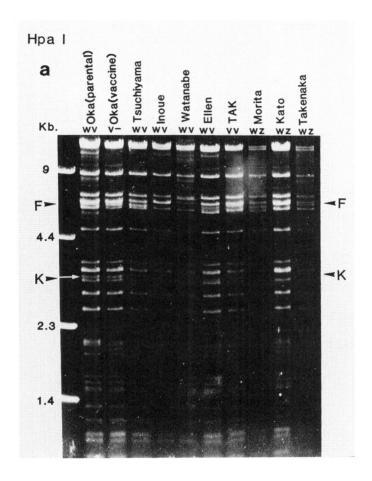

Fig. 13.1 Left: Profiles of DNA cleavage by restriction endonuclease Hpa I. DNAs from 10 strains of VZV are shown: seven wild-type strains, the Oka parental strain, the Oka vaccine strain, and one strain (TAK) recovered from a vaccine recipient. From Hayakawa et al (1984)

Table 13.5 shows the immune response to Oka vaccine over a four-year period. Note that both antibodies and cellular responses appeared regularly after vaccination and showed good persistence although cellular responses have begun to fade.

With regard to prevention of chickenpox after exposure, the Oka strain has proven to be highly effective. Table 13.6 lists pre-exposure efficacy studies that have been performed. In the double-blind, placebo controlled study of Weibel et al (1985) Oka showed excellent efficacy during the two years post-vaccination

243

in which the population was observed. In addition, uncontrolled data showed that more than 90% of exposures in vaccines failed to result in clinical disease (Arbeter et al, 1984; Horiuchi, 1984; Asano et al, 1984; Katsushima et al, 1984).

Table 13.6 Studies of protective efficacy of Oka vaccine

Investigator	Type of study	No.	Efficacy
Weibel	Pre-exposure controlled	486	100
Arbeter	Pre-exposure uncontrolled	154	94
Arbeter	Post-exposure controlled	13	90
Horiuchi	Pre-exposure uncontrolled	854	98
Asano	Pre-exposure uncontrolled	179	97
Asano	Post-exposure controlled	37	100
Katshushima	Pre-exposure uncontrolled	205	94
Andre	Pre-exposure uncontrolled	*	95

* Several hundred children.
54 Episodes of close exposure.

Of special interest is the possibility of preventing varicella by post-exposure immunization. Asano et al (1984) immunized 34 children within three days of household exposure to varicella with 500 or more pfu and followed an additional 28 non-immunized children similarly exposed. Clinical varicella developed in all of the non-immunized children but in only two of the vaccinated children, a protection efficacy of 94.2%.

Our post-exposure trial with the Oka-Merck vaccine was placebo controlled and double-blind. The protective efficacy was 90% for those who received vaccine within three days of onset of rash in the index case, and the efficacy for protection plus modification was 100% (mild rash with fewer than 50 pocks), even up to five days post-exposure (Table 13.7). This study requires confirmation, because post-exposure prophylaxis could be useful before immunization of the population with varicella vaccine becomes routine.

Table 13.7 Post-exposure efficacy in healthy children (8,700 pfu/dose)

	Vaccine	Placebo
Varicella (60–600 lesions)	0	12
Mild varicella (1–50 lesions)	4	0
No disease	9	1
Total	13	13

$p = <0.003$.

An interesting by-product of varicella vaccine studies is the discovery that subclinical reinfection occurs frequently in both naturally immune and vaccinated individuals (Arvin et al, 1983; Gershon et al, 1984b). This may be a mechanism for maintaining varicella immunity, and it will be interesting to see what happens when such boosts are less common.

COMBINED VACCINATION

Since children are now routinely vaccinated against measles, mumps and rubella in one combined vaccine, the advantage of adding a fourth live vaccine is obvious. Merck and SK-RIT have each prepared experimental quadrivalent vaccines which have had limited testing. Just et al (1985) found some interference with varicella responses when the four vaccines were combined, unless a large dose of varicella was used. In our studies (Table 13.8), responses were good to a vaccine containing only a moderate amount of varicella (Arbeter et al, 1986). However, at one year, two of ten children lost antibody to VZV.

Table 13.8 Proportion of children responding with antibodies who were given tetravalent measles-mumps-rubella-varicella (MMRV) vaccine or MMR + varicella separately

	Post-vaccination	
	6 week	1 year
MMRV		
Measles	16/16	12/12
Mumps	15/16	12/12
Rubella	16/16	12/12
Varicella	13/13	8/10
MMR + V		
Measles	7/7	4/4
Mumps	8/8	4/4
Rubella	7/7	4/4
Varicella	8/8	5/5

Brunell et al (1988) have also reported good results with MMRV vaccination, and it is probable that with some juggling of content, a successful quadrivalent vaccine will be developed.

IMMUNOCOMPROMISED CHILDREN

Considerable effort has been expended on vaccination of leukaemic children, for several reasons:

(1)   Children with ALL have a high rate of morbidity and mortality after natural chickenpox, for which they need protection (Feldman et al, 1973). The use of VZIG has been only partly successful in preventing disease and antiviral treatment may come too late (Zaia et al, 1983).

(2) Children with ALL undergo chemotherapy which induces immunosuppression. Thus, as they need vaccine, one can determine vaccine safety by observation of their vesicular rashes immediately post-vaccination. In addition, because of immunosuppression, they have a high incidence of zoster. Latency of the vaccine virus will be detected by the occurrence of zoster post-vaccination.

(3) Children with ALL form the largest group of children with cancer, and they will certainly be on the list of patients for whom vaccine is indicated.

Children with leukaemia have been vaccinated in Japan (Ha et al, 1980), Europe (André, 1985), and the United States (Brunell et al, 1982), where the largest study has been a collaborative one conducted by Gershon (Gershon et al, 1984a, 1986). In this study several hundred children have been vaccinated and followed. The protocol which has evolved is to select children who are 12 months or more post-induction of chemotherapy, and to interrupt their chemotherapy for one week before and one week after vaccination. Eligibility for vaccination requires the presence of at least 700 lymphocytes/mm^3 and an intact proliferative response of white blood cells to phytohaemagglutinin or pokeweed mitogen.

The results of this study have been as follows:

(1) Although in general Oka has been well tolerated by leukaemic children, about 40% have developed vesicular rashes, in rare cases with sufficient number of lesions to convince clinicians of the need for acyclovir treatment.

(2) The vesicular rashes in these children may contain infectious vaccine strain viruses, and transmission to contacts occurs about 10% of the time. Fortunately, transmission to normal siblings was not accompanied by symptoms.

(3) Antibody responses of children with ALL have been slightly poor relative to normal individuals, with 90% seroconverting after one dose and 95% after two doses. Moreover, antibody disappears more often than in normal children.

(4) Protection of leukaemic children by the vaccine was imperfect, as only 80% was protected. However, nearly all breakthrough disease were mild.

(5) The incidence of zoster in vaccinated leukaemics was not higher than after natural disease (see below).

(6) The interruption of chemotherapy for ALL did not lead to a greater relapse rate of leukaemia.

Children with solid tumours (excluding lymphomas) were vaccinated by Heath et al (1987) in London. Seroconversion was noted in only 62% of 39 children, and 78% of seroresponders lost antibodies within two years. Nevertheless, none of nine exposed children, including non-responders, developed varicella.

VACCINATION OF ADULTS

The high complication rate of varicella among adults, and the problem of health care workers who develop varicella exposing immunocompromised patients, make vaccination of adults interesting. We have had experience with vaccination

246

of 21 young adults, 19 (90%) of whom seroconverted after one inoculation of vaccine. However, two lost antibody during the first year post-vaccination.

Gershon et al (1988) have recently analysed a larger series of varicella vaccinations in adults. Like us, they found that the vaccine was well tolerated, but induction and persistence of antibody response were not as good as in children. Of 187 vaccinated adults 82% responded with antibody to one dose and 94% to two doses (Table 13.9). From one to six years after a single dose, about 25% of previous seroconverters lost antibody. Persistence of antibody was a significant protective factor, in that four of five adults who lost antibody experienced varicella after exposure, compared with none of eight who retained antibody. Vaccine efficacy over a mean period of 28 months was only about 50%. However, the breakthrough illnesses were all mild.

Table 13.9 Seroconversion of seronegative adult to Oka VZV vaccine†

Number of doses	Seroconversion
1	151/184 (82%)
2	141/150 (94%)
	19/28* (68%)

* Failed to respond to first dose.
† From Gershon et al (1988).

A similar experience was reported in the UK by Ndumbe et al (1985), who vaccinated paediatric nurses. They found seroconversion in 94% of the nurses, but subsequent loss of antibody in one third over two years. Nevertheless, the protective efficacy of the vaccine was 83%, and varicella was mild when it occurred (Table 13.10).

Table 13.10 Results of exposure of seronegative nurses to varicella (Ndumbe et al, 1985)

	Varicella
Vaccines	2/13 (15%)
Unvaccinated	6/7 (86%)

In summary, vaccination of adults is feasible, although two doses are necessary to attain the highest seroconversion rate. There may be little advantage to a second dose, however, since modified illness follows exposure even in those who have lost antibody. Perhaps persistence of T-memory cells explains the partial protection afforded by prior vaccination.

ZOSTER IN VACCINE RECIPIENTS

The chief remaining issues that cloud widespread acceptance of varicella vaccine are the development of zoster and the persistence of immunity. Perhaps these are Janus faces of the same issue: if vaccine strain virus persists there will be immunity but also zoster from vaccine, whereas if it does not there will be neither zoster nor immunity.

In any case, we have now observed zoster in two normal children vaccinated with Oka (Plotkin et al, 1988). In addition, many vaccinated leukaemic children have been reported to have developed zoster (Williams et al, 1985; Hayakawa et al, 1984) and in some cases there has been confirmation by restriction-endonuclease analyses that the virus causing zoster was the vaccine strain. Are these cases indicative of a greater risk from vaccine than from natural disease? Thus far, the answer is in the negative.

To calculate comparative rates of zoster in normal children we used the data obtained in Olmstead County, Minnesota, the home of the Mayo Clinic. The rate of zoster for normal children after natural varicella was 7.7/10,000 person years (Ragozzino et al, 1982; Guess et al, 1985, 1986) compared with a calculated rate of 2.1/10,000 person years for normal vaccinees (Plotkin et al, 1988).

More crucial, perhaps, are the data obtained in leukaemic subjects. Because of their immunosuppression, leukaemic children who have had varicella have a high rate of zoster. Thus, one can compare rates of zoster in these children after vaccine and after natural disease. Several studies have been reported, and all showed a lower rate after vaccine (Brunell et al, 1986; Yabuchi et al, 1984; Lawrence et al, 1988). The most recent study was one performed by Lawrence et al (1988): this was the product of the large collaborative study led by Gershon. In that study; children with ALL were followed from the time of vaccination and compared with other leukaemic children who had natural varicella either prior to the onset of malignancy or after the diagnosis, and who were matched for age and other characteristics. Fig. 13.2, taken from their paper, shows that, in fact, reactivation as zoster was less likely after vaccine than after natural varicella, although the difference was not yet statistically significant.

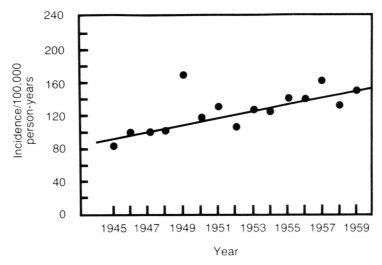

Fig. 13.2 Probability of remaining free of zoster in the entire group of 84 matched pairs of vaccinated and control children. Time zero denotes the acquisition of both risk factors: (1) primary varicella-zoster virus either by immunization or by natural infection, and (2) the diagnosis of leukaemia; the end points are the development of zoster, death, or the end of the study (March 1986). Log-rank and Gehan tests revealed no statistically significant difference between the two curves. From Lawrence et al (1988)

Since the other published studies have all shown the same tendency—i.e. lesser reactivation after vaccine than after natural disease—we can assume that vaccine will not increase the rate of zoster. The mildness of the post-vaccine zoster is also comforting, but will it always remain so? As severity of zoster increases with age, it may not be possible to answer this question for many years.

One point which makes this problem even more difficult is that superinfection with wild virus may occur in vaccinees. Infection of immune individuals exposed to varicella is known to occur with some frequency, although the vast majority of times the infection is subclinical (Arvin et al, 1983). Re-infection in vaccinees may also be subclinical, but evidently the re-infecting strain may also establish itself (Gershon et al, 1984b). This fact was confirmed using restriction-endonuclease analyses by Gershon et al (1986). The basis for this work was the demonstration that strains isolated in the USA had different R-E patterns than those isolated in Japan, such as the Oka vaccine strain, and that Oka itself could be differentiated from wild strains in Japan. The differences, though not great, permitted the identification of some cases of zoster after vaccination as being vaccine-caused, and at least one case was identified as being caused by a non-vaccine strain that presumably infected after vaccination. In this connection a clinical point should be made. Physicians see many mild vesicular rashes in children, which if only present as a few lesions, are unlikely to be diagnosed as varicella. Thus, mild varicella may often go undiagnosed and this must be true in vaccinees as well as children who have had prior natural disease.

PREVENTION OF ZOSTER

Another side of the coin is the possible use of an immunogen to prevent reactivation of naturally acquired virus. After all, zoster is probably the result of a loss of specific cellular immunity to varicella. This has been shown by the demonstration of declining positivity with age in skin tests using varicella antigen and in lymphocyte proliferation to varicella antigen (Miller, 1980; Burke et al, 1982). On the other hand, antibody to varicella does not seem to be deficient in those who get zoster even in old age. The rates of zoster with age are shown in Fig. 13.3, which was obtained from a population based study performed in Olmstead County, Minnesota (Ragozzino et al, 1982). Clearly, immune debility becomes important after the fifth decade of life, and it is therefore worth asking if a vaccine could be delivered at that age which would boost V-Z specific cellular immunity.

Duchateau et al (1985) previously reported antibody boosts in seropositive adults after Oka vaccine and we recently completed a study in which individuals in their 50s, 60s, or 70s who had low VZV-specific lymphocyte proliferation responses and never had zoster, were given Oka vaccine (Table 13.11). Interestingly, lymphocyte proliferation responses were boosted by vaccination of individuals under 70 years of age, and such boosted responses were maintained for at least nine months. In contrast, individuals older than 70 years failed to respond immunologically to the vaccine. As the rate of zoster is too low to consider a large vaccine trial without a previously demonstrated immune

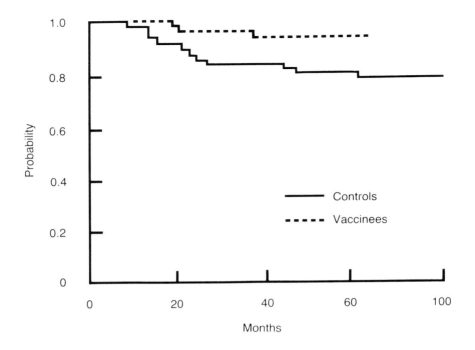

Fig. 13.3 Incidence per 100,000 person-years of herpes zoster among residents of Rochester, Minnesota, 1945–1959, by age and sex. From Ragozzino et al (1982)

effect, further progress in this field must depend on the identification of an immune function that is important in preventing reactivation and the demonstration that vaccine elicits that function. Larger vaccine doses should also be tried in older individuals.

Table 13.11 Proportion of elderly adults who developed significant lymphocyte proliferation responses to varicella antigen

Age (years)	Responders
50–59	10/11
60–69	5/7
> 70	0/5

PERSISTENCE OF IMMUNITY

Fears have been expressed that a varicella vaccine might provide only temporary immunity, and that vaccinees would again become susceptible at ages when they would also be more prone to complications of the disease. Several lines of evidence can be brought to bear on this question, although a definitive answer cannot be given.

First there are data on persistence of antibody from Japan (Asano et al, 1984)

showing the presence of antibody for as long as 10 years post-vaccination. Table 13.12 provides data on American children followed for five years after vaccination with Oka.

Table 13.12 Persistence of antibody and geometric mean titres among healthy children and adolescents who received Oka/Merck varicella vaccine

Assay	Time range (month)	Midpoint of range	Persistence rate	GMT*
FAMA	0–3	6 wks.	125/125 (100%)	36.6
	6–18	1 yr.	110/110 (100%)	17.0
	18–30	2 yr.	17/17 (100%)	20.4
	30–42	3 yr.	28/29 (97%)	>11.7
	42–54	4 yr.	39/39 (100%)	>9.1
ELISA	0–3	6 wks.	572/572 (100%)	>15.3
	6–18	1 yr.	102/107 (95%)	>10.2
	18–30	2 yr.	122/122 (100%)	16.3
	30–42	3 yr.	—	—
	42–54	4 yr.	15/15 (100%)	26.4
	54–66	5 yr.	9/9 (100%)	58.8

* Comparison of geometric mean titres over time is inappropriate since the same individuals were not bled at each time point.

Second, there are data on actual protection on exposure to varicella years after vaccination. Unfortunately, controlled data on protection, from the study done in suburban Philadelphia, extend only to two years. In that study, protection was 100% for one year and 95% for two years (Weibel et al, 1984; Weibel, personal communication).

Uncontrolled data from Japan are available in various populations over four to ten year periods, and are summarized in Table 13.13 (Asano et al, 1984; Horiuchi, 1984; Ozaki et al, 1984; Naganuma et al, 1984; Katsushima et al, 1984).

Table 13.13 Persistence of protective efficacy over four to 10 years in uncontrolled Japanese trials of Oka vaccine*

Varicella cases among vaccinees	40/854 (4.7%)
Varicella after known exposure	28/367 (7.6%)

* From Asano et al (1985), Horiuchi (1984), Ozaki et al (1984), Naganuma et al (1984).

PUBLIC HEALTH CONSIDERATIONS

What if a varicella vaccine is licensed for normal children? How would it best be used? Some guesses can be hazarded (Table 13.14).

Certainly the vaccine would be used to protect immunosuppressed seronegative individuals. Children with ALL, children with other cancers, children receiving steroids or aspirin for chronic conditions, and perhaps those with chronic disease even not receiving steroids. For example, those with chronic skin disorders would be candidates for vaccination.

Table 13.14 Target groups for varicella vaccine (1988)

Children with leukaemia
High risk children (cystics, diabetics, nephrotics, asthmatics)
Normal seronegative adolescents and adults especially history-negative medical personnel
Normal children, pre-exposure

With regard to normal children, public health considerations argue for the use of combined quadrivalent MMRV vaccine. Currently, measles, mumps and rubella vaccines are administered in most countries at the age of 15 months. Since transplacental antibodies to varicella do not last as long as measles antibody, earlier vaccination against varicella would be feasible. However in the USA only 2.4% of chickenpox occurs before the age of one year (Preblud, 1986), and it is likely that varicella will be proposed for infants 12 to 15 months of age. Another reason for not advancing the age is that congenital immune deficiencies which would increase the risk of complications of vaccination may not be detected until later in life. Here the spectre of HIV infection raises its head, but there are as yet no data on VZ vaccination of HIV infected children. Very likely, as with measles, HIV infected children who are not severely immunocompromised will tolerate the vaccine while those who are frankly symptomatic will have significant reactions. Nevertheless, some safety data will be obtained in this group by accidental immunization. No doubt there will be an indication for vaccination of those over 15 years of age who have never had varicella. Currently in the USA, that group comprises 6.5% of individuals, but sustains 37.3% deaths (Preblud, 1986). Vaccination of that older age group would also avoid the annoying problem of varicella during pregnancy (Plotkin, 1985).

A specific induction for childhood vaccination will be for siblings of immunocompromised children, in order to protect them from household exposure.

Vaccination of health care workers will be an important indication for varicella vaccine. One American hospital (Weber et al, 1988) recently estimated its costs for varicella prevention during a single year. The total cost was $55,934, comprised of about $40,000 for work furloughs, $10,000 for serologies, $4,300 for isolation costs, $2,000 for infection control personnel time and $150 for varicella zoster immune globulin.

KILLED VACCINE

This review would be incomplete without some word concerning inactivated vaccine. As is frequently the case in virology these days, information on the molecular structure of VZV far exceeds information on the biological function of the various proteins. The genome has been sequenced by Davison et al (1986) and several envelope glycoproteins have been identified (Davison and Scott, 1986) (Table 13.15). However, linkage between protein structure and cellular immune responses is lacking, and we can only speculate as to the proper composition of a subunit vaccine. African green monkeys, which are susceptible to varicella, have been immunized with individual glycoproteins, and feeble protection was demonstrated with gpII and III in these preliminary experiments (Soike et al, 1987). Manufacture of a glycoprotein vaccine would be feasible now, but may be set aside until the results of vaccination with Oka are clear.

Table 13.15 Principal varicella glycoprotein complexes

Glycoprotein	Molecular weights ($\times 10^3$)
gpI	98/88/62
gpII	140/66
gpIII	118

REFERENCES

André F E 1985 Worldwide experience with the Oka-strain live varicella vaccine. Postgraduate Medical Journal 61: 113

Arbeter A M, Starr S E, Preblud S R et al 1984 Varicella vaccine trials in healthy children: A summary of comparative and follow up studies. American Journal of Diseases in Children 138: 434

Arbeter A M, Baker L, Starr S E et al 1986 Combination measles, mumps, rubella, and varicella vaccine. Pediatrics 78 (Supp): 742

Arvin A M, Koropchak C M, Wittek A E 1983 Immunologic evidence of reinfection with varicella-zoster virus. Journal of Infectious Diseases 148: 200

Asano Y, Nagi T, Miyato T, et al 1984 Persistence of protective immunity after inoculation with live varicella vaccine (Oka strain). Biken Journal 27: 123

Balfour H, Suarez C, Kelly J, Crane D, Amren D 1986 Adverse effects and immunogenicity of simultaneously adminstered varicella and measles-mumps-rubella (MMR) vaccines. Twenty-sixth Interscience Conference on Antimicrobial Agents and Chemotherapy. Abstract 315: 154

Brunell P A, Geiser C, Shehab Z, et al 1982 Administration of live varicella vaccine to children with leukemia. Lancet 2: 1069

Brunell P A, Novelli V W, Lipton S B, Pollock B 1988 Combined vaccine against measles, mumps, rubella, and varicella. Pediatrics 81: 779

Brunell P A, Taylor-Wiedman J, Geiser C et al 1986 Risk of herpes zoster in children with leukemia: Varicella vaccine compared with history of chickenpox. Pediatrics 77: 53

Burke B L, Davis R C, Marmer D J et al 1982 Cellular immune responses to varicella-zoster (VZ) in the aged. Archives of Internal Medicine 142: 291

Davison A J, Edson C M, Ellis R W et al 1986 New common nomenclature for glycoprotein genes of varicella zoster virus and their glycosylated products. Journal of Virology 57: 1195

Davison A J, Scott J E 1986 The complete DNA sequence of varicella-zoster virus. Journal of General Virology 67: 1759

Duchateau J, Vrijens R, Nicaise J et al 1985 Stimulation of specific immune response to varicella antigens in the elderly with varicella vaccine. Postgraduate Medical Journal 61: 147

Feldman S, Hughes W, Kim H 1973 Herpes zoster in children with cancer. American Journal of Diseases of Children 126: 178

Fleisher G, McSorley H W et al 1982 Life-threatening complications of varicella. American Journal of Diseases of Children 135: 896

Gershon A A, Steinberg S P, Gelb L et al 1984a Live attenuated varicella vaccine: Efficacy for children with leukemia in remission. Journal of the American Medical Association 252: 355

Gershon A A, Steinberg S P, Gelb L 1984b NIAID Varicella Vaccine Collaborative Study Group. Clinical reinfection due to varicella-zoster virus. Journal of Infectious Diseases 149: 137

Gershon A A, Steinberg S P, Gelb L et al 1986 NIAID Varicella Vaccine Collaborative Study Group. Live attenuated varicella vaccine in immunocompromised children and healthy adults. Pediatrics 78: 757

Gershon A A, Steinberg S P, LaRussa P et al 1988 NIAID Varicella Vaccine Collaborative Study Group 1988 Immunization of healthy adults with live attenuated varicella vaccine. Journal of Infectious Diseases 158 (1): 132

Guess H A, Broughton D D, Melton L J, et al 1984 Chickenpox hospitalizations among residents of Olmstead County, Minnesota, 1962 through 1981. American Journal of Diseases of Children 138: 1055

Guess H A, Broughton D D, Melton L J et al 1985 Epidemiology of herpes zoster in children and adolescents. A population based study. Pediatrics 76: 512

Guess H A, Broughton D D, Melton L J, Kurland L T 1986 Population-based studies of varicella complication. Pediatrics 78 (Suppl): 723

Ha K, Baba K, Ikeda T, Nishida M et al 1980 Application of live varicella vaccine to children with acute leukemia or other malignancies without suspension of anticancer therapy. Pediatrics 65: 346

Hayakawa Y, Torigoe S, Shiraki K et al 1984 Biologic and biophysical markers of a live varicella vaccine strain (Oka): Identification of clinical isolates from vaccine recipients. Journal of Infectious Diseases 149: 956

Heath R B, Malpas J S, Kangro H O et al 1987 Efficacy of varicella vaccine in patients with solid tumours. Archives of Diseases in Childhood 62: 569

Hediard B, Burguiere A M, Devillechabrolle A et al 1983 Preliminary study of an attenuated varicella-zoster vaccine (Webster strain) in 27 children with uncompromised immunity (French). Annales Pédiatrie 30: 440

Horiuchi K 1984 Chickenpox vaccination of healthy children: Immunologic and clinical responses and protective effect in 1978–1982. Biken Journal 27: 37

Just M, Berger R, Luescher D 1985 Live varicella vaccine in healthy individuals. Postgraduate Medical Journal 61: 129–132

Katsushima N, Yazaki N, Sakamota M 1984 Effect and follow-up study on varicella vaccine. Biken Journal 27: 51

Lawrence R, Gershon A A, Holzman R, Steinberg S P 1988 NIAID Varicella Vaccine Collaborative Study Group 1988 The risk of zoster after varicella vaccine. New England Journal of Medicine 318: 543

Martin J H, Dohner D E, Wellinghof W J, Gelb L D 1985 Restriction endonuclease analysis of varicella-zoster vaccine virus and wild type DNAs. Journal of Medical Virology 9: 69

Miller A E 1980 Selective decline in cellular immune response to varicella-zoster in the elderly. Neurology 30: 582

Naganuma Y, Osawa S, Takahashi R 1984 Clinical application of a live varicella vaccine (Oka strain) in a hospital. Biken Journal 27: 59

Ndumbe P M, Cradock-Watson J E, Heath R B, Levinsky R J 1985 Live varicella immunization in healthy non-immune nurses. Postgraduate Medical Journal 61: 133

Neff B J, Weibel R E, Villarejos V M et al 1981 Clinical and laboratory studies of KMcC strain live attenuated varicella virus. Proceedings of the Society for Experimental Biology and Medicine 166: 347

Ozaki T, Matsui T, Ichikawa T et al 1984 Clinical trial of the Oka strain of live attenuated varicella vaccine on healthy children. Biken Journal 27: 39

Plotkin S A 1985 Clinical and pathogenic aspects of varicella-zoster. Postgraduate Medical Journal 61: 7

Plotkin S A, Starr S E, Connor K, Morton D 1988 Zoster in normal children after varicella vaccine. Journal of Infectious Diseases, in press

Preblud S R 1986 Varicella: Complications and costs. Pediatrics 78 (Suppl): 728

Preblud S R, Arbeter A M, Proctor E A, Starr S E, Plotkin S A 1984 Susceptibility of vaccine strains of varicella-zoster virus to antiviral compounds. Antimicrobial Agents and Chemotherapy 25: 417

Ragozzino M W, Melton L J, Kurland L T, Chu C P, Perry H O 1982 Population based study of herpes zoster and its sequelae. Medicine 61: 310

Soike K F, Keller P M, Ellis R W 1987 Immunization of monkeys with varicella-zoster virus glycoprotein antigens and their response to challenge with simian varicella virus. Journal of Medical Virology 22: 307

Takahashi M 1986 Clinical overview of varicella vaccine: Development and early studies. Pediatrics 78 (Suppl): 736

Takahashi M, Otuska T, Okuna Y et al 1974 Live vaccine used to prevent the spread of varicella in children in hospital. Lancet 2: 1288

Takahashi M, Hayakawa Y, Shiraki K, Yamanishi K et al 1985 Attenuation and laboratory markers of the Oka-strain varicella zoster virus. Postgraduate Medical Journal 61: 37

Weber D J, Rutala W A, Parham C 1988 Impact and costs of varicella prevention in a university hospital. American Journal of Public Health 78: 19

Weibel R E, Neff B J, Kuter B J et al 1984 Live attenuated varicella virus vaccine: Efficacy trial in healthy children. New England Journal of Medicine 310: 1409

Weibel R E, Kuter B J, Neff B J et al 1985 Live Oka/Merck varicella vaccine in healthy children. Further clinical and laboratory assessment. Journal of the American Medical Association 254: 2435

Williams D, Gershon A, Gelb L, Spraker M, Steinberg S, Ragab A 1985 Herpes zoster following varicella vaccine in a child with acute lymphocytic leukemia. Journal of Pediatrics 106: 259

Yabuchi H, Baba K, Tsuda N et al 1984 A live varicella vaccine in a pediatric community. Biken Journal 27: 43

Zaia J A, Levin M, Preblud S R, Leszczynski J, Wright G et al 1983 Evaluation of varicella-zoster immune globulin: Protection of immunosuppressed children after household exposure to varicella. Journal of Infectious Diseases 147: 737

Discussion of paper presented by Stanley Plotkin

Discussant: Max Just

It is rather difficult to summarize the European experiences with chickenpox vaccine after the paper given by Stanley Plotkin's American group.

European experience is only marginally different from the American one, any small discrepancies probably being explained by differences in the two chickenpox vaccines. European experience is based on the vaccine produced by SK-RIT in Belgium (Andre et al, 1985) and most of the US experience has been with a vaccine produced by MSD. Although both vaccines are produced in a similar way and use the same seed virus from Takahashi, there might be small differences.

In Switzerland the vaccine is licenced with a recommendation that it should be used especially in at-risk groups. This might be one reason why no further large studies have been done with the SK-RIT vaccine since 1985. Our group in Switzerland has most experience with the vaccine in children and in a few adults, all of whom were normal and healthy. I will therefore concentrate on immunologically normal individuals.

One difference between the US and our experience, in normal children, is that we saw no side effects. This might be because of small differences in the vaccine batches used or because we used a different approach to the evaluation of side effects. Our studies were done in out-patients, mostly by private paediatricians working from their own offices and not in a hospital environment, and parents were asked to call the paediatrician in case of an unexpected reaction. As a result some slight fever reactions or a few papules may not have been regarded as unusual by the parents and therefore not mentioned to the paediatrician or to us. For an unbiased evaluation of side effects, a placebo-controlled study similar to the one done with measles + mumps + rubella in the Finnish twin study ought to be carried out (Peltola and Heinonen, 1986).

Dr Plotkin mentioned that chickenpox vaccine induces not only humoral antibodies but also specific cell-mediated immunity and I would like to emphasize this point. Importantly, specific cell-mediated immune reactions to varicella-zoster (VZ) virus can be detected even before the increase in humoral antibodies.

According to the US experience it was more difficult to immunize seronegative adults than seronegative children; in our experience it was difficult to find VZ seronegative adults. In those we found, about 10% showed no seroconversion

256

or only low antibody titres could be induced. In three students we could demonstrate that they developed a VZ-specific cell-mediated immune response but no humoral antibodies. My hypothesis about the reasons for the lower seroconversion rate or the lower antibody titres in seronegative adults is that at least some of them had a cell-mediated immunity against VZ resulting from a previous natural subclinical infection.

Although we did not carry out a formal trial, none of our adult VZ-vaccinees complained of clinical symptoms of chickenpox. I personally see no reason why a vaccine which is effective in children should not protect young non-immune adults. When we gave the live VZ vaccine to seropositive adults, we could induce a booster reaction. This was rather unexpected with an attenuated vaccine, but could be the result of the rather large amount of inactive VZ particles in the vaccine preparations.

We observed lower seroconversion rates when using the chickenpox vaccination together with measles + mumps + rubella (MMR) vaccine, but only when all four vaccines were given in the same syringe. When the MMR vaccine was injected in the right arm and the chickenpox vaccine in the left, or vice versa, there was no such interference (Table 1).

Table 1 Combined vaccination, VZ/M + M + R (Pluserix)

	Seroconversion	Rate
VZ alone		
High dose	94%	122/130
Low dose	76%	29/38
VZ/M + M + R combined (Different syringe)		
VZ High dose	93%	67/72
Low dose	75%	24/32
VZ/M + M + R combined (Same syringe)		
VZ High dose	79%	77/97
Low dose	42%	15/36

In a recent study, in which a reduced amount of live measles virus in the MMR vaccine was used, we detected no interference between MMR and chicken pox vaccines, even when all components were administered in the same syringe.

I return to the problem of cell-mediated immune reactions to VZ antigen in adults. When normal adults, all with humoral VZ antibodies, of the age of 20–40 years were tested, most showed rather strong VZ specific cell-mediated immunity reactions. Normal individuals in the age group of 55 to 65 yielded 23% negative cell-mediated VZ immune reactions, despite the fact they all had humoral VZ antibodies. In a group of healthy individuals older than 65 years the percentage of negatives in VZ cell-mediated immune tests was even higher. We selected 33 individuals with positive VZ humoral antibodies (FAMA tests) but with negative VZ cell-mediated immune reactions and gave them a VZ vaccine booster. With the exception of five, all reacted positively in the CMI tests. Two years after the VZ boostering, seven out of 15 were still positive and, after three years, two out of four. Everybody working with such transformation tests knows that they are rather difficult to standardize. However, we used criteria for considering the test positive which may have been too strict. We would like to do a large clinical trial to test the hypothesis that VZ-boostering for enhancing cell-mediated immunity might offer the possibility of preventing zoster in the elderly. Such testing would require a large patient sample and would therefore be rather expensive.

For the following reasons, VZ vaccination should not only be used in leukaemics but also in normal seronegative children and adults:

(1) The vaccination has no side-effects.
(2) It induces humoral as well as cell-mediated immune reactions.
(3) It protects against chickenpox disease.
(4) Japanese experience shows a long lasting protection.
(5) The VZ vaccination can be done together with the MMR vaccination and together with the diphtheria-tetanus and a polio booster immunization.

At present we face the problem of a very high price for the vaccine. Since, at least in leukaemics, it is now proven that the vaccinees have no greater, and probably a reduced, risk of getting zoster at an advanced age, the vaccine-related zoster problem is no longer a very important issue.

In Journal of the American Medical Association published at the end of December 1987 it was suggested that chickenpox vaccine will be licensed in the USA in 18 to 24 months. Is JAMA correct?

REFERENCES

Andre F E, Heath R B, Malpas J S 1985 Active immunization against varicella. Postgraduate Medical Journal 61, Suppl. 4: 1–171
Peltola H, Heinonen O P 1986 Frequency of true adverse reactions to measles-mumps-rubella vaccine—a double-blind placebo-controlled trial in twins. Lancet 939–942

Discussion: Varicella

Stanley Plotkin and Max Just

The role of different areas of immunity in determining whether a monodermatomic 'normal' zoster, or a multi-dermatomic zoster affiliated with an immunocompromised state occurs, was discussed. The difference appears to involve cell-mediated and not humoral immunity. However, there may be qualitative differences in the defect of cell-mediated immunity. Thus recurrent monodermatomic zoster has been seen in AIDS patients. In general the reactivation of varicella occurs at a much lower rate than that seen for reactivation of herpes simplex.

Vaccine strains have been characterized by restriction enzyme analysis. This technique does not reveal any difference between the Smith, Kline and French (European) Takahashi strain and the Merck, Sharp and Dohme (US) strains. The virus strains have been considered to be homogenous even though a splitting of bands was observed.

It has been proposed that there may be a slight difference in the complication rate after the use of European and American vaccines. However, no such difference was considered to be adequately documented. It was not considered necessary to give aspirin for the mild fever sometimes seen in connection with vaccination.

The duration of immunity after vaccination was considered. Plotkin speculated that possibly no life-long immunity was obtained. In fact re-infections may be relatively common. The antibody response after such an infection appears quantitatively and qualitatively like the response after 'mild' varicella. The risk for development of serious disease in adults was considered negligible. Sufficient immunity was expected to remain to mitigate the disease. It was inquired whether Rye's disease might occur in connection with vaccination. This is not known at present since the rarity of this complication does not allow it to be detected in phase I-III trials. As already mentioned the use of aspirin in vaccinated children should be avoided.

Since the vaccine is used in leukaemic children the relation of immunization to treatment with cytotoxic drugs was discussed. Such a treatment does pose limitations. Oncologists generally want to consolidate chemotherapy and wait at least nine months before vaccination. Chemotherapy is interrupted for a week before vaccination and one week afterwards. The relapse rate does not appear to be increased by this procedure.

The final topic discussed concerned whether it might be appropriate to modify the current restrictive attitude towards use of different live attenuated vaccines in immunocompromised patients. It was commented that CDC and ACIPP, a US public health services committee, recently recommended measles vaccine to be given to HIV-infected children, even those with systemic infection, since two HIV-infected children in the US have died of measles, whereas no severe disease was seen in children, both in the US and Africa, inadvertently immunized with live measles vaccine. Each live vaccine should be administered individually, however. Further it was considered advisable not to give varicella vaccine to a child with systemic HIV infection, since it is known that this vaccine may cause disease in immunocompromised leukaemic children.

Guest Lecture

14. Lessons from Lassa—a brief review and perspective

Stuart C. Glover

INTRODUCTION

The viruses which have a propensity to cause haemorrhage as a clinical manifestation or complication in a previously immunocompetent host are known as the *haemorrhagic fever viruses*. This broad description is rather unsatisfactory since the viruses which cause these various infections belong to a variety of viral families: some are transmitted by different arthropod vectors and they all have quite distinct geographical and epidemiological features. In addition, haemorrhage is an early and regular feature of some of these infections, namely Ebola and Marburg virus disease, while bleeding is a late and relatively uncommon feature of Lassa fever. The major viral haemorrhagic fevers and their causative agents are summarized in Table 14.1.

The viral haemorrhagic fevers are widely distributed in Africa, Asia, Europe and Oceania, and sporadic cases occur in travellers who have recently visited these endemic areas. Most of these viral haemorrhagic fever viruses cause no public health concern in the United Kingdom as there is no evidence of airborne or respiratory droplet spread, the arthropod vectors responsible for transmission are absent in the United Kingdom, and there is no indigenous non-human host likely to act as a reservoir of infection. Unfortunately, four of these viral haemorrhagic fever viruses—Lassa fever, Ebola virus, Marburg virus and Congo-Crimean haemorrhagic fever viruses—are capable of person-to-person transmission through close contact with infected blood and other body secretions.

Medical and laboratory staff in hospitals in endemic areas have been shown in previous studies to have been at increased risk as witnessed by several outbreaks of nosocomial infection with Lassa fever and Congo-Crimean haemorrhagic fever. Fortunately, the numbers of confirmed cases of imported viral haemorrhagic fever in the United Kingdom are extremely small: 10 cases of proven Lassa fever have been managed in the United Kingdom since 1969, and one case of Ebola fever, contracted by accidental self-inoculation, has been documented. What is more clinically pressing and relevant is the large number of travellers both native and expatriate, who are suspected of having a viral haemorrhagic fever.

The objective of this paper is to outline salient features of the most common viral haemorrhagic fever, namely Lassa fever, to summarize the current guidelines for the isolation and management of suspected cases, and to indicate some of the practical and logistical problems associated with the High Security Trexler Tent Negative Pressure Isolation.

Table 14.1 The viral haemorrhagic fevers

Disease	Virus family	Virus group	Vector	Natural host reservoir	Geographical distribution
Dengue haemorrhagic fever	Togaviridae	Flavivirus	Mosquitoes	Man Monkeys	Africa Oceania South-east Asia Central and South America
Yellow fever	Togaviridae	Flavivirus	Mosquitoes	Primates	Africa Central and South Africa
Omsk haemorrhagic fever	Togaviridae	Flavivirus	Ticks	Small mammals ? Muskrat	USSR
Kyasanur forest disease	Togaviridae	Flavivirus	Ticks	Rodents Monkeys	India
Rift Valley fever	Bunyaviridae	Phlebovirus	Mosquitoes	? Rodents ? Sheep: Camels	Africa
Congo-Crimean haemorrhagic fever	Bunyaviridae	Nariovirus	Ticks	Small mammals	USSR Africa Central–West Africa
Haemorrhagic fever with renal syndrome	Bunyaviridae	Hantaan virus	—	Rodents	Asia Europe Africa
Lassa fever	Arenavirus	Lassa virus	—	Rodents Multimammate rats	West Africa
Argentinian haemorrhagic fever	Arenavirus	Junin	—	Rodents	Argentina
Bolivian haemorrhagic fever	Arenavirus	Machupo	—	Rodents	Bolivia
Marburg	'Filoviridae'	Marburg	—	Unknown	East and Central Africa
Ebola	'Filoviridae'	Ebola	—	Unknown	East and Central Africa

LASSA FEVER

Lassa fever was first described in 1969 when three missionary nurses in Northern Nigeria were sequentially infected by person-to-person spread of a virus (Frame et al, 1970). Subsequent investigation identified the cause as a virus morphologically and antigenically similar to *lymphocytic choriomeningitis (LCM) virus* and the viruses causing haemorrhagic fever in Bolivia (Machupo virus) and Argentina (Junin virus) (Buckley & Casals, 1970).

By 1970 these viruses and six other related viruses from South America were categorized in a new taxon—family Arenaviridae; genus, Arenavirus. Currently, the Arenavirus genus contains 13 viruses of which three, *Lassa, Toure* and *Ippy* are found in Africa, including two antigenic varients of Lassa virus which have been described in Central and Southern Africa.

The early nosocomial outbreaks of Lassa fever in medical and nursing staff in missionary hospitals in Nigera and Liberia carried a case fatality rate of 50% and generated a sinister reputation for Lassa fever. These outbreaks also allowed investigators to establish the incubation period, to describe the signs and symptoms of the clinical illness and to demonstrate that direct contact with an infected patient or accidental inoculation of blood and tissue fluid was usually required for person-to-person spread (Monath et al, 1973). Mild and asymptomatic Lassa fever infections were identified retrospectively by sero-epidemiological studies of both hospital staff, concurrent inpatients and in-habitants of villages from which the index cases had arisen. A further investigation of Lassa fever in Panguma Hospital, Eastern Province, Sierra Leone, revealed a total of 63 cases over a two year period, that less than 10% of the cases were nosocomial and that the case fatality rate was less than 5% (Fraser et al, 1974). To the scientific and medical communities at least, the spectre of the highly infectious image of Lassa fever was beginning to wane. The next link in the chain of knowledge about Lassa fever was the isolation of Lassa fever virus from a high proportion of multimammate rats (*Mastomys natalensis*) trapped in village households in Sierra Leone (Monath et al, 1974).

At this stage a group from the Centers for Disease Control (CDC), Atlanta, led by Karl M. Johnson and later by Joseph B. McCormick and aided by the government of Sierra Leone, was established to study the epidemiology, ecology and clinical manifestations of Lassa fever. This unit is currently based in Segbwema, in Eastern Province of Sierra Leone and close to the diamond mining area of Tongo fields. This team of investigators rapidly showed that Lassa fever was responsible for 10–16% of all adult medical admissions and for 30% of adult medical deaths in two study hospitals (McCormick et al, 1987a). Little, however, is known about the morbidity of Lassa fever in other areas of West Africa. As patients admitted to hospital represent a highly selected population, McCormick has studied Lassa fever in rural Sierra Leone villages where serological conversion occurs at a rate of 2% per annum. Only a quarter of these seropositive individuals could recall an acute illness consistent with Lassa fever (McCormick et al, 1987b). In this particular study, the case fatality ratio of 1–2% was much lower than the case fatality ratios amongst ill hospitalized patients. Another tantalising observation made in this study was the eight-fold increase in the titre of specific Lassa fever virus antibody in 1–18% of the antibody positive population, suggesting re-infection with Lassa fever virus. Whether such re-infection with Lassa fever results in clinical disease, a less severe clinical outcome or virus excretion remains moot.

One explanation for the occurrence of asymptomatic infections and re-infections, and one which may account for the variability of illness seen in hospitalized patients, is the possibility of strains of Lassa fever virus with different virulence. Jahrling and his colleagues have found that strains of Lassa fever virus from Liberia exhibit a spectrum of virulence for strain 2 and 13 guinea pigs. Antigen variation between strains of Lassa fever virus from Sierra Leone, Liberia and Nigeria has been demonstrated (Jahrling et al, 1985a).

Clinical manifestations

The incubation period of Lassa fever may be as short as five or as long as 21 days but is usually between 10 and 14 days. The illnesss begins insidiously with fever with associated malaise and myalgia. Many infections remain subclinical or very mild. More severe cases progress to develop pharyngitis characterized by erythematous lesions on the palate and fauces, occasionally associated with central white exudates and pain. Diarrhoea, headache, cough, and chest and abdominal pain are not uncommon. Patients appear anxious, toxic, prostrated and may exhibit mild facial oedema, conjunctival inflammation and bradycardia. A major feature of Lassa fever infection is capillary leakage and this manifests as flushing of the skin, crepitations in both lung fields and pleural effusions. Neurological signs are uncommon but include altered consciousness, meningeal irritation, coma and convulsions. Petechiae are uncommon and difficult to see in dark skinned patients but frank haemorrhages including haematemesis, melaena, vaginal bleeding and oozing from venepunture sites occurs in up to 20% of patients.

Such haemorrhage portends a poor prognosis. Lassa fever patients die in the second and sometimes third week of their acute illness, the adverse clinical signs being increasing capillary leakage, haemorrhage, and the development of clinical shock, often associated with intense facial and body oedema. The complications of Lassa fever include nerve deafness which may be bilateral in 5–8% of patients. This is often permanent. Pericarditis occurs in both non-fatal and fatal infection. Other complications include uveitis, orchitis and transient hair loss.

Lassa fever in pregnant women is a particularly difficult and serious problem. Abortion and still-birth are common and maternal mortality is increased. The prompt delivery of a Lassa fever virus infected pregnant woman has been recommended as part of the management strategy for these patients.

Given the relatively non-specific nature of the onset of Lassa fever, there is a wide differential diagnosis associated with such febrile patients in West Africa. This differential diagnosis is summarized in Table 14.2.

Table 14.2 Differential diagnosis of viral haemorrhagic fevers

---

Malaria
Bacterial septicaemia
Enteric fevers — typhoid and paratyphoid
African trypanosomiasis (*Trypanosoma rhodesiense*)
Rickettsial infections (tick typhus)
Viral hepatitis
Epstein-Barr virus infection
Streptococcal pharyngitis
Leptospirosis
Other viral infections

The best clinical predictor of a fatal outcome is the combination of fever, sore throat and vomiting while patients having a viraemia of at least 10^4 $TCID_{50}/ml$ and levels of aspartate aminotransferase of greater than 150 IU had a case fatality rate of 81%; 85% of patients without either laboratory abnormality survived (Johnson et al, 1987).

Further studies from the CDC Lassa fever group have shown that patients with the risk factors of viraemia and raised aspartate aminotransferase, who received intravenous Ribavirin within six days of the onset of fever, experience a significant reduction in mortality. Apart from inducing a reversible anaemia, intravenous Ribavirin is well tolerated and safe (McCormick et al, 1986).

The Lassa fever virus is present in high concentration in the blood of all patients at the onset of the illness and can be isolated from the throat and urine of most patients. The virus grows rapidly in the Vero cell cultures and can be confirmed within 72 hours. This work, however, must only be done in a designated laboratory with category 4 biocontainment facilities. Serological diagnosis is confirmed by demonstration of a rising titre of Lassa specific IgM by indirect fluorescent antibody test (IFAT). As two thirds of the patients have detectable IgM antibodies to Lassa fever virus at the time of admission to hospital, a diagnosis of Lassa fever can be supported by the immunofluorescent antibody test for Lassa specific IgM. For those patients who do not have specific antibodies at the time of admission, the availability of a Lassa antigen detection immunoassay would be very helpful. Such a system remains to be refined (Jahrling et al, 1985b). One of the enigmas of Lassa fever is the observed inability of the infected human host to clear viraemia and prevent viral replication in tissues by means of either humoral antibody or cell mediated immune responses. It remains to be seen what the host specific and virus specific variables are and how they relate to Lassa fever severity.

Approach to a suspected case of viral haemorrhagic fever

From the clinical descriptions of Lassa fever given above, it is clear that it is impossible to make a definite diagnosis on clinical grounds. The doctor, be he general practitioner at home or in his surgery, the casualty officer, the admitting house physician or house surgeon or port doctor, must be aware of this rare but important disease so that an informed travel history and detailed epidemiological history can be taken. It is my practice to brief new house staff on Lassa fever and to provide them with a checklist of questions to be asked (Table 14.3). The most important questions are:

(1)   Where has the patient been?

(2)   What time has passed between the patient's presence in an area with endemic viral haemorrhagic fever or since exposure to a person with viral haemorrhagic fever and the onset of the illness?

(3)   What did the patient do when in a country with endemic viral haemorrhagic fever?

(4)   What are the current symptoms and signs?

Table 14.3 Vital information when assessing probability of Lassa fever

Patient's name, age, address
General practitioner's name, address and telephone number
Location of patient (for example, home, casualty department)
Which countries has the patient visited
How long since the patient left the endemic area?
Reason for presence in Africa (for example, recreation, work)
Any known contact with ill people
Did the patient take antimalarial chemoprophylaxis, and type of chemoprophylaxis
What are the current symptoms and signs?

Clearly, it is impossible and unreasonable to take strict precautions with all patients who develop a pyrexia of unknown origin (PUO) before or within three weeks of arrival from an area endemic for Lassa fever.

Nonetheless, a very small number may have Lassa fever and therefore their blood and secretions pose a real hazard to laboratory and hospital staff. Given the strictness and the inherent dangers of High Security Trexler Tent Negative Pressure isolation it is essential that only those at very high risk of actually having an infection are isolated.

The Memorandum on the Control of Viral Haemorrhagic Fevers, 1986, published by Her Majesty's Stationery Office on behalf of the DHSS, sets out the guidelines for action when considering a diagnosis of Lassa fever (Memorandum on the Control of Viral Haemorrhagic Fevers, 1986). It must be remembered that Lassa fever is a notifiable disease under the Public Health Infectious Diseases (Amendment) Regulations, 1976.

Risk groups

Having identified a febrile patient, recently returned from a Lassa endemic area, it is essential that the clinician seeks the help and advice of a specialist in infectious diseases or tropical diseases, some of whom will be in charge of one of the designated high security infectious diseases units. The specialist will also give immediate advice on the appropriate investigation and treatment of malaria which is a common cause of PUO in travellers from Lassa endemic areas. That specialist will also assist in categorizing the febrile patient into one of three risk groups outlined in the Memorandum on Control of Viral Haemorrhagic Fevers. Those risk groups are: (1) strong suspicion; (2) moderate suspicion; (3) minimal suspicion, and they determine the immediate isolation management of these patients.

Strong suspicion
The following patients fall into this category:

(1)   Patients presenting with a PUO who have been in rural areas or large towns where Lassa fever is known to be endemic.
(2)   Medical and nursing staff from country hospitals in these areas.
(3)   Laboratory workers who handle Lassa fever virus, both in the United Kingdom and abroad.
(4)   Febrile contacts of confirmed cases.

These high risk patients must be admitted directly to a designated high security infectious diseases unit. No blood specimens or body secretions/sputum, or urine, should be sent to the routine laboratory. Specific protocols for the ambulance transportation of these patients exist and the immediate arrangements are made by the clinician in charge of the receiving high security infectious diseases unit. The Medical Officer for Environmental Health (MOEH) is informed and he informs the Public Health Laboratory Service Communicable Diseases Surveillance Centre (CDSC). The CDSC holds the responsibility for national co-ordination of infectious diseases, including Lassa fever. The MOEH identifies close contacts and places them under surveillance and liaises with the other medical officers for environmental health and the CDSC on the identification of contacts in other health districts.

Moderate suspicion
Patients who have been in small towns or country districts not known to be associated with viral haemorrhagic fever can be viewed with less suspicion. The case details must be discussed with a specialist in infectious diseases or tropical medicine who will advise on the appropriateness of submitting blood for malaria parasite examination. Blood must not be submitted to the laboratory without first discussing the differential diagnosis with the clinician in charge of the laboratory. If these blood films are negative or if the onset and course of the febrile illness are consistent with a viral haemorrhagic fever, then the patient should be transferred to a high security infectious diseases unit. No further blood, urine or sputum specimens must be submitted to the routine laboratory. The MOEH must be informed as with the strong suspicion group.

Minimal suspicion
Patients who have come from major cities where the risk of Lassa fever is minimal are regarded with minimal suspicion. If there is no immediate threat to life and malaria has been excluded, the patient may be managed at home. It is prudent, however, to admit the patient to an isolation bed in a district general hospital or to an infectious diseases ward where the patient is isolated under 'enteric precautions', that is, taking precautions with stools, urine and blood. The ambulance control officer must be informed that 'enteric precautions' are required by his men when transporting such a patient.

Every effort must be made to avoid admitting patients who are catagorized as high or moderate suspicion to hospitals or departments without isolation facilities. Accident and emergency departments not infrequently admit patients with PUO from countries such as Africa. Ideally, these patients should be assessed in a single room until the necessary epidemiological details have been collected. It is essential that an infectious diseases physician is contacted and the risk category assessed. No blood samples must be submitted without first discussing the request with the consultant in charge of the relevant laboratory.

Laboratory investigations
Given the high level of viraemia occurring in Lassa fever, patients' blood is the major hazard. All specimens from suspect patients must be taken and handled

with extreme caution. Falciparum malaria is the most likely and imperative diagnosis in febrile patients recently returned from Africa. Falciparum malaria is unpredictable and a potentially fatal medical emergency. Consideration of this diagnosis requires prompt examination of blood films for malarial parasites. A 4 ml sample of blood is placed in a potassium EDTA container. Every effort must be made to avoid external contamination of the specimen container. The labelled sample is placed in an intact plastic bag containing absorbent material. The request form must not be put in the same bag as the specimen. Blood cultures for typhoid and other septicaemias may be taken at this stage and sent to the microbiology laboratory under the same stringent precautions. All specimens must be clearly labelled to indicate the level of clinical suspicion and carry a biohazard warning sticker.

The plastic bag containing the specimen is then enclosed in a stout sealable container or box marked with a biohazard warning label and a warning 'not to be opened if found' also applied. This container is transported by a responsible person directly to the appropriate laboratory whose senior staff have already been advised and have agreed to accept the specimen. In the laboratory the thick and thin films are made in a microbiological safety cabinet and rendered safe by fixing in 10% buffered formalin and methanol.

Specimens for specific viral haemorrhagic fever investigation are taken only after malaria has been excluded. This is the responsibility of the physician in charge of the high security infectious diseases unit. These specimens are sent under secure conditions to the PHLS Viral Zoonosis Laboratory at Colindale, London for virus culture and serological testing. Clinical management tests such as routine biochemistry and haematology can only be ordered by the physician in charge of the high security infectious diseases unit and can only be performed in a laboratory which complies with the requirements for containment level four. An alternative arrangement is to perform these investigations inside a flexible film isolator mini laboratory within the high security infectious diseases unit housing the Lassa fever patient.

THE FUTURE

In 1976 the DHSS issued a memorandum on Lassa fever which outlined strict guidelines for the isolation of patients and the surveillance of their contacts. Since then much has been learned about the epidemiology of Lassa fever and the other dangerous viral pathogens. This new knowledge is incorporated in the Memorandum on Control of Viral Haemorrhagic Fever (1986), which includes guidance on Ebola, Marburg and Congo-Crimean haemorrhagic fevers. The stringent surveillance advice has been relaxed to include close contacts only. The relaxation in the definition and surveillance of close contacts is welcome as it recognizes the growing awareness amongst clinicians and scientists, with extensive experience of Lassa fever, that the infection is transmitted from man to man by needlestick injury and close contact with blood and blood contaminated secretions. The respiratory/droplet route of infection is rare and perhaps confined to those patients with overt pneumonia. Evidence supporting this opinion has recently been produced from Sierra Leone where simple barrier nursing precautions are used. In that study the Lassa fever antibody prevalence rates amongst staff from hospitals looking after Lassa Fever patients were no greater than those of people from nearby village populations (Helmick et al, 1986). Frame et al (1979) found that the prevalence of Lassa fever antibodies among those with patient contact was the same as that among those without patient contact. These studies support the opinion that nosocomical respiratory spread of Lassa fever occurs infrequently and can be prevented by sound barrier nursing techniques.

It also, of course, begs the question of the appropriateness of Negative Pressure Trexler Tent Isolation which is an extremely efficient method of preventing airborne infection. Unfortunately, the transportation of sick patients and this incarceration in the Trexler Isolator, may not only be unnecessary but also be to the disadvantage of the patient, attendant staff and the community. The Trexler Tent severely impedes medical and nursing care and supportive therapy; it increases the hazard of needlestick injury by making simple procedures awkward; and it perpetuates the mystique and fear of these viral infections in the lay and professional mind alike.

It is ten years since the first memorandum on Lassa fever was published. It is to be hoped that the current recommendations will be updated as soon as additional and reliable information about the infectivity of this virus becomes available. In the meantime, however, it is important that physicians are aware of this rare but serious viral infection and are not slow to ask the vital question 'Where have you been and when did you return?'

REFERENCES

Buckley S M, Casals J 1970 Lassa fever, a new virus disease of man from West Africa. III. Isolation and characterization of the virus. American Journal of Tropical Medicine and Hygiene 19: 680–691
Frame J D, Baldwin J M, Gocke D J, Troup J M 1970 Lassa fever, a new virus from West Africa. I. Clinical description and pathological findings. American Journal of Tropical Medicine and Hygiene 19: 670–676.
Frame J D, Casals J, Dennis E A 1979 Lassa virus antibodies in hospital personnel in Western Liberia. Transactions of the Royal Society for Tropical Medicine and Hygiene 73: 219–224.
Fraser D W, Campbell C C, Monath T P, Goff P A, Greig M B 1974 Lassa fever in the Eastern Province of Sierra Leone, 1970–1972. I. Epidemiologic studies. American Journal of Tropical Medicine and Hygiene 23: 1131–1139.
Helmick C G, Webb P A, Scribner C L et al 1986 No evidence for increased risk of Lassa fever infection in hospital staff Lancet 2: 1202–1204
Jahrling P B, Frame J D, Smith S B, Monson M H 1985a Endemic Lassa fever in Liberia. III. Characterization of Lassa virus isolates. Transactions of the Royal Society for Tropical Medicine and Hygiene 79: 374–379
Jahrling P B, Niklasson B S, McCormick J B 1985b Early diagnosis of human Lassa fever by ELISA detection of antigen and antibody. Lancet 1: 250–252
Johnson K M, McCormick J B, Webb P A, Smith E S, Elliott L H, King I J 1987 Clinical Virology of Lassa Fever in hospitalized patients. Journal of Infectious Diseases 155: 456–464
McCormick J B, King I J, Webb P A et al 1986 Lassa fever. Effective therapy with ribavirin. New England Journal of Medicine 304: 20–26
McCormick J B, Webb P A, Krebs J W, Johnson K M, Smith E S 1987a A prospective study of the epidemiology and ecology of Lassa fever. Journal of Infectious Diseases 155: 437–444
McCormick J B, King I J, Webb P A et al 1987b A case-control study of the clinical diagnosis and course of Lassa fever. Journal of Infectious Diseases 155: 445–455
Memorandum on the Control of Viral Haemorrhagic Fevers 1986 London HMSO

Monath T P, Mertens P E, Patton R et al 1973 A hospital endemic of Lassa fever in Zorzor, Liberia, March-April 1972 American Journal of Tropical Medicine and Hygiene 22: 773–779

Monath T P, Newhouse V F, Kemp G E, Setzer H W, Cacciapuoti A 1974 Lassa virus isolation from Mastomys natalensis rodents during an epidemic in Sierra Leone. Science 185: 263–265

Discussion: Lassa fever

Stuart Glover

On a question about the natural course of the Lassa virus infection in the multimammate rat, Dr Glover responded that the rats are subclinically infected and that about 60% of rats caught in Segbwema, Sierra Leone, excreted the virus.

The risks for nosocomial outbreaks of Lassa fever were discussed. The experiences from the Lassa unit in Segbwema and from other places, including those in Western countries which have treated Lassa patients or handled laboratory samples from such patients, clearly indicate that prevention from blood contact is the crucial factor in preventing such outbreaks. This can be achieved by wearing gloves and masks. Among laboratory technicians, one case of nosocomial Lassa fever has been described from New York. It was also pointed out that strict isolation becomes more important for cases of Ebola and Marburg virus infections because of the high mortality in those conditions. It was agreed that these patients should optimally be cared for in air conditioned rooms with negative pressure and that preventative measures should concentrate on avoiding blood contaminations. Plastic tent isolation, which is today used in the UK, seems not to be necessary, causes considerable problems for the hospital staff and problems, psychologically for the patient.